Models and Critical Pathways in Clinical Nursing

Liz Herring
April '99

Models and Critical Pathways in Clinical Nursing

Conceptual Frameworks for Care Planning

(Second edition)

Mike Walsh PhD, BA(Hons), RGN, PGCE, Dip N
Reader in Nursing, University College of St Martin, Lancaster, UK

with contributions by

Joy Duxbury
Nursing Officer, Salus Health and Safety,
Hillhouse International, Thornton, Lancashire and Part-time
Lecturer in Mental Health, University College of St Martin, Lancaster, UK

Miriam Rowswell
Formerly Nursing Lecturer at St Christopher's Hospice, Sydenham,
Kent, UK

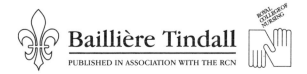

Baillière Tindall
PUBLISHED IN ASSOCIATION WITH THE RCN

Baillière Tindall   24–28 Oval Road
London NW1 7DX

The Curtis Center
Independence Square West
Philadelphia, PA 19106–3399, USA

Harcourt Brace & Company
55 Horner Avenue
Toronto, Ontario, M8Z 4X6, Canada

Harcourt Brace & Company, Australia
30–52 Smidmore Street
Marrickville
NSW 2204, Australia

Harcourt Brace & Company, Japan
Ichibancho Central Building
22–1 Ichibancho
Chiyoda-ku, Tokyo 102, Japan

First published 1991
Second edition 1998

A catalogue record for this book is available from the British Library

ISBN 0–7020–2188–1

Typeset by J&L Composition Ltd, Filey, North Yorkshire
Printed and bound in Great Britain by Bath Press, Bath

Contents

Preface

Evidence-based practice has become a major principle of modern nursing and I have therefore based the revision of this book on the evidence that has accumulated since its first edition in 1991. This evidence has been very critical of the nursing process as a means of planning care while nursing models in their original form, have failed to make a significant impact in the real world of nursing within the UK. This book is therefore much more than an update to the original *Models in Clinical Nursing* book; it is more a sequel or successor rather than a second edition.

A great deal has changed in the last six years, not least of which is the way care is planned and documented, and the thinking that underpins that care. As a result of the need to reflect changes such as the spread of critical pathways and the increasing criticism of the nursing process, this book explores new areas in care delivery and the conceptual frameworks that support nursing care. It also critiques the influential work of Pat Benner and questions the growing orthodoxy that sees nursing as more intuitive rather than rational and evidence based.

The reader is introduced to critical pathways and their role in getting rid of time-wasting documentation is examined. Pathways have been shown to have the potential to greatly increase multidisciplinary working and patient involvement in care whilst making a major contribution to quality enhancement. Research on the nursing process has been discussed at the same time as the early evidence from the USA on critical pathways. There does seem to be a great deal of potential in their use but as practice should always be evidence based, there is a need for some serious and rigorous UK evaluative trials of critical pathways.

Of even more importance is the thinking that lies behind care planning and documentation: the conceptual frameworks that guide care. The original nursing models explored in this text have been retained and revisited but not with the 'cook book' approach that characterized so much early writing in this field. The first edition called for flexibility and creativity in the use of models not the dead hand of blanket uniformity. The standard nursing model imposed everywhere in a rather unimaginative and ultimately token way was criticized in the 1991 edition, and here I continue to argue with even more conviction that this is not the way for nursing to develop.

We should be seeing models as frameworks to guide, or philosophies to underpin, care. They make the care plan or critical pathway patient-centred and offer principles to help the nurse deal with the infinite range of complexities that patients present. This text argues for objective reality, i.e. there is a real world inhabited by patients and nurses and within that world there is right and wrong. This may seem like stating the obvious, but the book takes serious issue with those nurse theorists who would argue that all things are subjective and knowledge is relative to the situation you are in. Nursing theory is therefore kept rooted in reality where some things are right and others are wrong. This approach to nursing requires practical conceptual models to guide care; it needs a good understanding of issues such as what it means to be an accountable practitioner and it also requires the nurse to be able to document care practically and reliably. These are all the key themes that are explored in a range of settings in this text, encouraging the nurse to always be asking 'What is the evidence upon which I am basing my care?'

This text therefore moves nursing models from the realms of another, rather abstruse, academic notion which nurses are too busy to do anything about towards the position where they can be seen as helping to provide the necessary principles and guidelines for care. Accountability is all about the justification of care given and by viewing nursing models as conceptual frameworks to help organize care, rather than in the 'cook book recipe fashion' that characterized their debut in the UK, this book argues they have a valuable place in nursing today. In order to keep a caring and holistic focus within the protocol-driven, multidisciplinary, cost-conscious climate of today, nursing needs all the help it can get. The conceptual frameworks of writers explored in this book, such as Roy and Orem, can keep the patient centre stage as a real human being, whatever new approaches to care organization and delivery may be introduced.

Acknowledgements

The case study material in chapter 11 was originally published in *New Rituals for Old, Nursing Through the Looking Glass* (1994) by Mike Walsh and Pauline Ford. It is reproduced here by kind permission of Butterworth-Heinemann Publishers and Pauline Ford.

I would like to say thank you to the library staff of the University College of St Martin at the Cumberland Infirmary, Carlisle, who have been very helpful in researching this edition.

It would also be very nice to say a big thank you to Birgit Evensen and all the staff and students in the department of Nursing at the Høgskolen i Tromsø, Tromsø, Norway, for showing me the true, international meaning of caring.

Glossary

ABGs	arterial blood gases
ACNP	acute care nurse practitioners
A&E	Accident & Emergency
ADL	activity of daily living
AIDS	acquired immune deficiency syndrome
ADL	activity of daily living
AL	activity of living
BMD	bone marrow depression
BP	blood pressure
BSE	breast self-examination
CBG	capillary blood glucose
CCTV	closed circuit television
CCU	cardiac care unit
CHF	congestive heart failure
COAD	chronic obstructive airways disease
CP	critical pathway
CVA	cerebrovascular accident
CVP	central venous pressure
DN	district nurse
DVT	deep venous thrombosis
DySSSy	Dynamic Standard Setting System
ECG	electrocardiograph
ET	endotracheal
FANCAP	Fluids, Aeration, Nutrition, Communication, Activity, Pain
FBC	full blood count
FHSA	Family Health Service Authority
GA	general anaesthetic
GP	general practitioner
GTN	glyceryl trinitrate
HCA	health care assistants
ICP	intracranial pressure
IM	intramuscularly

INR	international normalized ratio
ITU	intensive treatment unit
IV	intravenously
IVI	intravenous infusion
JCAHCO	Joint Commission on Accreditation of Health Care Organizations
L	left
LMP	last menstrual period
MI	myocardial infarction
MSU	midstream specimen of urine
NAD	nothing abnormal demonstrated
NBM	nil by mouth
NG	nasogastric
NHS	National Health Service
NP	nurse practitioner
NVQ	National Vocational Qualification
OPD	Outpatients' Department
OT	occupational therapy
P	pulse
PAMS	professions allied to medicine
PCA	patient-controlled analgesia
PE	pulmonary embolism
PFH	patient-focused hospital
PHCT	primary health care team
prn	as required
Pt	patient
p.u.	pass urine
PVD	peripheral vascular disease
R	right
RCN	Royal College of Nursing
RGN	registered general nurse
RLT	Roper, Logan, Tierney
RN	registered nurse
RR	respiratory rate
RTA	road traffic accident
Rx	treatment
s/c	subcutaneously
SNO	senior house officer

SOB	short of breath
S/S	signs and symptoms
T	temperature
TED	graduated compression stockings
TENs	transcutaneous electrical nerve stimulation
TTO	to take out
U&E	urea and electrolytes
UKCC	United Kingdom Central Council
UTI	urinary tract infection
VAS	visual analog scale
VS	vital signs
WHO	World Health Organization

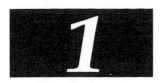

What is the Basis for Nursing Practice?

Theory is the poetry of science. Levine (1995)

What are models of nursing?

Nursing models developed initially in the USA as nurse academics attempted to formulate a basis for nursing practice that went beyond following medical instructions. They became widely publicized in the UK during the late 1980s as British nurses also joined in the quest for the holy grail of differentiating nursing from medicine. Unfortunately, the terms *model*, *conceptual framework* and *nursing theory* have been used loosely and interchangeably in casual conversation while the confusion this has caused has been compounded by various nurse authors using the terms in different ways also.

Dubliners usually console a person trying to find a difficult location with the words 'Well if that's where you're going, I wouldn't start from here'. This piece of Celtic wisdom emphasizes the importance of starting out on the right foot and so following in the tradition of my Dublin grandfather, let us look at exactly where we are starting out from on this journey in search of nursing models, conceptual frameworks or theories. This requires us to start with some definitions and discussion of what these terms mean.

In defining models it is best to think of them as simplified ways of representing reality, as ways to facilitate understanding. Models are used extensively in this way and we are all familiar with the physical models that represent a simplified version of human anatomy. The real thing is much more complex as any nurse who has worked in theatres will testify. Models in this sense are descriptive of the way things are or ought to be, but do not claim the power to make predictions about the future based upon the way various things interact. As we shall see, theories carry with them the power of explanation and prediction.

Models can be constructed from sets of theories in such a way as to achieve predictions. These models do not exist in the physical world like the contents of an anatomical model, but they exist in the abstract, such as the complex numerical models that are used by the Meterological Office computers to predict the weather or the Treasury to predict the behaviour of the economy.

Nursing models exist in the abstract, only they rely on words rather than numbers to express their simplified description of how things ought to be in the world of nursing. They do not, however, consist of a set of theories with predictive power, which makes them different from the computer-based models used by scientists. When reading the word 'model' it is therefore very important to know which of these three meanings is being attached to the term as they are very different.

The term 'conceptual framework' overlaps with model and is very similar to the last description of a model given above. A concept is an idea, therefore a conceptual framework is a framework of ideas constructed around a key area of activity, in this case nursing. Therefore, it too is a description of the ideal, a set of ideas, but it does not claim predictive power.

Models and conceptual frameworks can be derived from observation of what actually goes on in real nursing, combined with ideas from some other allied discipline such as the social sciences. They are therefore practice based. An alternative approach is to start off from the abstract world of philosophy and theories and then construct a model by logical deduction of how the author thinks nursing should be carried out. This latter approach is reminiscent of the methods of Aristotle and a whole school of Ancient Greek philosophers and led to the Aristotelian view of all matter being composed of earth, air, water and fire and a whole host of other incorrect statements about the world we live in, including its place at the centre of the universe with the sun orbiting around it. These views lingered on into the Middle Ages before being eroded and then finally displaced by the scientific revolution that accompanied the Renaissance. One of the key elements of this revolution was the emphasis upon observation of the real world and active experimentation aimed at discovering the truth rather than logical deduction conducted in a vacuum. Even so, Galileo could show people the moons of Jupiter orbiting that planet but found it very difficult to persuade people of the truth because this contradicted the tradition of Aristotle. Theorizing in a vacuum, without recourse to reality, is flawed by its lack of engagement with that reality.

There is therefore a clear parallel and a warning for those who would construct models of nursing: ignore reality at your peril!

Departing from the reality of everyday nursing life may result in abstract ideas which have little relation to the real world, producing ivory tower pseudoscience reminiscent of the psychobabble normally associated with the west coast of the USA. The approach taken in this book is derived from experience of what nurses actually do, and is firmly rooted in the real, practical world of nursing which nurses identify with and can see the relevance of. Does this approach reject the importance of philosophy in nursing? We return to this later.

Theories can also be constructed from ideas but they are much tighter structures than models or conceptual frameworks because they try to explain relationships between concepts in a deterministic way; that is, if this happens then that will follow. There are therefore law-like elements of generalization and prediction involved in theories which are absent from models or conceptual frameworks.

This is the classical meaning of theory as used in the natural sciences and we need to remember this in asking: how does theory relate to models and conceptual frameworks?

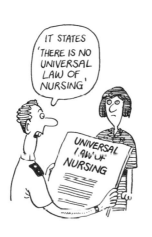

Nursing is not, however, quite like the natural sciences such as physics or geology because it involves human beings. The ability to generalize with universal laws that will predict outcomes is lacking in nursing. As Roy (1995) observed, this is due to the context-dependent nature of nursing. In simple English, no two patients are the same and, additionally, there are lots of other factors at work which influence the outcome. In scientific language, there are a multitude of intervening variables which mediate between cause and effect and so produce a wide range of possible outcomes besides the one we would expect on the basis of our theory. Roy (1995) therefore points out the need for nursing to be concerned with the key questions: to whom can any theory be applied and under what circumstances? There are no universal laws of nursing out there waiting to be discovered. Theory is only predictive with a given degree of probability. Uncertainty is introduced by the complex nature of patients, health and the world of nursing.

The implication of this is that as nurses we must recognize that when we use a piece of theory to guide our actions, we can never be certain of the outcome. We might place a patient with a certain Waterlow Pressure-Sore Risk Score on a pressure-relieving mattress because theory predicts that it is *probable* that this person will develop a pressure sore and that the use of a pressure-relieving mattress will *probably* prevent sore formation. We need to forget the old certainties of the procedure manuals as they were naïve and simplistic and come to terms with a world in which we are managers of uncertainty. The natural sciences operate in this way and so does medicine. It is all about balancing the probabilities, thus a doctor prescribes a certain antibiotic because he or she thinks it is the *best chance* of curing an infection, a surgeon operates upon a cancer because he or she thinks it is the *best chance* of improving the patient's life.

The patient and their environment are therefore central to trying to apply any nursing theory, a point elaborated upon by Roy (1995) who reminds us that the setting within which care occurs sets the context within which communication takes place. This context is characterized by a major power imbalance with the patient having least power, the doctor most and the nurse somewhere in between. Models, as simplified representations of reality, have tried in varying degrees to reflect this problem and sought to correct it by concentrating on the nature of the nurse–patient relationship.

Theory in nursing is not therefore a grand generalized explanation of everything but it does seek to predict outcomes with certain probabilities depending upon the circumstances. This is different from a conceptual framework (or model) which, as Fawcett (1992) explains, seeks to describe global ideas about individuals and groups that are of interest to a discipline whereas theory has much greater specificity. Theory therefore is a practical tool that allows the nurse to deal with specific problems such as a patient at risk of developing a pressure sore or a client with alcohol abuse problems. This practical bias to theory is advocated by Levine (1995) who pours scorn on the expectation of some nursing academics that theory can only be theory if it is obscure and difficult to understand. Many North American nursing scholars stand guilty of producing a dense fog of incomprehensible jargon under the banner of theory, none more so than Martha Rogers (1970) whose unitary forecefield view of human beings was dismissed by Stevens (1979) in the following terms:

Rogers may be the recipient of esteem from those nurses who mistakenly assume that any theory must have merit if they cannot understand it.

The position taken in this book therefore is that models and conceptual frameworks are very similar, consisting of sets of ideas which establish a framework to guide nursing practice. If they are to be given credibility by nurses and therefore be of any value, they should be based in and derived from practice. Theory on the other hand is a more focused approach which seeks to explain relationships between concepts and permit prediction of likely future events, but only within certain probability limits. There is no such thing as certainty in theory when applied to nursing, or medicine for that matter. Part of the skill of nursing is being able to manage that uncertainty. The good nurse can improvise when things do not work out as expected and learn from that situation; this is known as reflection in action and is a topic we explore later.

The problems associated with differing uses of the terms 'model' and 'theory' are exemplified by Benner and Wrubel's description of a model as something which consists of measurable constructs which can be causally related (Benner and Wrubel, 1989). This leads these authors to dismiss models as mechanistic and of no value. What they have described is, of course, a theory not a model. When such an influential nurse scholar as Benner uses terms in this confusing way, it is small wonder that others also become confused. To dismiss theory and the value of causal relationships in this way is a serious flaw in Benner and Wrubel's work and undermines the credibility of nursing in the eyes of most other professional groups. It also reveals a lack of understanding of how science works, as it is not as mechanistic as these authors suggest.

Paradigms, world views and the origin of theory in nursing

Nurses tend to have a bias for action and getting on with things; consequently, philosophy is not everybody's cup of tea. However, increasing numbers of nurse authors are justifying their views by recourse to philosophy and we cannot afford to take these justifications for granted. Ford and Walsh (1994) have written extensively of the problems nursing has had with unthinking, uncritical acceptance of new ideas; the 'flavour of the month' syndrome. It is important therefore that theories and conceptual frameworks are subjected to critical scrutiny, rather than passively accepted. This requires dipping into philosophical waters in order to examine the foundations claimed for some of these ideas.

Traditionally, there have been two approaches to gaining knowledge which have been divided into quantitative and qualitative. This leads to two different world views with the former identified with tried and tested scientific method which emphasizes testing hypotheses, developing predictive theory, empirical observation, and a belief in an objective reality which exists independently of the observer. The latter approach stems from a belief that human activity is too complex to be measured and reduced to abstract theory, therefore emphasis is placed upon descriptions of the world and interpreting the meaning of events to individual participants as they see them. In this view objectivity is discounted and subjectivity is recognized and valued.

These two views are compatible with each other and good research draws upon both traditions according to the demands of the problem being investigated. Unfortunately, some authors have chosen to champion one approach as the *only* way to gain knowledge, rejecting the other out of hand. It is not difficult to recognize the quantitive methodology as underpinning medicine. As nursing has tried recently to establish itself as a separate independent profession, moving out from under the shadow of medicine, it is not surprising that nurses have been tempted to reject quantitative foundations of knowledge and unfortunately this has led to a situation where many nurse writers have rejected an objective foundation for nursing (e.g. Rogers, 1970; Watson, 1988; Newman, 1994).

A third recent world view to arrive on the scene and which is of relevance in the social sciences has been the critical social theory perspective which is concerned with uncovering the hidden power imbalances that are contained within the social world, setting itself an agenda of empowerment (Robinson and Vaughan, 1992). This approach is increasingly being studied by those concerned with developing nursing's independence (Ford and Walsh, 1994).

Critics of the objective, quantitative approach to discovering knowledge argue that the world of nursing is too complex for mechanistic determinism, while pointing out that, in practice, science cannot proceed in such an ideal objective way. In reality, science does not subscribe to this view either; it is a simplification and a caricature of science that has been portrayed by those who would argue against the quantitative approach. Scientists should not be likened to fictional characters such as *Star Trek*'s Mr Spock! They are human and consequently science does proceed in illogical ways at times. This was recognized by writers such as Lakatos (1978) who drew attention to the social factors involved in the development of scientific ideas while others such as Feyerabend (1975) proposed that there were no rational set of rules which could guide scientists in their choice of theories, leading to his anarchistic argument that astrology, mysticism, witchcraft and the like, were as equally valid and deserving of public esteem and resources as science. For Feyerabend, nurses could just as readily base their practice upon witchcraft or astrology as pathology and pharmacology.

It is fashionable for many nurse authors to discuss philosophy by writing about the notion of paradigms and their associated changes or shifts (it was years before somebody explained the pronunciation of this word to me, so if you as the reader are puzzled, it is pronounced *paradime*). This is an issue that has been argued about considerably in the realms of the philosophy of science and has recently surfaced in discussion about nursing theory. It is an issue therefore worth briefly attempting to clarify as many authors attempt to justify their theories about nursing in terms of a paradigm shift.

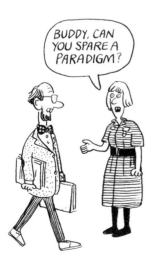

BUDDY, CAN YOU SPARE A PARADIGM?

The notion of a paradigm originated with Kuhn in the 1960s. His thesis was that scientists (including social scientists) work within a broad set of ideas and assumptions about the world that are widely shared by most scientists (Kuhn, 1970). This constitutes the prevailing paradigm and it allows us to interpret the world and make sense of the observations we make. It has been likened to a pair of spectacles through which we view the world. If we put on a new pair of spectacles, or adopt a new paradigm, we see the world as a very different place. This opens up a key philosophical question for as Casti (1989) points out, this suggests that there is no such thing as a measured fact, as we see *by interpretation* and the interpretation of what we measure depends upon the prevailing paradigm that we have adopted. For example, a person who is hearing voices and seeing visions would, according to one paradigm, be defined as mentally ill and suffering some biochemical disorder in the brain. However, another paradigm might define that person as a religious visionary, a saint or even a prophet. Within the former paradigm, epilepsy is a disease that can be treated but in another paradigm, it is evidence of possession by the devil best treated by being burnt alive rather than a course of anti-convulsants. Truth, knowledge and reality have now become relative rather than absolute and it all depends upon your paradigm. The scientific researcher can no longer be independent and objective about whatever they are researching as the paradigm notion entwines the researcher and influences whatever it is they see or measure.

Kuhn (1970) went on to argue that paradigms do change, but often in a revolutionary way and as a result of irrational factors such as group affiliations and faction fighting rather than the cool logic of scientific progress.

Kuhn's ideas have influenced many nurse academics who have adopted them and replaced the scientist with the nurse, arguing that indeed truth is relative as it is different for each patient and nurse. This also opens up the notion of a paradigm shift away from the biomedical paradigm to some new nursing paradigm that seeks to define itself by rejecting objective science and embracing subjectivity and holism. This presents many difficulties which will be explored in the rest of this chapter not least of which is the rejection of knowledge and truth which is objective. Planning the care, however, of patients in a multidisciplinary care environment, who are in pain, deeply distressed or suffering life-threatening conditions, does require a factual base of objective knowledge.

It is worth noting that there have been many critics of Kuhn's ideas led by Shapere (1971) who argued that Kuhn reduced science to a series of trendy fads dressed up to look presentable. Would Shapere say the same about some of the 'new nursing' that is claimed to flow from the paradigm shift away from the medical model I wonder? He homed in on the spectacles analogy by pointing out that spectacles may affect the colouring of what is seen if they have tinted lenses; they may also distort or even invert the image, but nevertheless the basic shape and structure of the object being viewed remain the same. In other words there is an objective reality.

This section started with a review of the quantitative/qualitative debate and the suggestion that many nurse authors had rejected the notion of objective reality in order to embrace the subjective and qualitative view of the world. Kuhn's work on paradigms is frequently cited uncritically by such authors, yet as we have seen here, it is open to serious criticism. Paley (1996) considers that much of the critique deployed by such writers against a quantitative, objective view is out of date and draws attention to writers such as Lakatos (1978) and Feyerabend (1976) among others, who post-date Kuhn and yet remain ignored by nurse critics of science. Those who philosophize about a new nursing paradigm, such as Watson (1988), are considered to be amateurish and ill informed by Paley who strongly urges nurses to go back to the original sources of ideas about science and knowledge and to recognize that thinking has moved on a long way since Kuhn's original ideas of 1970.

There is therefore a significant critique of those who claim a philosophical justification for developing a new nursing independent of the natural and biomedical sciences. However, there is an even bigger and more pragmatic problem than any such critique, which can be summed up by the simple question; does philosophy make any difference? To explore the role of philosophy in shaping nursing theory or conceptual frameworks, it is worth looking at the natural sciences as a good analogy. According to Casti (1989), the level of contact between philosophers of science and practising scientists is zero and therefore the effect that philosophers have on day-to-day science is minimal: it goes on without them. Casti put it this way:

As far as most practising scientists are concerned, there's nothing more dangerous than a philosopher in the grip of a theory. Casti (1989, p. 48)

There are probably many clinical nurses who would agree with the sentiments behind this statement when thinking about nurse academics or philosophers. Nurses, like scientists, are practical people who like to get on with the job. If they are to give ideas credibility, they have to see the practical connections to their real world, which is not often easy in philosophy. So while we might occasionally have the time to step back and wonder what is the meaning of reality, in practice such ponderings have little impact upon the work of the clinical nurse.

This discourse into the realms of paradigms and paradigm shifts suggests that while they may interest philosophers and academics in nursing, their impact upon the real world of nursing care has been limited. However, there has undoubtedly been some movement away from the traditional medical view that was prevelant perhaps 20 years ago as nurses increasingly attempt to care for the whole person rather than a piece of pathology. Sometimes, however, lack of time and resources makes such a whole-person approach very difficult to practise.

It remains then to move on and look at the notion of theories, whether we wish to accept the concept of paradigms or not. A key question that has to be addressed is: where does theory come from? We have already seen that models have either been derived from observation of the real world or developed from the world of abstract philosophical ideas and assumptions about human beings. Newman (1994) describes how Martha Johnson worked with this latter approach as she rejected practice-based methods and with them the social and biological sciences as valid foundations for nursing. It was argued that this represented a paradigm shift. Instead, she called for a new discipline of nursing science that embraced her holistic concept of the human being and unitary energy fields (whatever they are!), dreaming up an approach to nursing that is divorced from reality and which has no foundation in the biological or social sciences. It is also incomprehensible, as Stevens (1979) earlier observed. Rogers' work should therefore serve as a cautionary tale to academics, about the dangers of straying too far from reality and current nursing practice.

The need to keep theory and practice closely linked has been emphasized by Rolfe (1993) who argued for theory generation out of practice in the reflective practitioner mode attributed to Donald Schon (1983). However, Rolfe argues for a redefinition of the word 'theory' to mean the informal theory that nurses use all the time in everyday practice rather than the conventional scientific meaning of the term. Without this informal theory that is embedded in practice, practice would degenerate into a series of random and meaningless acts. Schon (1983) argues that practitioners build up a situational repertoire of knowledge to allow them to deal with a range of situations. This repertoire is continually being expanded and is enhanced by reflection in action. This is consistent with Benner's differentiation between 'knowing how' and 'knowing that' which implies that knowing how to do something may not require the abstract form of knowledge, 'knowing that', which can be demon-strated by writing down a reasoned case that justifies and describes the action to be taken (Benner, 1984). This latter point opens an interesting angle on the accountability debate that follows later. For now we stay with Rolfe's rejection of the conventional under-standing of theory in favour of this new idea which says that the knowledge and meaning are embedded in the situation and are therefore unique to the individual practitioner.

Rolfe (1993) justifies this departure on the grounds that the normal understanding of theory implies prediction and this is impossible with any certainty in the world of nursing. As we have seen, pre-diciton is only possible within limits of probability due to all the intervening variables of situation and context. Rolfe argues that in the natural sciences this probability problem is not there, therefore this approach to theory is appropriate in considering the properties of a steel girder, but it is not appropriate for nursing. However, there is a flaw here for the natural sciences have also realized that theory cannot predict with certainty, so there is no justification for the rejection of theory on these grounds. The history of science in the

20th century has been characterized by the destruction of certainty. It started in the exotic world of quantum physics with the Heisenberg Uncertainty Principle and has now spread through Chaos Theory to embrace meteorology, biology and economics among others. The physical world is now recognized as a chaotic place and the notion of scientific theory predicting exactly what will happen next with 100% certainty is redundant. The whole of science, including medical science, embraces uncertainty and in looking to nursing theory we have to accept that, in common with other disciplines, it can only predict what will happen with a given degree of probability. It is worth harking back to the point made earlier about some nurse authors presenting an oversimplification of science (or maybe just failing to understand it?) for Rolfe appears to have done just that in his failure to acknowledge chaos and probability theory.

It is not helped by mainstream nursing research texts falling into the same trap. For example, we find the following misleading oversimplification in Polit and Hungler (1995) as they write about objective reality, completely ignoring the lessons of chaos theory:

A related belief is that natural phenomona are basically regular and orderly. Polit and Hungler (1995, p. 17)

Rolfe was right to stress the importance of practice informing theory and the notion of nurses learning by reflecting critically on their care, but wrong to reject the normal view of theory in favour of this personalized experiential version of theory. What happens when a nurse encounters a particular situation for the first time and has no situational repertoire to draw upon? Theory in the normal sense of the word equips the nurse to make a start at solving the problem; theory in this new sense of the word leaves the nurse guessing as s/he has no previous experience of the situation. What price accountability then?

The personal nature of knowledge derived in this way opens up the question: which nurse's theory is correct? Presumably, all are equally valid – in which case we have the problem of relativism and subjectivity replacing theory and knowledge. This important issue has already been alluded to in the discussion on paradigms and it is returned to later.

Theory is only of any value if nurses can use it in practice to deal with patient problems. Nursing models or conceptual frameworks paint the broad picture of how we would like nursing to look, and Wright (1986) was probably correct to assert that every nurse has their own individual model of nursing in their head. Such informal, individualistic 'models' do, however, have strong elements in common concerned with basic beliefs on the one hand and plain common sense on the other. Nursing theory, however, introduces agreed objective truth which allows us to carry out the work of nursing; it illuminates the darkness of not knowing what to do when confronted by a patient in pain or who is emotionally distressed. We do not have to make up our own completely individual pattern of responses from zero because we know that theory will predict that if we do certain things they will probably lead to a better outcome than others. That theory though needs applying correctly to individual patients and it is in individualizing the theory to meet the patient's needs, that we find high-quality nursing care.

Levine (1995) wrote that poetry is a collection of known words which only spring into life with the ability to inspire and amaze when assembled in a certain way by the poet. In the same way, Levine wrote that theory is the poetry of science as it also takes known facts and assembles them together in a new way to inspire and motivate, to provide insight into insoluble problems and allow the practitioner to see the way ahead. If theory is unclear and obscure, it is bad theory for it serves no useful purpose.

The terms discussed so far all depend upon knowledge and some idea as to the nature of nursing. Conceptual frameworks, models and theories all use these elements as their basic building blocks. The study of knowledge is called epistemology and if we are to make sense of nursing models and theory, we have to undertstand something about knowledge in nursing.

Knowledge for nursing

Whether we are dealing with models or theories, they are both intimately concerned with knowledge about nursing. Robinson and Vaughan (1992) point out that the nurse must access this extensive knowledge base before being able to practice and recommend the classic description of the origins of nursing knowledge attributed to Carper (1978) who described four ways of knowing in nursing:

- *Empirics.* That which can be observed and measured is empirical knowledge. This forms the basis for much of the knowledge drawn from the social and biological sciences and also nursing research. This is the knowledge that Benner would call 'know that' (Benner, 1984).
- *Ethics.* Moral judgements about what is right or wrong have long played a part in nursing as evidenced by the UKCC Code of Professional Conduct. As nurses learn to be more accountable for their actions, the spotlight will fall increasingly upon ethics.
- *Aesthetics.* Nursing has a side that cannot be written down in the normal way; this is what Benner (1984) alludes to in her view that nurses know more than they can tell: the 'know how' of nursing. Vaughan and Robinson (1992) consider this leads to the need to interpret meaning from action. Benner also considered that sometimes expert nurses appear to act by intuition as there was no evidence of knowledge underpinning action – the knowing was in the action. This elusive quality is the art of nursing or aesthetics.

● *Personal knowledge.* Self-awareness is crucial because it influences everything that we do and makes us all different. The nurse has to know him or herself and recognize the implications this has for practice. This is a major problem for Rolfe's view of nursing theory as the self will influence knowledge derived in this way, leading to the issue of subjectivity raised on p. 10.

In understanding how nurses have tried to uncover nursing knowledge, where they are starting out from in other words, these four types of knowledge should be borne in mind. There are discernible influences upon the way nursing models or conceptual frameworks have been shaped according to the preferences of authors for Carper's four types of nursing knowledge. Some have placed great emphasis upon the empirical side of nursing, having built their model from observation of practice (e.g. Roy, 1995; Orem, 1990), while others have started in the practice field but have then been more concerned with the aesthetic dimension, seeing nursing knowledge as a personal, increasingly intuitive activity. The work we have already encountered by writers such as Benner (1984) and Rolfe (1993) falls into this category but their concerns are more with models of how nurses learn to be nurses rather than models of what nursing itself is. As we have seen, there are others such as Rogers (1970) and Newman (1994) who have rejected empirics altogether to develop a view of nursing from moral philosophy and the interaction of the nurse with the patient who is conceptualized as a holistic being. This is therefore drawing heavily upon the ethical and personal self areas of knowledge and this rejection of empirical knowledge is claimed by these authors to constitute what Kuhn (1970) would call a paradigm shift.

In reviewing the origins of nursing knowledge, Bradshaw (1995) considers that a major trend in recent years has been to try and construct an understanding from the lived experiences of those involved, citing Benner (1984) and Benner and Wrubel (1989) as the prime exponents of this approach in the USA but also acknowledging the work of people such as Robinson (1993) in the UK who also pointed out that there can be no such thing as a general theory of nursing. There are parallels here with the approach recommended by Rolfe (1993), drawing heavily upon the nurse's reflections in action to build up knowledge about nursing. Bradshaw argues at length that this more subjective approach, which does not fit the normal methodology of the natural sciences upon which nursing is based, is taking nursing down the wrong road. It will also act as a hindrance to developing closer working relationships with other professional groups who remain loyal to the notion of objective reality.

Benner's seminal work described how nurses progress and learn as they grow from novice, through advanced learner, competency, proficiency and on to expert (Benner, 1984). She considered that nurses start off as novices in a state of confusion, only seeing fragments of the picture because of their lack of experience. As they progress they exhibit heavily rule-bound behaviour, utilizing received wisdom and knowledge to work methodically and logically in an explicit problem-solving approach to achieve competency (the newly qualified nurse) before moving on to more advanced stages. At these levels the rationales for decisions become implicit and the nurse's actions according to Benner become more intuitive. They are less able to explain why certain courses of action are pursued, the knowledge is in the doing rather than separate and therefore able to justify the doing.

It is this view of advanced nursing knowledge that characterizes the expert nurse which has stirred up considerable controversy. Many nurses seem able to identify with it and recognize it in practice, leading to widespread support. However, as Bradshaw (1995) points out, it does lead to several serious difficulties as a foundation for nursing knowledge – the same sort of difficulties we encountered with Rolfe's (1993) views about generating knowledge out of practice. The problem is that if knowledge is intuitive, it is subjective, therefore how can it be tested as right or wrong?

The work of Benner and others is derived from phenomenology, a qualitative research method that acknowledges that we each see things differently and attach our own meanings to events. A patient refusing treatment may be exercising their rights as a human being to one nurse while to another that same patient may be acting selfishly because of the impact on the rest of the family of their continuing illness, while a third nurse might see the patient as simply lacking knowledge and in urgent need of health education. The same event has three different meanings to three different nurses and of course a fourth meaning – that which the patient attaches to the situation. It may also have different meanings to other professionals involved in that care and, as care is becoming increasingly multiprofessional, we cannot ignore the issue of different professional as well as personal perspectives. This approach leads to the denial of absolute objective truth and its replacement with relativism. Bradshaw (1995) goes further and argues this view also denies the validity of absolute codes of conduct as 'it all depends upon the situation', therefore the nurse is operating a form of moral relativism at odds with absolute standards such as those set by the UKCC Code of Conduct for example.

Benner's work has also been subjected to critique by Cash (1995) who echoes these criticisms of intuitive and therefore subjective knowledge. This leads Cash to suggest that Benner's work is a major obstacle to the development of nursing knowledge and practice as it '. . . retreats into the validation of practice by authority and tradition'. The point is that, if a sister does things a certain way, and is challenged as to why, she can claim to be an expert and justify her actions accordingly. Benner's view of nursing therefore offers a convenient bolt hole for authoritarian nurses to avoid the challenge of justifying their actions. The claim that the knowing is in the doing absolves the nurse from having to produce the evidence to justify their practice. Benner's ideas, which on the one hand can be seen as a great liberating influence upon nurses in the clinical environment (Ford and Walsh, 1994), can also be something of a double-edged sword as they can be used to justify outdated and ritualistic practices.

Benner's ideas touched off a particularly illuminating debate about the state of nursing theory between English (1993) who voiced various criticisms similar to the ones discussed above and Darbyshire (1994) who defended Benner vigorously. Darbyshire's defence was based upon an outright attack upon the notion of objective rationality as a basis for nursing, one of the main thrusts of English's paper. A fascinating analysis of this at times rather acrimonious exchange has been offered by Paley (1996) who seeks to clarify the fog of war which surrounded this conflict. Paley is of the view that both protagonists got certain key ideas wrong and sets out to clarify them while pointing out that at times the level of debate was rather juvenile. English (1993) is accused of caricature as he describes the expert practitioner as a 'blessed practitioner initiated into the knowledge of some secret society' while Darbyshire is considered to be guilty of self-conscious posturing in his account of dominant worldviews!

Paley is right to move the debate about scientific philosophies on from the time warp of the 1960s and early 1970s where it appears to have become fossilized and also right to point out the futility of this polemic debate between quantitative and qualitative methodologies in underpinning nursing knowledge and models. Paley also makes some interesting new points about Benner's ideas such as asking how we recognize expert practice? Darbyshire (1994) claims from his relativistic stance that there are no explicit criteria, only the judgement of the relevant community. Paley rightly asks who are the relevant community because, if this only means other nurses, what about the views of doctors, patients and NHS managers? As patterns of working become increasingly multidisciplinary, we need to recognize that other professional groups also have a valid point of view concerning nursing expertise. We can end up with four different groups, all with different views about expert practice if Darbyshire's views on Benner are adhered to. They cannot all be correct as the result would be contradictory and unsafe. This is the morass that relativistic thinking leads into.

Existentialism is the touchstone of many current nurse academics and leads to the philosophical positions we explored earlier. It is a philosophy which proposes that each individual is a free human being, free and responsible for determining their own destiny. This underpins ideas about developing the nurse–patient relationship, self-actualization as the main goal of the patient, and the nurse making sense of the lived experience of the patient. The recognition of the patient as a person in this way and the way this has changed the traditional nursing approach is most welcome. It is a short step from here, however, to the subjective, intuitive approach to knowledge that we have discussed so far, leading to the view that knowledge is what each expert nurse says it is. This is intellectual relativism and complements the moral relativism discussed earlier. This is the basis of Bradshaw's critique of much contemporary thinking about nursing knowledge (Bradshaw, 1995).

Bradshaw develops her thesis by reminding us of where we actually have come from: the ideas of Florence Nightingale, who advocated a sense of absolute goodness and objective reality, no relativism there! Medicine also grew up in the same framework of an absolute sense of good and right coupled with an objective truth about the world of disease and treatment. The nurse–patient relationship took place within this framework and developed in such a way as to reflect the reality of the unequal nature of that relationship. The patient is very vulnerable and not in possession of the knowledge, authority and good health that the nurse has. That is reality, whatever the views of modern theorists. Bradshaw's arguments culminate in her call for nursing to pause and reflect upon where it is going. She feels nursing has lost contact with the practical reality of nursing, which is founded upon technical skills, objective scientific truth and an absolute code of moral conduct. Instead, we have been seduced by the social sciences and as a result the subjective, personal, intuitive side of nursing is receiving too much attention compared with the practical, technical, science-based aspects of care (Bradshaw, 1995). It is this that allows Newman (1994) to claim that theory is lived by the nurse rather than being an abstract entity which is applied by the nurse to patient care.

This critique may look like a call to abandon current nursing education in favour of the traditional task-based apprenticeship system, with the old procedure manual restored to its rightful place at the altar at which all staff worship and receive their daily quota of ritual. But Bradshaw has a point, for if we walk away from the objective reality of science, we ignore the reality of clinical nursing. This is particularly crucial today because we are seeing an increased realization that good patient care is collaborative care involving medicine and all the other professions such as physiotherapy, occupational therapy, radiography, etc. More than ever, the need is for a common language and a common basis for care rather than nursing pulling up the drawbridge behind a rejection of the objectivity that underpins all other professional groups. We should also remember

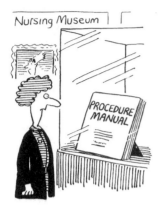

that the UKCC Code of Conduct is an absolute code of ethics which does not permit moral relativism.

Perhaps the pendulum has simply swung too far in the existentialist's direction and what is needed is a return to reality, but certainly not to any rose-tinted spectacle vision of matrons and back rounds. We can leave the procedure manual as part of our history along with impractical uniforms and frilly caps. However, we have to acknowledge that patients have a right to expect the increasingly technical nature of their care to be performed promptly and with expertise, they have a right to expect care to be based upon sound evidence and for nurses to be approaching their work with a knowledge base that is rooted in reality. Patients also have a right to be treated like human beings, so remembering the old wisdom about babies and bathwater, we need to strike the right balance between the social and the biological sciences as the basis for nursing knowledge. That balance is not about rejecting the whole of biomedicine in favour of a new paradigm or pseudoscience of nursing as those such as Newman would argue (Newman, 1994). It is better to heed Roy's warning that nurses have a built-in bias for action but tend to forget there is someone on the other side of that action, the patient; therefore, we must have an understanding of the patient to make the best of our actions and interventions (Roy, 1995). We must avoid a return to thinking of patients as diagnoses and bits of pathology or as collections of tasks to be performed in accordance with the procedure manual. We also need to realize that our actions produce unintentional as well as intentional effects for the patient and real nursing expertise is in understanding of both these sets of consequences, but within a framework of objective reality, truth and falseness, good and bad (Roy, 1995).

Behi and Nolan (1995) rightly point out that nursing has to draw upon the wealth of biological and social science knowledge that is available as the foundation for the body of theory that makes nursing practice possible (empirics). However, that is not enough for as Rolfe (1993) reminds us – while the scientist may discover knowledge, it is the engineer who has to apply it. Nurses are acting as engineers in this sense and it is the application of this empirical knowledge that requires use of the other three areas of knowledge that Carper (1978) articulated: ethics, aesthetics and personal. The need is to incorporate all four areas of knowledge into practice but not to exclude empirics as some modern writers would advocate nor to relegate the latter three areas to their former position of relative insignificance.

If this approach is adopted, nursing research can be seen as research in the application of knowledge to nursing and therefore helps to inform evidence-based practice. The body of knowledge that develops around the application of biological and social sciences knowledge to caring becomes nursing knowledge and remains rooted in reality – a reality which nurses can recognize and therefore identify with, rather than the mysticism which has come to envelop some theorists' writings. Because it is reality, it is open to scrutiny and objective testing, which is essential if we are to conform to the famous dictum of Nightingale and the UKCC Code of Conduct and do the patient no harm (and preferably some good!).

Benner's views have influenced many nurses, including the current author who can readily identify with her first three stages of learning (novice, advanced beginner and competency). There is a groundswell of recognition for her more controversial final two stages of proficiency and expertise but there are significant criticisms that we have explored in this chapter to do with the subjective nature of her description. It is necessary to make explicit the objective knowledge that lies within her account of these levels of practice or else those who operate with a more objective framework (e.g. medicine) will never take expert nursing seriously. Cash's comment that intuition may be a necessary condition of expertise, but not a sufficient one, rings true in this regard (Cash, 1995). Perhaps the view of Noyes (1995) that Benner's ideas explain the rapid recognition of problems by experts, rather than describe a true problem-solving process, helps place Cash's comment in context.

Research aimed at replication of Benner's findings in nursing is urgently needed to help clarify this argument. Can we identify her stages of development in the way nurses work? Little seems to have been published in this field although Greenwood and King (1995) have carried out one study which failed to find any evidence of different ways of thinking when looking at expert and novice nurses in the clinical situation. These authors reported significant issues with their methodology, which involved nurses talking out loud as they were thinking their way through problems, and are now repeating the study using improvements gained from experience in the first exercise. Kitson *et al.* (1993) also failed to find any significant difference in acceptable knowledge between novices and experts when looking at one specific aspect of care: post-operative pain management. This is a single issue investigated in one study, therefore too much should not be read into this finding either. It is true to say though that little work has been done in nursing to replicate Benner's original research and the two studies cited above failed to achieve replication.

The theory–practice gap: reality or illusion?

If knowledge is discovered from such wide areas of academic activity and is able to provide the theory on which we can base nursing practice, why is there the famous 'theory–practice gap' that nurses have been talking about for so long? The analogy of scientists and engineers alluded to earlier provides part of the answer (Rolfe, 1993). If nurses are the 'engineers' then it is easy to argue that there will always be a gap between knowledge and how we apply it in practice. However, engineers make it their business to be as up to date as possible about the science they seek to apply. Before building a bridge over a river, an engineer will have thoroughly researched the strengths and properties of the materials of his bridge; they will also know about the rainfall and runoff patterns of the river so that they can make predictions about the likely size of major floods that the bridge will have to cope with. In short, their practice will be evidence based. This has been the problem with nursing for so long in the past – the evidence has been there but it has been ignored in favour of ritual and tradition (Walsh and Ford, 1989). The solution lies in shifting the way nurses think about practice and the need for evidence upon which to base it, coupled with research into the most effective ways of applying knowledge to nursing situations. This in its turn may generate new knowledge which could be called uniquely nursing knowledge.

The issue of the theory–practice gap is explored further by Levine (1995) who takes educationalists to task for helping to propagate and widen this gap. She initially points out that if educationalists lack understanding and conviction about the use of theory, students can hardly be blamed for failing to recognize the importance of theory to practice. It is a short step from here to question the extent to which educationalists actually believe in what they teach. Do they really believe for example in the value of exploring a range of conceptual frameworks and models? If they lack recent clinical involvement, it will be difficult for them to see the links between the theory they espouse and practice in the real world. This undermines their conviciton and understanding of theory.

The main target of Levine's fire, however, is the way academics have tried to develop a separate language of nursing, rather than use widely understood terms, simply because they were medical (Levine, 1995). How many students were taught that they cannot use medical terms in a nursing care plan a few years ago? This is seen in extreme form in the North American Nursing Diagnosis terminology and in the language used by various proponents of nursing models. As Levine points out, communication is hampered by the use of a theoretical language that practising nurses do not understand and which cannot be superimposed on the workplace. Care is becoming increasingly multidisciplinary with different professions sharing the same plan of care such as the development of critical pathways (CPs). This is explored in a later chapter but for now it is obvious that interprofessional co-operation will be enhanced by the development of a common language of care rather than nursing seeking to go it alone.

Similar observations about language and research publications also apply. Many authors write up their findings only for other researchers, utilizing an arcane and jargon-riddled language, rather than write in plain English for the practising nurse. A typical finding is that of Walsh (1997) who discovered that the biggest single group of problems cited by both hospital and community nurses as perceived barriers to research implementation were to do with the difficult way the research was written up and published.

Accountability and nursing knowledge

Several allusions have been made to the term 'accountability' in this chapter so far. This is a concept that has taken on a high priority in recent years, thanks to a series of key papers from the UKCC, culminating in the *Scope of Professional Practice* document (UKCC, 1992). Nurses have been used to being responsible for their actions, but accountability is something different – even though used loosely as an interchangeable term with responsibility.

Accountability means literally to be able to give an account of your actions; in other words, why you did what you did. For the nurse to be accountable, therefore, s/he has to be able to justify the actions taken. This justification requires knowledge upon which to base actions and the ability to show what other courses of action were considered before deciding upon the one carried out. Nurses also need the authority to do what they have decided to do, otherwise they may be overridden by others and are then merely following orders. In this latter case, they are responsible but not accountable.

If we reflect back upon the existentialist school of thought that leads to theory being lived by the nurse, rather than an abstract and objective truth, then there is a difficulty emerging here. To talk of expert nursing knowledge being in the doing, being intuitive, known to only the doer and therefore subjective means that it cannot be objectively scrutinized. There is no standard of what constitutes correct nursing care in any given situation except that which each individual nurse says it is. How then can the nurse be accountable for his/her actions other than by saying 'I did it my way'?

To be accountable, more than this is needed as the nurse is accountable not only to his/herself. The nurse is accountable to the patient both morally and in the eyes of civil law, the employer and the UKCC. When faced by such an authoritative panel all sitting in judgement upon the nurse by holding him or her accountable, is it really good enough to say 'Well it seemed a good idea to me at the time'? Yet the subjective and relativistic approach to theory espoused by many leads to this predicament as shown by Benner's statement that:

There is no higher court than the expert's reading of a particular situation. Benner (1984, p. 177)

Setting aside the question of who decides whether a nurse is an expert or not, this statement throws up some interesting possibilities not least of which is the thought that this places the nurse above the

UKCC or the civil law. The nurse's interpretation of a particular situation determines action, but that action must be justifiable in the world of objective reality if the nurse is to be truly accountable. It will also help the nurse to avoid being on the wrong end of a lawsuit for negligence while practising safely, legally and within the UKCC Code of Professional Conduct. The nurse should not be lulled into a false sense of security by the siren call of being labelled an expert.

Accountability also needs objectivity to supplement knowledge and authority. The demands of the UKCC Code of Professional Conduct and documents such as *The Scope of Professional Practice* therefore make it mandatory that there should be an objective and realistic base for nursing theory, models and conceptual frameworks.

Do models and conceptual frameworks really matter?

In the chapter so far we have explored the meaning of the terms 'models' and 'conceptual frameworks', showing that they are closely allied but operate in a loose way to set a framework within which nursing takes place. Theory has a different meaning as it guides practice by giving the nurse the ability to generalize and predict, but only with a given probability and usually depending upon the circumstances. Theory therefore should concern itself with the practicalities of care and be rooted in the real world, possessing objective reality and a sense of absolute right and wrong.

Much recent nursing debate about theory has become lost in the subjective world of existentialism leading to a multitude of versions of the truth with each nurse having their own personal version of theory. The enthusiasm for talking of paradigms and a paradigm shift to a 'new nursing' has been questioned in light of the debate which has raged elsewhere. Subjectivity and relativism lead to major problems of accountability, may compromise working with other professions and have also seen the development of theory which has little relevance to, and therefore credibility with, clinicians. Relativism and subjectivity are rejected in favour of objective reality and a re-affirmation of support for the traditional scientific approach to knowledge which feeds into a need to restore the balance between clinical and social skills in nursing. The development of models for nursing must reflect these principles and the increasing reality of multidisciplinary care in a rapidly changing health service.

This brief resume of the chapter so far leads up to the key question: does it all matter? After all we have been nursing since the days of Nightingale without models of nursing, so why do we need them now? Hardy (1986), for example, wrote that models were unhelpful as they would lead to incomprehensible jargon, encourage tramlines thinking where nurses see only what the model tells them to see, and that models suffer from subjectivity as they are only the author's point of view.

Nursing, of course, has always had jargon and the general UK population seem quite adept at coping with the American version of the English language, if TV-viewing figures are anything to go by. Hardy has a point, however, as we have seen already how some American authors have relished a fog of obscure language.

Tramlines thinking was an issue raised by Walsh and Ford (1989) in their review of ritualistic nursing practice but this had much to do with nurse training and the balance of power within health care and little to do with nursing models. It is true that the strict use of a rigid assessment schedule denies the patient the opportunity to talk about their priorities, but that schedule could come from anywhere, not necessarily a nursing model, and the problem is in the implementation of the assessment rather than the actual assessment itself. Without a structured assessment to guide the nurse, major areas of health concern may be missed. Any worthwhile assessment scheme must include the patient's view of their health problems, whether it be based on a mainstream nursing model or not.

As a model becomes part of the wider nursing community, it should be open to scrutiny, critique, evaluation and amendment. Ford and Walsh (1994) have shown, however, that nursing has in the past had a tendency to accept new ideas uncritically, reflecting its authoritarian background, professional immaturity and the weaknesses in traditional nurse training. Nursing models such as the Roper Logan Tierney model were, in the 1980s, subject to uncritical adoption with little input other than from their authors, making the charge of subjectivity a valid one at that time. However, the process of scrutiny and evaluation should reduce substantially the subjective element as more nurses have an input, and it is an input derived from the harsh world of practice where things either work or they do not. What may start out life as a subjective view of nursing can be tested against objective standards in practice and either rejected or amended accordingly, thereby substantially reducing subjectivity.

We have dwelt at length upon the issue of subjectivity in terms of theory which predicts outcome, identifying this as a major weakness. However, a model is not a theory predicting outcomes of care. As we have seen, it is a framework of ideas to guide practice, just as George Washington and the Founding Fathers had their model of a constitution in mind when they established the USA and Churchill had his own democratic model in mind when he led the UK in standing alone against Nazi tyranny. A framework of ideas may be subjective in that it is one person's vision but it can be tested against a moral framework of right and wrong which will determine its acceptability and value. In this way the charge of moral relativism is avoided. And so it is with nursing models – as long as they can be objectively tested and accepted or rejected accordingly, the charge of subjectivity does not hold.

Models really do matter because they are the stuff of nursing. If we are to argue that nursing is a profession in its own right, then we need to be able to work out the boundaries of nursing so that we can recognize our legitimate field of practice. If nurses wish to be able to deliver the quality of care that they feel patients deserve, they must first of all know what that care is and how it should be delivered in order that they can fight for the necessary resources to carry out that care. The struggle for resources has become an increasingly dominant feature of the UK health scene in recent years and nursing care is the biggest consumer of those scarce resources.

Arguments about skill mix and staffing levels on wards revolve around what needs to be done and who is the most appropriate person to carry out that care. Can wards be run with one registered nurse and the rest of the staff acting as care assistants without a professional qualification? If not, why not? What is the stuff of nursing that says this cannot be, that it needs several qualified staff to care for these patients or that patients in the community must be visited by registered nurses? In attempting to answer these sort of questions we are trying to define that which is uniquely nursing, for which a professional education and qualification is necessary. Models of nursing are trying to do the same thing.

Field (1987) has argued along these lines, pointing out that models indicate the area of practice that is nursing as distinct from that of other allied health professionals. Nursing of course draws on these allied areas such as medicine or the behavioural sciences, but the nurse needs to take such knowledge and interpret it in nursing terms for it to be of benefit to the patient. Thus, Field rightly cautions that nursing models alone do not provide a sufficient knowledge base for nursing care, rather they set the framework for knowledge from a range of disciplines to be synthesized into effective nursing care. Nursing models are thus essential as they map out the boundaries of nursing and facilitate the bringing together of knowledge from a wide range of other disciplines to supplement the core nursing knowledge required for quality nursing care.

It is only possible to defend something when its boundaries are known, and today we need to defend nursing from the threats of de-skilling and take-over by a whole range of technicians, and other ancilliaries. Models define those boundaries and help us organize our delivery of care to suit the patient's needs.

Luker (1988), in asking whether models will work or not, raised the question that they may be red herrings. Nurses might say they have implemented a model, leading to the belief that change has occurred and gaining academic kudos in the process. This could be an illusion though and in reality very little has altered apart from using different bits of paper and introducing some new jargon. The obvious analogy with the implementation of the nursing process is discussed later. For now we should observe that introducing a model requires a fundamental re-examination of the way we think and carry out nursing care. Anything less is merely academic window dressing and cannot be given credit as really tackling the challenges presented by nursing models.

Do models matter? If having ideas which influence practice matters, then yes they matter. Torres (1986) pointed out that just as models of teaching or psychology influence the practice of these disciplines, so too it is with nursing, while Botha (1989) considers that the influence of theories of nursing upon practice is so self-evident that it no longer needs argument. This sweeping statement cannot be left unchallenged and Kristjanson and Tamblyn (1987) indeed take issue with this view, arguing that the literature contains no evidence that different conceptual frameworks produce differences in practice. Work by Faucett (Faucett *et al.*, 1990) does, however, suggest that implementing a model of nursing, in this case Orem's self-care model (1990), does produce changes in practice and for the better. A fuller consideration of Faucett's work is found later. For now the case is argued that, as practice cannot be divorced from a conceptual framework in any discipline, models of nursing do matter!

References

Behi R & Nolan M (1995) Sources of knowledge in nursing. *British Journal of Nursing*, **4**(3), 141–142, 159.

Benner P (1984) *From Novice to Expert. Excellence and Power in Clinical Nursing Practice*. Menlo Park, CA: Addison Wesley.

Benner P & Wrubel J (1989) *The Primacy of Caring*. Menlo Park, CA. Addison Wesley.

Botha E (1989) Theory development in perspective: The role of conceptual frameworks and models in theory development. *Journal of Advanced Nursing*, **15**, 49–55.

Bradshaw A (1995) What are nurses doing to patients? A review of theories of nursing past and present. *Journal of Clinical Nursing*, **4**, 81–92.

Carper B (1978) Fundamental patterns of knowing in nursing. *Advances in Nursing Science*, **1**(1), 13–23.

Cash K (1995) Benner and expertise in nursing: a critique. *International Journal of Nursing Studies*, **32**(6), 527–534.

Casti J (1989) *Paradigms Lost*. London: Abacus.

Darbyshire P (1994) Skilled expert practice: is it all in the mind? A response to English's critique of Benner's novice to expert model. *Journal of Advanced Nursing*, **19**(4), 755–761.

English I (1993) Intuition as a function of the expert nurse: a critique of Benner's novice to expert model. *Journal of Advanced Nursing*, **18**(3), 387–393.

Faucett J, Ellis V, Underwood P, Naqvi A & Wilson D (1990) The effects of Orem's self care model in a nursing home setting. *Journal of Advanced Nursing*, **15**, 659–666.

Fawcett J (1992) Conceptual models in nursing practice: the reciprocal relationship. *Journal of Advanced Nursing*, **17**, 224–226.

Feyerabend P (1975) *Against Method. Outlines of an Anarchistic Theory of Knowledge.* London: New Left Press.

Field P (1987) The impact of nursing theory on the clinical decision making process. *Journal of Advanced Nursing*, **12**, 563–571.

Ford P and Walsh M (1994) *New Rituals for Old: Nursing Through the Looking Glass.* Oxford: Butterworth Heinemann.

Greenwood J & King M (1995) Some surprising similarities in the clinical reasoning of 'expert' and 'novice' orthopaedic nurses; report of a study using verbal protocols and protocol analysis. *Journal of Advanced Nursing*, **22**, 907–913.

Hardy L (1986) Identifying the place of theoretical frameworks in an evolving discipline. *Journal of Advanced Nursing*, **11**, 103–107.

Kitson A, Harvey G, Hyndman S & Yerrell P (1993) A comparison of expert and practitioner derived criteria for post-operative pain management. *Journal of Advanced Nursing*, **18**, 218–232.

Kristjanson L & Tamblyn R (1987) A model to guide development and application of multiple nursing theories. *Journal of Advanced Nursing*, **12**, 523–529.

Kuhn T (1970) *The Structure of Scientific Revolutions*, 2nd edn. Chicago: University of Chicago Press.

Lakatos I (1978) *The Methodology of Scientific Research Programmes.* Cambridge: Cambridge University Press.

Levine M (1995) The rhetoric of nursing theory. Image. *Journal of Nursing Scholarship*, **27**(1) 11–14.

Luker K (1988) Do models work? *Nursing Times*, **84**(5), 27–29.

Newman M (1994) Theory for nursing practice. *Nursing Science Quarterly*, **7**(4), 153–157.

Noyes J (1995) An explanation of the differences between expert and novice performance in the administration of an intramuscular injection of an analgesic agent to a patient in pain. *Journal of Advanced Nursing*, **22**, 800-807.

Orem D (1990) *Nursing: Concepts of Practice*, 3rd edn. New York: McGraw Hill.

Paley J (1996) Intuition and expertise; comments on the Benner debate. *Journal of Advanced Nursing*, **23**, 665–671.

Polit D & Hungler B (1995) *Nursing Research: Principles and Methods*, 5th edn. Philadelphia: Lippincott.

Robinson J (1993) Problems with paradigms in a caring profession. In Kitson A (ed.) *Nursing Art and Science*, pp. 72–84. London: Chapman & Hall.

Robinson K & Vaughan B (1992) *Knowledge for Nursing Practice.* Oxford: Butterworth Heinemann.

Rogers M (1970) *An Introduction to the Theoretical Basis of Nursing.* Philadelphia: Davies.

Rolfe G (1993) Closing the theory–practice gap: a model of nursing praxis. *Journal of Clinical Nursing*, **2**, 173–177.

Roper N, Logan W & Tierney A (1996) *The Elements of Nursing*, 4th edn. Edinburgh: Churchill Livingstone.

Roy C (1995) Developing nursing knowledge: practice issues raised from four philosophical perspectives. *Nursing Science Quarterly*, **8**(2), 79–85.

Schon D (1983) *The Reflective Practitioner – How Professionals Think in Action.* London: Temple Smith.

Shapere D (1971) The Paradigm Concept. *Science*, 172, 706–709.

Stevens B (1979) *Nursing Theory. Analysis, Application, Evaluation.* Boston: Little Brown.

Torres G (1986) *Theoretical Foundations of Nursing.* Norwalk, CT: Appleton Century Crofts.

UKCC (1992) *The Scope of Professional Practice.* London: UKCC.

Walsh M (1997) How nurses perceive barriers to research implementation. *Nursing Standard*, **11**(19), 34–39.

Walsh M & Ford P (1989) *Nursing Rituals, Research and Rational Action.* Oxford: Butterworth Heinemann.

Watson J (1988) *Human Science and Human Care: A Theory of Nursing.* New York: National League for Nursing.

Wright S (1986) *Building and Using a Model of Nursing.* London: Edward Arnold.

2 Choosing a Model of Nursing

In the first chapter we saw that the terms 'model of nursing' and 'conceptual framework' are largely interchangeable and both are different from nursing theory. This chapter seeks to explore steps along the way to choosing a model or conceptual framework.

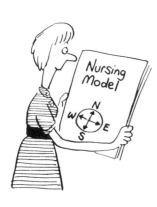

A model of nursing offers us a way of thinking about nursing. It is rather like a map and compass in that it maps out the terrain of nursing; it gives the nursing–patient interaction structure and allows us to find our way around this complex topography. Work with models so far leaves us at the stage of having carried out the first rough survey of the ground; we have only a sketch map showing a major river here and a mountain there, but we are awaiting the Ordnance Survey to come along and give us a reliable, detailed map that will allow us to confidently trust any chosen nursing model. It is up to ourselves as nurses to be our own surveyors, however, and not allow others to map out our territory for us; we must be our own Ordnance Survey.

The reliable charting of the model will only come from nurses working with the model, trying it out, questioning it and suggesting adaptations and improvements. Models are not set in tablets of stone, but rather are loose frameworks of ideas whose aim is to facilitate care, not to get in the way. Wright (1986) has written about the way a model of nursing evolved on his care of the elderly unit from the ideas of Virginia Henderson coupled with the development of existing practice by the unit staff. This is an excellent example of the usage of nursing models.

This approach involves starting out with a framework of ideas and putting them into practice, and observing how they perform before adapting them to try to achieve better results. This is known as inductive reasoning, whereby generalizations and knowledge are generated from observation (Pollit and Hungler, 1995). Thus, Orem's self-care model (1990) leads us to expect that patients with diabetes would wish to learn how to manage their diabetes for themselves; however, observing real patients shows this is sometimes not the case, therefore we must think why not? What causes these exceptions? How can we adapt this model of nursing to accommodate this observation and help patients who are poorly controlling their diabetes to manage their health more effectively? This is inductive reasoning working within a nursing model to adapt and refine that model.

Is it possible to generate a model of nursing from pure observation with no preconceived ideas? The answer is no, because such an inductive system needs an original framework of ideas and concepts, for as Hammersley and Atkinson (1983) point out, it is impossible to discover the nature of the social world without some method to guide our practice. Nursing models, with their views about the nature of people, how nurses and patients interact, the environment surrounding this interaction and the nature of health and illness, serve to provide this framework.

Field (1987) has developed this idea and argues that as long as any model includes these four key elements plus a method of systematic problem solving then it can rightly be considered a nursing model. What will differ, however, is the way in which the database is organized; that is, how the assessment differs, leading to a range of approaches to care. Field therefore argues that differing nursing models will lead to differences in care and illustrates her case with reference to a comparison of Orem's, Neuman's and Roy's models.

Field sees nurse theorists as thinkers who on the basis of years of practical experience have tried to break nursing down into the constituent parts that go to make up the whole and in this way give nursing a theoretical framework. There is a danger here and, as Botha (1989) points out, the theorist may come to deal only in the abstract, leading to the risk of reductionism. Thus, the theorist loses touch with reality as the complexities of everyday life become broken down into convenient, easy to handle packages and the human factor becomes lost. Rourke (1990) is very critical of the Roper model from this point of view because it leads to ritualistic nursing as the patient is dehumanized into a series of biological systems, some of which are seen as failing. Roper's model is therefore constructed in such a way that it only focuses on negative physical attributes, leading to patient labelling and ignoring the psychological and social aspects of the person.

Nursing models, therefore, are not watertight theories, but rather sets of ideas about the way patients and nurses interact. The dangers of reductionism and losing touch with reality are such that model development must take place with at least one foot in the real world of practical nursing care. Model development and nursing practice should therefore be closely related by continual feedback, and both should never lose sight of the person as a holistic integrated being.

The benefits of choice

It is necessary to look first at the different types of model that are available before considering how to choose between them.

In Chapter 1 we saw that there will never be a single general theory of nursing that explains everything, nor will there be a universal model that is equally valid in all situations. Human behaviour is too complex for that and if theorists try to develop increasingly abstract and general models in an attempt to explain everything, they will end up explaining nothing (Miller 1985 in Wright, 1986). This therefore means that inevitably there will be many different types of model from which the nurse has to choose.

This is a healthy state of affairs for any discipline, as competing approaches to problems stimulate debate, enquiry and research, whereas a single solution leads to minds being closed against alternatives and the triumph of the procedure manual over individualized, creative nursing care. Botha (1989) has argued passionately for the development of a variety of models as in her view the proliferation of theories opens up any discipline and equips its practitioner to deal with a wide range of situations. As Kristjanson and Tamblyn (1987) point out, the adoption of a single universal model of nursing stultifies critical appraisal of that model and leads to a single approach to nursing being used that is lacking in evidence to support its validity.

Hardy (1986) has described the parlous state of affairs that can arise when a single model of nursing is adopted to the exclusion of all others, leading to a situation where lip service only is paid to the model, which nobody actually believes in. She reminds us of the work of Peters and Waterman (1982), who wrote a classic account of what makes for a successful business. They found it was the avoidance of rigid management models and instead a bias for action out of which creativity could flow, emphasis on the importance of people and 'staying close to the customer' to provide service of the highest quality.

In terms of using models of nursing, therefore, we must beware the zealots who would have one model only to the exclusion of all others. Sadly, UK nursing seems to show signs of this approach with the blanket implementation of the much criticized Roper model. Nursing must avoid reducing models to ritualistic exercises in bureaucracy; rather, clinicians must have the freedom to develop and evolve models in the light of practical experience; only in this way can the notions of creativity and staying close to the customer

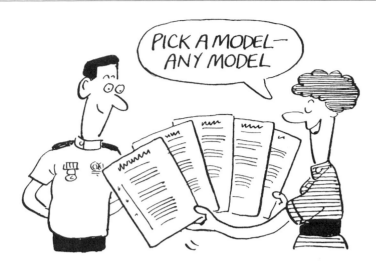

espoused by Peters and Waterman work to the full benefit of all concerned.

It must also be said that, in view of the immature state of many nursing models, the more they are used and compared with each other, the better will be the likely outcome as inductive reasoning and reflection in action are used to develop and refine each model in turn. Cross-fertilization can also occur as nurses borrow concepts and ideas from one model and apply them to another. Field (1987) has defended models from the charge of incompleteness in these very terms, arguing that attempting to negate the role they can play in nursing is an unfortunate and uninformed attitude when what is needed is constructive usage.

It can, however, be a daunting prospect for the nurse to be confronted by a dozen or more different models of nursing and to have to decide which ones are suitable for her or his own clinical area. It might help nurses, therefore, to stop and think in broad terms about what type of model would be most applicable to their nursing situation before getting into the detail of individual models. At this broad strategic level the writings of Aggleton and Chalmers (1987) are most useful as they show that models can be grouped under three broad headings: developmental, systems and interactionist.

A developmental model will focus on how a person is developing and how nursing is needed when normal development is threatened or actually impaired. Development refers to more than the obvious physical aspects of human behaviour and also includes psychological and social processes. Peplau (1952) is an example of a developmental approach, but strong developmental strands can be found in other models such as that of Orem (1990).

The systems approach is concerned not only with physiological systems but also with psychological and social systems, and how they all interact. Notions of maintaining balance between systems run through such models as the body strives for homeostasis; consequently, nursing is seen in these terms; that is, helping the person achieve equilibrium or a balance of functioning in their everyday life. Roy and King (1981) are examples of systems models, although the latter has a strong interactionist component.

An interactionist view of nursing centres around how humans communicate with each other and the meanings that are attached to such communication. Striving to see the other person's point of view and understand the role they are playing are essential ingredients of such models as patients are seen to have health problems deriving from self-perception and the roles they are adopting in living their life. Riehl (1980) and Orlando (1961) have offered models of nursing based upon these interactionist principles.

The problem of subjectivity was discussed in Chapter 1 and it is clear that the interactionist type of model is a very subjective approach to care as it involves interpreting the meanings that the patient attaches to the world around him/her. The systems models tend to be more rooted in objective reality while it is usually possible to arrive at a reasonably objective consensus regarding developmental aspects. This is not to decry the use of an interactionist approach, but rather it is a word of caution to the nurse to recall the difficulties of subjectivity in the interpretation of another person's world and experience. As we shall see, there will be situations when insight into the patient's perspective is necessary but the nurse should be very aware of her or his own world view in making such interpretations. Carper's notion of personal self as one of the four ways of gaining nursing knowledge is very important here (Carper, 1978) as the nurse's own perspective may significantly affect the way the patient's experiences are interpreted. The aesthetic source of knowledge will be tapped into frequently by the nurse using an interactionist model. Systems and developmental models owe much more to empiricism but, like interactionist models, are still bound by ethical knowledge.

Aggleton and Chalmers (1987) emphasize that these three broad categories of models are not mutually exclusive. A nursing model can lie largely in one area, but still borrow ideas from the others. Thus, Orem sees the need for self-care as the core of her model and requires the nurse to assess the patient's self-care ability in a physiological systems manner, but her model also requires an assessment of the patient's developmental status, as this clearly affects self-care ability. The model may also be enhanced by asking the nurse to consider how the patients see their self-care requirements – their point of view may be very different from the nurse's. For example, while the nurse may consider smoking as harmful to health and therefore a self-care failure, the patient may see this as helpful to self-care as it is perceived to reduce stress.

If an integrated and holistic approach to nursing is to be developed, it seems logical not to rely exclusively on just one of the types of model identified by Aggleton and Chalmers (1987). We have already seen how concentration on systems leads to a reductionist and dehumanizing approach in the case of Roper, yet if only an interactionist approach were used, how might this be applied to a patient capable of little or no interaction with the nurse, for example an unconscious patient? In developing and applying models of nursing it is therefore essential that we recognize the need for the three dimensions – systems homeostasis, developmental status and nurse–patient interaction – to be incorporated into any working model. The nurse may start out with a model that is, for example, predominantly systems oriented, but should aim to incorporate into its application a developmental and interactionist perspective. For example, in assessing the patient after choosing a sytems model, the nurse may choose to consider for each topic the effect of the patient's age and position on the continuum of life and also how the patient sees and interprets events. In this way a more rounded picture of the patient emerges.

In practice, however, the nurse can only choose from what is on the menu and that means choosing an established model that will have a strong bias towards systems and homeostasis, developmental status or interactionism. The nurse therefore needs to consider how much his or her nursing practice is about restoring equilibrium and balance to permit everyday living, or whether the prime objective is to foster development and growth or to help a person understand how their perceptions of life and the roles they choose to act may be contributing to their health problems. These broad strategic aims and the sort of patients that are going to be cared for need to be thought through before homing in on any one group of models. The nurse therefore needs to work out a philosophy of care and the models must be matched to the philosophy, not the other way round. Nursing care cannot be forced into models like square pegs in round holes.

Arriving at a philosophy of care

In Chapter 1 we explored the impact of philosophy on science and nursing at the macro level. As we saw, there is a certain amount of scepticism about philosophy. However, it is necessary for all nurses to have some sort of belief system about nursing and patients within which they can operate. The UKCC Code of Professional Conduct offers one set of guidance on matters moral and ethical and the point was made that we cannot afford moral relativism in nursing. We need to try and accommodate a wide range of points of view, but there have to be some common denominator principles that all members of a nursing team can sign up to. This points up the need for a shared philosophy of care based upon the beliefs and aspirations of the nursing team. Such beliefs depend to some extent on the way we see life in general and also the way we see the delivery of health care. A philosophy of care might cover a ward, a unit or a community team and should be derived from the views of all the staff who work in that area and, wherever possible, the patients as well.

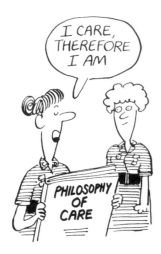

Wright (1986) has given a good account of how his unit developed their philosophy out of a series of meetings that involved all the staff on the unit as well as the views of the patients. For example, part of the philosophy states that each patient is seen as an individual entitled to the highest-quality skilled nursing care on an equal footing with any other person regardless of race, colour or creed and also entitled to freedom of choice in determining that care.

In determining a philosophy, general principles such as this need to be combined with the more specific needs of patients. Thus, patients in a hospice for the terminally ill will have some different needs from patients in a unit for the mentally ill, while acute hospital patients will have some different needs from community patients. The nurse can think of many different care settings and see that while there may be a common core to a philosophy involving the sort of values we cherish in a Western democracy such as those outlined by Wright above, there will also be some more specific elements dependent upon the type of care setting.

It is essential to enter a word of warning here, however. Supposing the patient does not subscribe to the nursing philosophy? An obvious example might be the way women are perceived in some cultures that is very different from the culture of northern Europe. Even within that latter culture there are many variations in how men, and women, see the woman's role.

To some extent this problem can be reduced by ensuring that patients are fully involved in drawing up a philosophy in the first place and by trying to make that philosophy as broad as possible to accommodate different points of view. However, it is still likely that there may be a problem of the nursing view being different from that of some patients. This philosophical problem underlines the need for the nursing team to look at the interactionist approach to nursing and grapple with the patient's point of view. Ultimately, we have to recognize certain fixed boundaries of care and these are laid down by the law of the land, the UKCC Code of Professional Conduct and whatever local policies may be in place. We simply cannot fall back on a relativistic 'anything goes' stance. However much we may value the individual's rights, that does not include the right to break the law nor the right to expect nurses to ignore employers' policies or the Code of Professional Conduct.

It must be emphasized that the philosophy should be derived from the efforts of all members of the care team. The increasing tendency towards multidisciplinary teamwork challenges us to embrace all the health professions in this process. Some of the more esoteric philosophies encountered in Chapter 1 have to be set aside in the interest of obtaining a common agreement. There is nothing more destructive than having different members of a team pulling in different directions or playing a game by different rules from everybody else. All team members must feel able to subscribe to a philosophy of care if it is to succeed, which means they must all be fully and equally involved in working out that philosophy. If each person feels that there is a little piece of his or herself in the philosophy, the team will come to own the philosophy; it will be seen as 'ours', which in turn helps to develop commitment and participation.

The philosophy should therefore reflect the patient's and care team's general views about human rights and health, and also ideas specific to the needs of the patient to be cared for, having been derived from the efforts of all staff and patients.

Matching the model to the philosophy

Once a clear idea has emerged of the nursing philosophy, the next step is to look at the types of models that are available before moving on to look at specific, individual models. As we have seen, models can focus on developmental aspects, on maintaining a balance between systems to ensure satisfactory human functioning or on interactionism, seeing things from the patient's point of view.

The three approaches discussed above may all appear equally attractive at first sight, but after careful consideration and discussion with colleagues and patients it should be possible to see one approach a little ahead of the others as being most appropriate. Having decided which of these three stratagems seems best, the nurse should not shut his or her mind to what the alternatives have to offer, but consider how much of these other approaches to nursing might also be taken on board. After all, a cake baked from flour, fat and water would be very dull and unsatisfactory, but add smaller proportions of some other very different ingredients such as chocolate and cream and the result is very different.

The next step is to try to pick a single model out from one of these three broad areas, always remembering what aspects associated with other types of models would be helpful also. This is essential as, when trying to make our chosen model work, we can adapt and change it accordingly. For example, we may have chosen a systems model such as Roy's, but the nursing team may feel it is very important to know the patient's point of view at all times, reflecting the interactionist approach. Arguments have already been deployed in favour of a multi-model approach to nursing, so the reader might detect a contradiction at this stage. The answer is that we should learn to walk before we run, as for most nurses the notion of models is a new concept, and therefore it is important not to be over-ambitious to start with. The aim should be to get one model of nursing working in a unit, then this can be adapted, changed and developed by reflection and the inductive process discussed earlier.

Parallel developments could see other models being introduced in other areas and perhaps, after a year or more the differing models would have been 'run in' sufficiently to allow nurses to ask two very important questions. First, has model X improved care in my unit? Second, what other models could be introduced from other areas into my clinical patch? Answers to these two questions depend among other things upon evaluation of the quality of care given.

The aim would be over a 2–3 year period to have several different models working in one care setting. Differing units may have each pioneered a different model on their own wards, but after this initial development period it is to be hoped that models would spread across wards and eventually any one ward may be able to offer several different approaches to care, selecting the one most appropriate to each individual patient.

At this stage it has to be acknowledged that it appears that a great deal of responsibility for developing and implementing nursing models is being placed upon clinical staff. Is this fair or realistic given all the other pressures staff face just to keep the service going? The disastrous implementation of the nursing process serves as a red light which should tell us to stop here and consider carefully exactly how staff on a busy ward or community patch can realistically be expected to implement a nursing model.

Implementing a model

Many writers have commented upon the disastrous way that the nursing process was foisted upon nursing in the UK (Walsh and Ford, 1989) with top-down implementation by a management that did not understand the basic concepts of care planning. Such a poorly managed change exercise guaranteed failure as the nursing process was greeted with hostility and scepticism. Laughlin (1988) and Lister (1987) are only two of many to draw an analogy with models, for if their attempted implementation follows the same pattern, the result will be equally disastrous. They argue that change should not occur for change's sake and that the imposition of models would be a great mistake. How right they are, for models will only find their way into nursing practice if nurses can see advantages in their introduction and can feel fully involved in their development.

This requires a bottom-up approach to models and not top-down implementation from either managers or academics. The original impetus towards introducing a model might come from a member of the ward team who develops an interest in the topic through a post-basic course or by attending a study day or reading a journal article or book. A new member of staff may join the ward who has studied models as part of an undergraduate training programme or the subject might be raised at a unit meeting. A key person in a ward or unit introducing a model of nursing is the charge nurse or sister, the acknowledged leader of the clinical team, and it is from within that team that the drive to change must be developed. Bellman (1996) offers a good example of this approach utilizing the Roper model, but her account contains salutory warnings of the problems in store when the medical team and outside change agent (researcher) are not in agreement with the ward staff.

The Project 2000 reform of education introduced models of nursing into the basic nurse curriculum, but do tutors have sufficient grasp of the ideas and concepts involved to be able to teach about different models? In Chapter 1 we saw how tutors divorced from clinical practice and with no real grasp of new concepts will only widen this theory–practice gap. This is a worrying gap in nurse education at present and one which it is hoped tutors and colleges will make strenuous efforts to close.

A recurring criticism of nurse education involves the fact that what students are taught in class often bears little resemblance to the reality of clinical areas. Teaching of models in colleges of nursing when they are not encountered in practice seems set to perpetuate this chronic problem. Morales-Mann and Logan (1990) offer interesting insights into the difficulties of designing a nurse education programme around models of nursing. They describe how the School of Nursing at the University of Ottawa decided to base its nursing curriculum upon a pluralistic approach to models, starting with the Roy model for the first year of the course. Before utilizing Roy's model, however, it was rigorously tested against the criteria of compatibility with the needs of the students, completeness as a model, practicality and feasibility. Only when it had met these criteria was the model chosen for use.

The use of Roy in this way required a fundamental rethink of the first-year curriculum, the teaching of supporting subjects to be congruent with Roy's model, the development of new teaching aids and a great deal of work to familiarize ward staff with the concepts involved. It was opposition from the ward staff that represented the greatest obstacle to change and presented the greatest difficulty to teaching the students Roy's model. Personal experience in teaching nursing undergraduates to use the Roy model (and other models) while working in clinical areas that adhere to traditional medical model nursing or that pay lip service to the Roper approach supports the views of Morales-Mann and Logan. Before departments of nursing implement a multi-model curriculum, a great deal of care and attention must be paid to thinking through which models are most appropriate to what areas of the course; recognition must be paid to the effects on how other areas of the course are taught as well as the effects on nursing teaching; and finally the problem must be addressed of how the students will cope with gaining experience on wards that are not using the models being taught in class.

This leads to the proposal that models need to be introduced in clinical practice with a bottom-up approach, and until they are working in at least a substantial part of the clinical field their value in pre-registration nurse education will be limited to that of an academic exercise. However, it is to be hoped that, as more nurses qualify with a knowledge of nursing models, implementation into clinical areas will accelerate so that eventually students will indeed be able to practise nursing in the way they have been taught in class.

One further impetus to model development might therefore be from within the department of nursing, as teaching models will only be good educational practice if they are being used in clinical areas. It would be wrong to say that unless a unit is using a model students will not be sent there for clinical experience and that therefore the unit must adopt a model immediately. Such a quick fix solution will lead to lip service only being paid to any model, like the nursing process, and the rationale for model choice will be expediency. The model chosen will represent the lowest common denominator that requires least understanding. The easiest model to understand is not always the best, after all it is much easier to understand that the earth is flat and that the sun goes around the earth, but both these models of the solar system are very wrong.

Nurse educators are therefore important change agents and along with clinical staff make up the two most likely sources for the impetus to introduce a model. However, to be effective they must be much more closely involved with the clinical field and work together with clinical staff in model development. We return to this point later.

Introducing a model to a clinical area is not a task to be undertaken lightly, as it involves fundamental changes in the way staff think and work. Luker (1988) has suggested that each nurse carries around their own informal model of nursing which guides their practice. It is probable that a formal model will be significantly different, although these differences can be minimized by full consultation and involvement with staff to ensure that the model chosen reflects their views of nursing as far as possible.

It is interesting to compare Luker's notion of each nurse carrying around their own personal model of nursing with the ideas of Benner (1984) which were discussed in Chapter 1. Many of Luker's experienced nurses with their own personal model contained in their head may be equated with Benner's expert nurse. The problem arises in that very often expert nurses cannot explain the process of their nursing, which has become based on this internalized personal model which, as Field (1987) points out, limits the development of the practice base of the profession. Two salient features emerge from these considerations. First, the development of expertise depends upon patterning of knowledge and experience; therefore to promote expertise we need to promote that patterning process. Models of

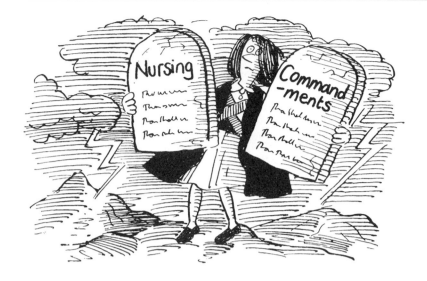

nursing help to provide a framework and pattern for nursing and therefore should be encouraged since they can assist a nurse's professional development. The second point addresses Luker's personal models: if every nurse has a different model of nursing, which as Benner argues will be largely implicit and appear intuitive, how can we share and develop nursing expertise? The need is for a common language or at least a common framework to allow clinical experts to share their knowledge with others rather than pursue their implicit, apparently intuitive, internal model of nursing.

The subjectivity problem inherent in Benner's work was extensively discussed in Chapter 1. There is a further point, however, that follows on from Luker's observation for if expert nurses have an internalized model of care which is unique to them, it is possible that they may have internalized some practices which are outdated, taken for granted or inappropriate (Paley, 1996) but which are never made explicit as their care is not based upon a commonly understood model of nursing. This notion of every nurse having their own model therefore can lead to the situation where outdated rituals can be propagated under the guise of expert practice. Having a series of explicit models whose aims and ideas are common knowledge, shared by all, opens up care to critical scrutiny in a way that is not possible if each nurse has their own private internal model.

Benner's concept of the novice nurse sticking closely to rigid rules is of relevance to educationalists and clinical staff who might be involved in a models-based, pre-registration educational programme. The author's personal experience in teaching on just such a course confirms Benner's view of how novices and beginners function, particularly with reference to models of nursing. Students seem to want a comprehensive assessment scheme that has a neat pigeonhole for every aspect of the patient, leading to difficulties in working with models such as Roy or Orem and particularly the FANCAP scheme (see p. 127), where the nurse is required to be flexible and interpret patient behaviour so as to assign it a place in the assessment scheme. A rigid, simplistic approach simply will not work and it must be recognized that the nurse has to move on along the scale of proficiency before being able to synthesize and analyse information in such a way as to make maximum use of any model.

Consider the example of pain; although there is no heading specifically entitled 'pain' under Roy, Orem or Roper, it still may be assessed. However, students frequently criticize these models because there is no such explicit heading in the assessment schedule, finding it difficult to see that the notion of body regulation and adaptation found in Roy's model directs the nurse to think of the nervous system, which in turn should lead to consideration of sensation and pain. Orem's health deviancy self-care category should also make the nurse enquire about pain, a very common symptom of 'health deviancy' to use Orem's slightly clumsy phrase. Pain can be seen as a dimension of Roper's activities of living, for example, it may be associated with mobilizing or breathing, and as such may be introduced wherever appropriate in the assessment. An assessment format that was as explicit as many junior students request would be totally unwieldy and fragment the patient beyond recognition in a battery of headings and subheadings.

It would therefore benefit students to introduce them early in their education to models that do have a more explicit assessment tool, such as Roper or Henderson, leaving other models until later. As students gain knowledge and experience they will be better able to interpret and use the more implicit assessment tools of other models which require higher-level functioning.

In developing models as a common language of nursing, creativity and individualism are to be encouraged and this is no argument for conformity in approaches to nursing. However, if nursing models were more used and well known, they could offer a common framework of ideas within which expert nurses could make more explicit the secrets of their success. A process of reflection, of looking at what the nurse does and placing successful care in a theoretical framework, could be of immense benefit to nursing. The experienced stoma care nurse may be able to benefit others by using Roy's model to try to understand how she successfully helps the patient to adapt to the stoma, while the experienced psychiatric nurse may be able to explain her success in helping a patient return to the home environment by analysing care using the concepts of King (1981). It is about interpreting the individual nurse's implicit model in terms of an explicit model that is in the public domain and has common meanings to most nurses.

Use of a model will also bring other changes in its wake, for, as we shall see in the next chapter, full implementation of individualized care planning will be necessary along with primary nursing. Care is now taking on an increasingly multidisciplinary approach as the old demarcation lines between different professional groups are being eroded away by the forces of change. It is essential therefore that in considering the use of nursing models, staff have to look at how they will fit in with other members of the care team. A nursing model which is not compatible with other professions will cause considerable problems and in the long run probably do more harm than good. The UKCC *Scope of Professional Practice* document (UKCC, 1992) also offers nurses new opportunities to expand their practice. We should take this opportunity and not hesitate to enrich or even stretch models and conceptual frameworks in response to these new-found freedoms. Major changes are also afoot in care planning and documentation, particularly as multidisciplinary working becomes more widespread. The linkage between any model and patient documentation must therefore be carefully considered.

Introducing a model is therefore a major exercise in changing attitudes and beliefs, as well as practice. Attitudes are very difficult to change, as people regard them as part of themselves, their own bit of property, consequently they tend to hang on to them. Nursing is very bad at letting people fail, yet to change and try out new ideas staff must feel able to fail, for mistakes are an inevitable part of the change process.

The social sciences offer us one method of changing attitudes that has been shown to work. It rejoices in the grand title of cognitive dissonance theory and it is really saying that people always tend to try to reconcile what they believe with what they know. Therefore, to change beliefs, the need is to change experience, for that determines what we know. The racial integration of American society in the 1960s was partly accomplished on the basis of this theory, which predicted that if white people came to experience and therefore know black people, they would be faced by the problem of reconciling their prejudiced old beliefs with a new reality that would often be very different. The way this might happen is by changing their beliefs to fit their new knowledge. To some extent this is indeed what happened and, while there is still a great deal of racial tension in the USA today, the situation is a lot better than it was 30 years ago.

This principle applied to nursing suggests that after a period of intensive debate and work involving all the staff, there has to come a time when a unit moves forward and implements its chosen model. Staff still displaying negative attitudes can experience working with the new system and, along with help and support, they will have to face reconciling a great deal of positive experience with their negative attitudes, which it is hoped will lead to a shift in attitude.

The introduction of change in nursing has been shown by Hunt (1987) to require a great deal of input from both management and educationalists; clinical staff alone do not have the resources, particularly in the present climate. The dissemination of knowledge about models has occurred mostly through qualified staff attending post-basic professional development courses such as the University of London diploma and part-time nursing degrees. Nursing has a professional responsibility to educate itself, and this process includes keeping abreast of model development. Thus, tutors and managers must keep up with clinical nurses in the field of professional development.

For a unit team to implement a model they need information about the various models in order that they can choose one that fits their philosophy, and they need the time and encouragement to discuss the relevant issues as well as the freedom to make any changes in working practice that are necessary. This demonstrates the importance of educational and managerial input, as the tutors can facilitate learning about models while it is the manager's responsibility to encourage and provide the necessary resources such as time. Meetings might not all take place during shift hours and the very fact that staff are prepared to meet and discuss their plans in their own time should act as a spur to management to spare no effort in helping clinical staff develop their practice.

Educationalists and managers can benefit from supporting clinical staff in this way. For the tutors it offers a way of overcoming the criticism that they teach in a vacuum and never work in the real world, hence the yawning theory–practice gap. By helping staff to learn about a model and being involved in its development in a real clinical situation, tutorial staff are bringing together theory and practice in a way that facilitates the requirements of good practice and also the teaching of models as part of the Project 2000 curriculum.

For the manager, developing a happy nursing team with a high degree of job satisfaction and commitment to their work must always be a prime goal. The sort of projects outlined here could achieve that goal by allowing clinical nurses to develop their own practice in their own way. In such a situation staff recruitment and retention could become a problem of the past along with high absenteeism rates and low morale.

The manager still has budgets to contend with and must be able to show that quality care is also cost-effective care. However, when the cost of treating avoidable complications such as pressure sores and wound infections is added to the cost of hiring temporary agency staff when there are high sickness rates, it becomes apparent that quality nursing can be cost effective.

The involvement of managerial and educational staff is therefore essential for the successful management of the major changes involved in introducing a nursing model. It would be beneficial to create some sort of forum within a Trust where staff from different clinical areas could meet and discuss their progress in model development. In this way mutual support could develop, solutions to problems could be shared and comparisons made between the different models under development in the district.

So far we have seen that for change to be successful it must come from within. The decision to introduce a model must be taken collectively by the clinical team, as must decisions about a philosophy of care and finally the actual choice of model itself. Before actually introducing the model the educational and managerial input that went into selecting the model must continue to allow staff to develop their knowledge base and to ensure a smooth change to new working practices. Staff have to become comfortable with the model and to have a common shared understanding of what is being attempted; this requires learning about the model. In addition there needs to be a careful review of what working practices will have to change, such as patient allocation becoming primary nursing.

An old adage in education is that it is not what is taught that counts, but what is learnt. It may seem a good idea to organize a series of lectures on Model X, but that is of limited value if little is learnt about how to apply the model in practice. An introductory lecture might serve to map out the ground, and readings from the literature will also be useful, but there is no substitute for active learning.

Staff need, therefore, to draw up an education programme to ensure that everybody has had the chance to learn how to use the model in practice. This means working in small tutorial groups, discussing how different terms and concepts within the model should be interpreted. Role playing is a valuable learning tool, with members of the team taking it in turns to play a patient while colleagues carry out an assessment and try to draw up a care plan based on the model. The finished care plan can then be reviewed by

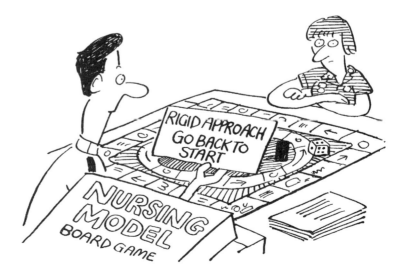

the 'patient' and feedback given to the planners. Observers may comment also. An innovative gaming approach to model development has been described by Hoon (1986) in which a board game may be developed to show how differing models might affect various patients. These sorts of methods constitute an active learning approach which can be recommended as it forms the basis for teaching models of nursing used by the authors of this book.

The emphasis in this learning period before model introduction should be on practical usage and ensuring that all staff have a common understanding of how the model will be used. Brainstorming sessions to suggest ways of adapting the model to the clinical area and also to agree documentation would be an integral part of this learning process. Group activity along these lines should help foster a feeling of team spirit and a sense that this model actually belongs to the staff who are going to work with it because they have all helped to put the project together. The views of all members of the nursing team should be given equal weight – there is nothing better than perceived hierarchies for destroying team spirit.

Once the appropriate changes in nursing systems have been made and the staff have a working knowledge, then it is time to launch the model in practice. It will not be plain sailing and nobody should expect it to be so; what matters is that mistakes are turned into positive learning experiences. Feedback should be sought at regular intervals from all the staff to allow the development and modification of the model in practice, while quality assurance monitoring is a desirable parallel development.

In an ideal world, a quality assurance programme would be in place pre- and post-introduction of the model to see whether it made any significant difference to the standards of care or to the way the staff felt about their work. Being realistic, it would probably absorb all the energies of the staff just to introduce the model and the new

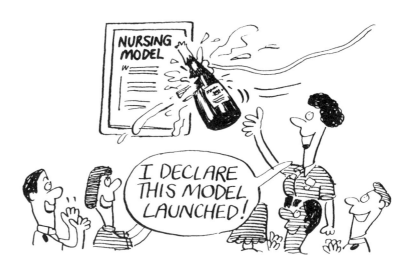

systems that might go with it. However, opportunities such as these almost demand that nurse researchers devote their energies to such investigations, for this represents innovative and creative nursing that is pushing at the very limits of the profession as we know it today.

Summary

In this chapter we have established that models of nursing really do matter because they represent a way of defining exactly what it is we mean by nursing, thereby mapping out the terrain for both education and practice. However, they are at present only collections of ideas about nursing, not theories in the scientific sense. In that form, though, they offer us a wonderful opportunity to be creative, for their application allows nurses to develop and refine these ideas in the light of experience gained in the clinical field.

The introduction of a model should be a bottom-up exercise being led by clinical staff with educational and management support. The unit team together with patients need to identify a broad philosophy of care and only then select a model to fit that philosophy. They should not be afraid to borrow bits from other models if appropriate. Introduction of a model needs careful preparation and education of all the staff involved, and patients where appropriate. Evaluation and feedback to modify the model are key points once it has been implemented. Finally, there is no place for a dogmatic single-model approach; students of nursing and care settings should be familiar with several differing models as such a range of care options is essential to reflect the variety in care needs of the patient population.

References

Aggleton PR & Chalmers H (1987) Models of nursing, nursing practice and nurse education. *Journal of Advanced Nursing*, **12**, 573–581.

Bellman L (1996) Changing nursing practice through reflection on the Roper, Logan and Tierney model: the enhancement approach to action research. *Journal of Advanced Nursing*, **24**, 129–138.

Benner P (1984) *From Novice to Expert*. Menlo Park, CA: Addison Wesley.

Botha E (1989) Theory development in perspective: the role of conceptual frameworks and models in theory development. *Journal of Advanced Nursing*, **14**, 49–55.

Carper B (1978) Fundamental patterns of knowing in nursing. *Advances in Nursing Science*, **1**(1), 13–23.

Field PA (1987) The impact of nursing theory on the clinical decision making process. *Journal of Advanced Nursing*, **12**, 563–571.

Hammersley M & Atkinson P (1983) *Ethnography: Principles in Practice*. London: Tavistock.

Hardy LK (1986) Identifying the place of theoretical frameworks in an evolving discipline. *Journal of Advanced Nursing*, **11**, 103–107.

Hoon E (1986) Game playing: a way to look at nursing models. *Journal of Advanced Nursing*, **11**, 421–427.

Hunt M (1987) The process of translating research findings into nursing practice. *Journal of Advanced Nursing*, **12**, 101–110.

King I (1981) *A Theory of Nursing*. New York: Wiley.

Kristjanson LJ & Tamblyn R (1987) A model to guide development and application of multiple nursing theories. *Journal of Advanced Nursing*, **12**, 523–529.

Laughlin M (1988) Modelled, muddled and befuddled. *Nursing Times*, **84**(4), 30–31.

Lister P (1987) The misunderstood model. *Nursing Times*, **83**(4), 40–42.

Luker K (1988) Do models work? *Nursing Times*, **84**(5), 27–29.

Morales-Mann E & Logan M (1990) Implementing Roy's Model: challenges for educators. *Journal of Advanced Nursing*, **15**, 142–147.

Orlando I (1961) *The Dynamic Nurse Patient Relationship*. New York: GP Putnam.

Paley J (1996) Intuition and expertise: comments on the Benner debate. *Journal of Advanced Nursing*, **23**, 665–671.

Peplau H (1952) *Interpersonal Relationships in Nursing*. New York: GP Putnam.

Peters TJ & Waterman RH (1982) *In Search of Excellence*. New York: Harper & Row.

Pollit D & Hungler B (1995) *Nursing Research*. Philadelphia: Lippincott.

Riehl JP (1980) The Riehl Interaction Model. In Riehl JP and Roy C (eds) *Conceptual Models for Nursing Practice*. Norwalk, Conn.: Appleton Century Crofts.

Rourke A (1990) Professional labelling. *Nursing Standard*, **4**(42), 36–39.

UKCC (1992) *The Scope of Professional Practice*. London: UKCC.

Walsh M & Ford P (1989) *Nursing Rituals: Research and Rational Actions*. Oxford: Heinemann.

Wright S (1986) *Building and Using a Model of Nursing*. London: Edward Arnold.

3 Using a Model in the Planning and Delivery of Care

Introduction

Models must be more than just academic exercises, they should be capable of use in the practical situation if they are to be of value. To facilitate practical usage it is necessary to review the way that care is planned and also the way the systems used to deliver that care are organized.

Care planning

Care was always planned long before the phrase 'nursing process' was coined; what has changed is the method of planning. In the traditional system of nursing, care was planned round tasks, with the nurse in charge allocating to each nurse a series of jobs. The planning of this care was then documented in the bath book, bowel book, dressings book, etc., and when the task had been completed this would be noted in the kardex as a record of care given. Nurses have therefore always planned care, documented their plans and recorded the results of carrying out their care.

There is nothing new, therefore, in the nursing process requiring nurses to plan, write down their plans and evaluate their care, it is something we have always done. The fundamental difference, however, is that the focus of care has changed from tasks to the patient, which has required nurses to consider the whole patient as a person and not just another wound that needs dressing or another section of constipated bowel that needs unblocking.

All the much-maligned nursing process is trying to do is to get the nurse to consider the whole patient and adopt a rational, problem-solving approach to planning care for that whole person, rather than seeing the patient as just another name in a list of people to be bathed or toileted. This of course means the nurse must start thinking and working things out from first principles rather than just following orders, and that is not so easy.

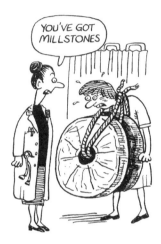

Following orders is one way of avoiding stress, a mechanism that Chapman (1983) argues leads to the perpetuation of much mindless ritual in nursing. Walsh and Ford (1989) agree with Chapman and point out that the traditional nurse training with its emphasis on getting tasks done and its lack of a questioning approach compounds the problem of getting nurses to think for themselves. There are also history and tradition hanging round nursing's neck like giant millstones, the history of female subservience and the tradition of obeying male, medical dominance. Given these powerful social forces acting on nurses, it is not surprising that the transition to a free-thinking, problem-solving approach has not been easy.

However, an individualized care planning approach is precisely what is required by models of nursing with their emphasis on the patient as a whole individual who is at the focus of nursing care. Whether a nursing model is based around helping a patient attain developmental goals, integrating and balancing the various physical and psychosocial systems of life or achieving an understanding of how roles and self-perception affect health, either way it is the whole individual that is involved. Such a coherent view of the individual person cannot be broken down into physical bits with a different nurse responsible for each. The *Mona Lisa* could have been painted if her arms had been painted by one artist, her eyes by somebody else and her smile by the 'smile artist', but would it have been the *Mona Lisa* of Leonardo Da Vinci? Just as great works of art and literature come from the integrated approach of one person, so caring for patients is best carried out in this integrated holistic fashion.

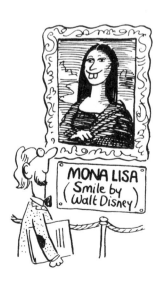

In this chapter and the next we examine the principal methods that have been used by nurses to plan and deliver individualized care, exploring how they interlink with conceptual models of what that care should consist of. This chapter focuses on the conventional nursing process approach and concludes with a critique of this method. In the next we examine some alternative ideas for care planning that are currently being developed.

The nursing process originated in the 1970s in the USA as a tool for teaching students how to plan holistic patient care. Its origins were therefore among educationalists and its intended field of usage was the classroom. Unfortunately, it was transposed with little involvement of clinical staff into the practice area and decreed to be essential for individualized care delivery. As a result in the USA the Joint Commission of Accreditation of Health Care Organizations (JCAHCO) made the written nursing process essential for Federal approval (and hence Federal funds!). The predecessor of the UKCC in England and Wales, the General Nursing Council, placed the nursing process on the UK nursing syllabus in 1977 and set in train its introduction in the UK. The implementation of the nursing process in the NHS that followed was a masterclass in the mismanagement of change. Many authors have catalogued the mistakes that were made in this top-down imposition of change (e.g. Mead and Bryar, 1992; Ford and Walsh, 1994). As a result something that was intended to improve patient care was seen by many as an unhelpful burden and met with much resistance.

It is important to separate out the written nursing process documentation from the nursing process itself, which is a way of thinking about nursing in a logical, problem-solving manner. Key points to remember, however, are that the nursing process is only *one problem-solving approach* amongst several (Hurst, 1993) and that the written care plan is a *tool of the nursing process* not the nursing process itself (Bellman, 1993). The nursing process is actually a way of thinking about nursing and helping the nurse to solve the problems presented by the needs of the patient. Documentation is a separate issue. This latter point goes back to the original idea behind the nursing process; that is, it was developed as a useful method of teaching students to plan care for a whole patient in an organized and logical way. It is this view that we work with in the next sections which review the various stages of planning care using the nursing process and the relevance of incorporating conceptual models into this approach. The chapter then moves on to review the criticisms that have developed around the nursing process and the cumbersome paperwork that has become associated with it in practice.

Assessment

Unfortunately, patient assessment is often poorly carried out. It is frequently lumped together with admission, to the point now that many wards talk of admitting rather than assessing a new patient. If it is seen as a chore to be done on admission, there will be little chance of on-going assessment, yet this is vital to monitor the success of care and to detect the emergence of new problems. When mixed up with the admission procedure, assessment tends to become delegated to a junior member of staff and interpreted as little more than a form-filling procedure for the kardex. Much vital information is missed and what is recorded lies unused in the care plan, ignored and forgotten.

Assessment must be seen as the beginning of nursing care and more than just a part of the admission procedure. Without a thorough assessment individualized nursing care cannot exist, as there is no knowledge base about the patient from which to identify problems and plan care. Care becomes standardized, routinized and impersonal as all patients are treated much the same with only their medical diagnosis having any influence on care. Nursing a patient recovering from a colostomy operation is clearly very different from nursing someone who has had a prostatectomy, but no two ostomy patients are the same either as they are unique people entitled to care tailored to their individuality. The only effective way this care can be delivered is if the nursing assessment has clearly established the individuality of the patient.

Different models have varying approaches to care and consequently seek to discover different types of knowledge about the patient and family. The nursing assessment therefore must reflect the model's philosophy. In practice the authors of models usually suggest detailed assessment schedules, which can be very helpful. An assessment schedule derived from a model has the strength of being as comprehensive as possible because the author will have thought a great deal about the assessment and tried to ensure that the nurse has the logical and consistent framework of knowledge necessary to plan care consistent with the model.

However, some notes of caution are needed. First, the nurse must see the assessment form as a tool which will enable staff to make the model work, it is not just another form-filling, box-ticking exercise. Assessment must therefore reflect the aspirations of the model. If, for example, the nurse is using Orem's self-care model and discovers that the patient has a self-care deficit in being unable to maintain continence, the assessment should not stop at ticking a box on a form. Gentle and tactful probing is necessary to find out whether this problem is associated with other events or time of the day, how frequently it occurs, what measures the patient takes to deal with the problem, whether others know of the problem and, if so, how they help, and of course how the patient personally feels about the continence difficulties. In this way the nurse is using the self-care concept to probe and discover as much as possible about how this continence problem affects the whole life of the patient, how the patient sees the problem and how the patient attempts to manage their self-care, rather than stopping at the simple statement that the patient cannot maintain self-care in terms of continence. Such an approach is consistent with the need to explore the patient's problems from varying points of view using interactionist, systems and developmental perspectives.

The second note of caution concerns jargon. If staff find the sorts of words used by the author of a model difficult to understand, then they should consider alternative wordings that are perhaps closer to commonly used English. The purpose of words is to convey rather than obscure meaning; if they fail to convey meaning they are of no value. Nurses should not be afraid, therefore, to change the language of models, including the key words used in an assessment schedule, as long as they retain the meaning. For example, Orem's 'self-care deficit' could be changed into 'self-care problem' or Roy's 'focal stimuli' might translate into 'principal cause of problem'.

A model-based assessment schedule should be only a tool in the hands of the assessor, it must not take over and rigidly determine the course of the assessment. This is a key point as it could be argued that by setting up an assessment schedule, a model precludes enquiry about other areas. It is also possible that the model has set up a list of items that nurses see as priorities, but which may not correspond to the patient's views about what is important. A model-based assessment schedule should therefore only be seen as a useful starting point to explore the patient's needs and not be viewed as a definitive and therefore exclusive picture of potential problems which the patient may have. The nurse must be free to explore detailed areas with patients that do not have headings on the assessment plan. It may well be that patients want to talk about things that do not neatly dovetail with the headings devised by the author of a model! Rather than try to force these areas into the assessment document artificially, it is better to leave a blank space for 'other issues' which might be raised in this way.

After using a model for some time it might be possible to go back over a series of patient assessments and see whether any recurring themes tend to crop up under 'other issues'. In this way the assessment schedule could be modified to incorporate areas that the model has overlooked, despite the author's attempts to make it comprehensive. For example, the nurse may note that patients' views of their illnesses are unrealistic or that many patients seem lacking in knowledge about their condition. As a result the assessment could be modified by borrowing from the interactionist approach to include a section which explored the patient's views of their illness in some detail. Alternatively, to use a more concrete example, if Roy's model were used on a surgical ward, staff might notice that there was no obvious heading under which to record essential information about a patient's wound or ability to maintain personal hygiene, and so modify the original assessment tool in this way. This is just one example of the way models can be developed and improved in practice.

There will be other situations when a thorough and comprehensive assessment is either not possible or is inappropriate and the nurse must recognize this possibility. Consider the patient brought to the A&E unit with multiple trauma after a road accident, or the patient who is having day surgery. In the former case, assessment should focus on life-threatening areas such as the ABCD of resuscitation, pain and fear, while in the latter case it may be very interesting to know the patient's hobbies, but of little relevance if the person is going to have surgery and be sent home all in the same day.

The message here is that just because a model has defined an area as worthy of assessment, it does not necessarily have to be assessed if the patient's condition indicates otherwise. Flexibility of thought and a little bit of plain common sense should ensure that the nurse only fills in the parts of the assessment document that are needed. This also helps deal with the criticism that the nursing process wastes time due to form filling; it is the nurse who often wastes time by recording information that is not needed. Assessment is an on-going process, and parts of the assessment schedule can be completed later as part of the reassessment process and as the patient's condition allows.

We have suggested that some thought about the depth of the assessment is needed. It is essential also for the nurse to think about how the assessment is carried out if the maximum amount of useful information is to be gathered. Any model's assessment schedule is only a tool, and like a saw or drill it has to be used correctly to get the best results that it is capable of. The following observations apply to assessment, whatever the model used.

The social sciences have taught us that first impressions really do count in human interactions (Hilgard *et al.*, 1987). This has two significant implications for a nurse assessing a patient, the first of which is that we should be careful how we approach the situation. An offhand manner or an initial appearance of disorganization (e.g. calling the patient the wrong name) may create an unfortunate impression that will last for days with the patient. Conversely, the nurse should beware his or her own first impression of the patient who may be very anxious and worried by their strange surroundings, leading to abnormal behaviour as a result of this stress.

The need for privacy and good communication skills in assessment was emphasized by McFarlane and Castledine (1982) and has been recognized by most authors since. The use of a clipboard and official-looking papers with the nurse scribbling away furiously in between stereotyped questions is not the way to make the patient relax and disclose what might be very sensitive and embarrassing information. It is worth considering a cultural point here; most models are American in origin and American society is on the whole more open than British. Is it possible that some models might seek information that American citizens might volunteer more readily than the more reserved British? Assessment is an on-going process and if the patient is to be under the nurse's care for a lengthy period, then there is time to explore more sensitive areas as the nurse–patient relationship develops. This two-stage view of assessment is supported by the research evidence of Hurst (1993) who also stresses the importance of the timing of the assessment in relation to the information it may yield. In short-stay care this in-depth assessment is obviously not possible and the nurse will have to make judgements about whether more personal information might be relevant to care before enquiring about matters that the patient may be unwilling to discuss with a comparative stranger.

Nursing models by their innovative and holistic nature may be exploring personal areas which nurses using the task-centred, medical model approach to nursing have traditionally stayed away from. When the cultural point raised in the preceding paragraph is taken into account also, the importance of privacy, sensitivity and good communication becomes apparent in a model-based assessment.

There seems little point in repeating questions which seek information that is readily available from admission documents and case notes, although such information can be stated to the patient who may then be asked to confirm that it is correct. In this way time is saved, the patient is not subjected to the annoying experience of having the same questions repeatedly asked, and the nurse demonstrates knowledge of and interest in the patient. It is always good policy to begin an assessment interview in this non-threatening factual way and it allows the patient to correct any inaccuracies such as a change of address or work. In this way the ice is broken and the patient can start to relax.

Patients' privacy must be respected at all times and if they show a reluctance to talk about an aspect of their health the nurse should not at this stage continue to push the matter. At a later time when the patient has gained more confidence, they may respond to a gentle prompt such as 'When we talked a couple of days ago you seemed a little unhappy at talking about . . .'. The assessment is not a one-off event, but rather an on-going process.

It is important for nurses who are going to work with models that they acquire good communication skills that will allow them to gently probe into sensitive areas that nursing has previously avoided. Roy's adaptation model, for example, seeks to discover a great deal about a person's self-concept and role function. Consider a woman who has been admitted for mastectomy and how she perceives herself and her role as both a woman and a sexual partner; assessment here requires more than a couple of questions with yes/no answers that allow the nurse to tick a couple of boxes.

The emphasis on introducing the social sciences into nursing education is well placed for a variety of reasons, not least of which is the hope that it might considerably improve nurses' communication and assessment skills. The need to link the assessment to patient care should be obvious. This involves two steps: a clearly recorded assessment and a plan of care that reflects the needs identified in the assessment. The use of a model provides a framework which should facilitate a well-recorded assessment that makes sense to another nurse looking at it a few days later which is the acid test of a good assessment. The work of Hurst (1993) confirms the need for a good assessment to show evidence of good data collection and organization of those data, both of which are helped by a model-based assessment framework. Models also require care to follow logically from the assessment as they give internal consistency to care delivery. If self-care requirements are the focus of assessment, then meeting self-care needs will form the crux of the care required.

Bearing in mind these statements, the findings of researchers such as Davis *et al.* (1994) are worthy of consideration. These authors carried out a study of nursing process documentation in a hospital which claimed to use the Roper Logan and Tierney model throughout its 11 wards. This blanket use of a single model has already been severely criticized as patients are far too complex to all conform to one single model. Davis *et al.* (1994) found that the assessment was consistently poorly recorded and had little resemblance to the care plan that followed. The psychosocial aspects of care were rarely identified and there was no logical connection between the assessment (such as it was) and the problems that were subsequently described.

This is a single study and therefore too much should not be read into these findings. They do, however, raise at least two key questions. Why after all these years of the nursing process do nurses appear to be failing to assess patients properly? In addition, is the Roper, Logan and Tierney model valid, if it leads to the omission of crucial psychosocial areas of care? We come back to these questions later, noting for now evidence that assessments may be little more than a cosmetic cover up for care that remains lacking in recognition of individual need. The care is documented in a standardized way regardless of the individual patient's assessment or whatever model is claimed to be in use. All that is assessed is not necessarily acted upon.

A model of nursing can therefore shape and guide the assessment process to ensure that data relevant to the person's individual care within the model's framework are collected. The nurse must also have an open mind and be aware of areas the patient wishes to discuss that are not detailed by the model assessment document. Good communication skills are essential to explore sensitive and personal areas with the patient.

Problems

The patient assessment should provide the nurse with sufficient information to begin working out the patient's problems. Regardless of the model used, some key points bear reiteration at this stage.

The problems identified must be patient centred and not nursing problems. A mistake commonly made is to write statements such as 'Patient needs enema' under the problem heading on a care plan. That is a nursing intervention, the organization of which might well be a problem; however, the patient's problem is (presumably) that he or she has not had a bowel movement for several days.

The fact that the problem is patient centred means that technical medical labels should be avoided if the care plan is to be shared with the patient. The nurse should try to imagine how the patient sees their problem, or better still, ask the patient to describe the problem. For example, a patient who has peripheral vascular disease (PVD) may be unable to walk more than 50 metres without developing severe calf pain. The *patient's* problem is 'severe pain on walking more than 50 metres', not a statement such as 'intermittent claudication' or 'PVD', neither of which will mean anything to the patient.

Problems also need to be prioritized in order that the most important are seen to first. Marriner (1979) suggested using Maslow's familiar hierarchy of needs as one method of prioritization, starting with physiological problems before moving on to problems associated with safety, love, esteem and self-actualization in that order. Roper *et al.* echo Maslow's views in describing their activities of living (ALs) model. Given the importance which has been ascribed to Maslow's work (Maslow, 1968) it is important to look at his views critically because there are substantial problems with transplanting them into nursing. Maslow's views about a hierarchy of needs stem from experimental work performed with white, North American college students in the 1950s. His subjects are therefore unrepresentative of the general population of the UK in the 1990s and it is questionable if his findings still apply. Further, Clark (1992) states that:

many of Maslow's concepts have not been precisely defined and his theories have not been sufficiently rigorously expressed to be testable. Consequently empirical evidence is not available to support many of his assertions. Clark (1992, p. 106)

Nurses will be aware that patients often place the higher needs in Maslow's hierarchy ahead of the lower needs (invalidating Roper *et al.*'s assumption that this is a valid basis for planning nursing care). For example, trauma nurses know that self-actualization leads people into a range of dangerous pursuits regardless of the lower safety need which it is suggested should be a priority, while belongingness and love needs may lead to unprotected sex, again regardless of safety. Nurses in the mental health field or working on medical wards will know that self-esteem needs can lead to substance abuse at the expense of both safety and physiological needs. Maslow's ideas belong to another era and another culture for as Clarke points out the America of Eisenhower at the height of the Cold War in the 1950s is a totally different place to the UK 40 years later. They do not form a reliable foundation for constructing models of nursing or even a framework for prioritizing patient needs.

It is possible, however, that the patient may see problem priorities very differently from the nursing staff. This may be resolved by giving information to help a middle-aged man understand why the nurse is so insistent on getting him out of bed the morning after his operation and performing deep breathing exercises when all he wants to do is lie in bed and go to sleep.

This example illustrates the importance of potential problems, for here it is extremely unlikely that the patient will understand the nursing care being carried out. The patient's priority might be the actual problem of feeling awful and just wanting to be left alone as a result, while the nurse's priority is the potential problem of respiratory and vascular complications, hence the active interventions. Wherever there are potential and actual problems, it is probable that priorities will differ between patient and nurse, although they can also differ when actual problems alone are considered. A noisy phone can be far more of a problem to a patient at night than the nurse could ever imagine! This raises the interesting point of what input night staff should have into planning care. Patients may have problems that are specific to night-time and therefore most appropriately dealt with by night staff.

Having made these general remarks about problems, it is necessary to look at how models affect this stage of the care planning process. A model reflects a definite philosophy of care and therefore the model will seek to define problems in such a way as to be consistent with its philosophy. The nurse should try to use the language of the model in stating problems, for this will reflect the ideas inherent in the model. When working with Orem, for example, this means seeing problems in terms of the inability to practice self-care, while with Roy's model a patient problem can be seen as an inability to adapt to a change in body structure such as the loss of a limb.

Is it possible that an aspect of human behaviour might be defined as a problem by one model but not by another? Given the different perspectives and conceptual frameworks employed by the authors of various models, this possibility raises itself and could be a source of significant difficulty in model development. If by simply changing from one model to another a patient's problem ceases to exist, then given our rejection of relativism in Chapter 1, we have a serious problem.

Perhaps one way forward is to set up a study which will analyse a sample of patients using a series of models. To some extent, problems will vary as the assessment tool itself varies, but is there a limit in the amount of variation that is tolerable, beyond which nurses may start questioning the model itself? We have earlier argued that there is truth and there is right and wrong, therefore if a model is seen as failing, it should be rejected.

One method of setting up a study might involve a panel of 'experts' independently assessing patient profiles drawn from real patients using differing models. This approach was attempted by Procter and Hurt (1994) and their work is described in the section on interventions (p. 59).

An interesting piece of research by Faucett *et al.* (1990) has shed some light on this area. These researchers studied two comparable

50-bed continuing care wards in a US veterans adminstration nursing-home care unit. In one ward a $2\frac{1}{2}$-year period of implementation of the Orem self-care model had taken place while the other ward had remained with the traditional nursing methods of the institution. The study took place in the final 6 months of this implementation period.

The researchers carried out a survey of patient care plans looking to see what differences in patient problems were identified and also interviewed the staff of the two units. They found that the documentation showed little significant differences, in that staff on both wards tended to identify the same problems with the same frequency and carry out the same interventions.

Interviewing showed that nurses on the ward using Orem showed more comprehensiveness in their approach to assessment and also had a greater degree of internal consistency in how they assessed patients. The use of the model, therefore, seemed to lead to a more integrated view of the patient, reflected in this more comprehensive approach. The latter point about internal consistency is relevant to the argument that models might improve nursing care by providing a framework to facilitate patterning of information as this seems to have happened here. The nurses using Orem also showed a greater interest in securing patient participation in the process of goal setting and were much more aware of the importance of the patient being actively involved in care. This places care on a stronger ethical footing.

In an attempt to understand why there appeared to be this paradox that nurses using the Orem model at interview showed a very different approach to care which was not reflected in the written care plans, the researchers constructed six patient vignettes from the data available to them. These were summarized versions of patient case histories and their nursing care. These vignettes were then sent to four independent expert assessors to see if they could tell which patients were on the traditional control ward and which were on the experimental Orem ward. The experts agreed unanimously and correctly on four vignettes but were split on the remaining two, one of which was from the control ward and one the experimental.

This suggests that it was possible to detect from the way care plans overall were written a difference between the ward using the Orem model and the traditional model. However, in terms of problem statements and nursing interventions for real patients the researchers conclude that the overall effects of the institution's policies and procedures has dominated the nursing documentation to such an extent that what is written about these aspects of care makes it impossible to differentiate between the Orem ward and traditional ward. This is despite clear differences in how the nurses talk about assessing their patients, goal setting and the involvement of patients in care.

Researchers are familiar with the differences between what people say, write and actually do. This study appears to have run into this problem and further direct observational study of the nursing care carried out would help resolve the argument about whether implementing a model of nursing makes any difference. Researchers and clinicians need to tackle this fundamental problem of measuring changes in nursing care before meaningful research can be carried out on the effects of nursing models in practice.

In the preceding section, models were identified as taking the nursing assessment into unfamiliar territory as more sensitive, personal areas may be explored. It follows from this that the sorts of problems that may be identified may also be unfamiliar to nurses. This has a clear knock-on effect for the rest of the care plan in terms of setting goals and deciding upon interventions. The use of models may lead British nurses into uncharted waters. This is no reason for not using them, but rather should serve as a stimulus for professional development in acquiring new skills to deal with the sorts of problems that have not previously been identified in traditional practice. It also underlines the need for increased levels of awareness concerning ethical issues.

Goals

Goals, like problems, should be patient centred. They are things we hope the patient will achieve, not the nurse. Davis *et al.* (1994) noted in their study that goals were written as things the nurses would do, showing little attention to patient behaviours. Writing '4-hrly obs' as a goal is a mistake, it is a nursing intervention. The relevant goal here might be 'Patient vital signs to stay within normal limits'.

This raises the question of what normal limits are and with it two more key points about goals: as far as possible they should be measurable and unambiguous. Thus, our goal statement might be better written with a qualification as follows: 'Patient vital signs to stay within normal limits; that is, systolic BP 90–130, P 70–80, RR 12–16, T 36–37°C. Perhaps this might be better broken down into a series of separate goals depending on the condition of the patient; the limits set should also reflect the patient. Thus, they would be very different if the patient was a 6-month-old baby. Similarly, a goal statement such as 'Adequate fluid intake' is unacceptable as it is too ambiguous – it can mean different things to different people. However 'Patient will have intake of 3 l fluid in 24 h' is patient centred, measurable and unambiguous.

In writing this goal, the nurse has added another ingredient of goal setting – a time scale, in this case 24 h. One of the main purposes of setting a goal is to set a standard by which we measure care, so a time limit must be set. Thus, if the nurse adds up the fluid balance chart and finds the patient only managed 2 l of fluid in the 24-h period, we know that the patient failed to achieve what was

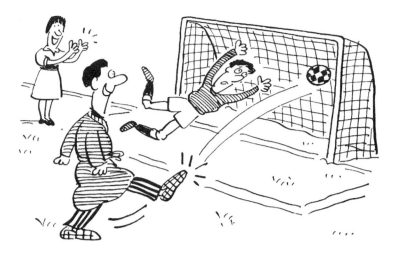

required and therefore we must ask what was wrong with the nursing care.

Goals can be set to different time scales varying from a few hours to weeks. Time scales must also be realistic. Thus, if a patient is severely overweight a goal of losing 5 kg is desirable, but unrealistic if the patient is only given 24 h to achieve it in. Realism is the next key ingredient in goal setting. However, supposing the patient does not wish to lose weight? The weight-loss goal could be written in a patient-centred, measurable, unambiguous, realistic, time-limited way, but come to nought if the patient does not share the goal with the nurse. Goals should therefore be negotiated with the patient.

How will the use of models ensure that these criteria for goals are met? By attempting to place the whole patient at the focus of care, they should ensure that goals are patient centred. The emphasis placed by some models on family and significant others should also help to bring these very important people into the goal-setting process, crucial in community care settings. Other models are based on the full involvement of the patient in care (e.g. King, 1981) and therefore should go even further in ensuring that patients are equal partners in goal setting.

Careful use of words in writing goals should avoid ambiguity and ensure that they are measurable in many cases. However, the use of models opens up a whole Pandora's box of unquantifiables such as fear, anxiety, self-concept and dependence. We cannot put numbers against such subjective properties, unlike a temperature reading, but that is no reason for slamming the lid shut on the box. Models and holistic care have helped liberate these aspects of our patients and we have to incorporate them into care planning.

Most patients have always had anxieties and fears. This fact has not just been recognized since models of nursing were introduced.

However, nursing models do raise nurses' awareness of such sub-jective areas and direct their attention towards the psychological and social aspects of care in a way that the medical model never did, legitimizing them in the process.

As an example, Roy's model may allow the nurse to identify under its self-concept and role-function headings the problem that the woman undergoing mastectomy is frightened that she will no longer be sexually attractive to her husband. How does the nurse set a measurable, unambiguous goal here? Clearly, any goal must be acceptable to the woman (negotiated with the patient) and might be seen as one small step along the road (short-term) to a long-term goal that the couple's sex life will return to its normal level before the surgery. For many nurses this is already unfamiliar territory. The first goal might therefore be that the man will look at his wife's operation site. However, even if this is achieved in a few days, the patient will be ready for discharge, leaving the surgical ward nurse's care plan hanging in mid-air.

This unsatisfactory example has several lessons. First, when we move outside physiology, not all goals can be as neatly packaged as a fluid-intake or weight-loss goal; second, the nurse needs to recog-nize that long-term goals may be very long-term with a rather roundabout route involving a lot of shorter-term goals on the way; and third, there needs to be a facility for transferring the care plan to community or specialist outpatient nursing staff to continue care directed at long-term goals. In such circumstances, attention should be given to the need to continue care along the lines of the model used in hospital, or whether a different model is now indicated. The converse is also true when a patient under care in the community is hospitalized.

In many areas of care, a goal might simply be that the patient will feel able to talk about something or will show a realistic view of their life situation when discussing a topic. Nurses in the field of mental health will be only too aware of this already, but now general nurses are coming to see goal setting in these terms also as they explore the more holistic aspects of care generated by the use of individualized care planning and models.

In conclusion, it remains to say that goals, like problems, should be worded in terms consistent with the philosophy of the model and have targets that reflect the model's view of nursing and health.

Interventions

It is crucial if a model is to be used that its philosophy should be felt in the field of practical nursing interventions. The use of a model should open up new areas in terms of patient problems and in this way influence itnerventions, although this brings with it the need for nurses to acquire new skills and knowledge. A model might also indicate new ways of dealing with old problems that would have been recognized with a more traditional approach.

Consider the example of a female patient who is obese and needs to lose weight. At present, a nurse may advise the patient that it is healthier for her to lose 10 kg in an attempt to encourage her to do so. That of course is correct, but it is a little vague and non-specific. If the nurse was working with Roy's adaptation model, he or she would be familiar with ideas such as self-concept in terms of both body image and self-worth, along with role function and interdependence; that is, how the patient relates to, and depends upon, others. Roy's model also emphasizes physiological aspects of nutrition and elimination. The nurse therefore has many more insights into human behaviour which could allow him or her to explore various strategies to help the patient lose weight other than simply saying that it is healthier.

One more example should suffice to demonstrate that the use of models can enrich nursing care. Consider an elderly male patient who has been admitted after an acute episode of heart failure. After making a recovery he will be discharged home on several different forms of medication which will continue the drug therapy he received in hospital. The traditional drug round will have ensured that he got the right medication at the right time, but it will not have taught him what the pills are for, how many to take and when, and what side-effects to look out for.

Research by Bliss (1981) showed that one admission in ten to elderly care units was due to iatrogenic, drug-related problems; that is, the patients had to be admitted to hospital because of the effects of the drugs they were on. If patients are taught nothing about their medication prior to discharge, this is hardly surprising. However, if Orem's self-care model was in use, then the emphasis would be on teaching the patient about their medication and where possible making them responsible for self-medication in hospital. It is reasonable to say that the patient is competent to manage medicines at home only after they have shown that they can self-medicate, under supervision, on the ward. The use of a model of nursing therefore could fundamentally change nursing practice by making patients responsible for self-medication, where able, on the ward.

Earlier in this chapter we asked whether different models might identify problems in different ways for the same patient and noted the possibility of research using patient profiles to see how different models might behave in their problem identification, goal setting and subsequent interventions. This would be an important test of their validity.

There are substantial difficulties with this approach, however, as Procter and Hunt (1994) described in their attempt to arrive at a professional definition of nursing based upon what it is that nurses do. Procter and Hunt (1994) were able to study a range of real patients and describe as a result, three levels of dependency (high, medium and low) with regard to nursing care. Key factors which determined dependency included mobility, communication and cognition and these authors comment that the picture of patient dependency that emerged was congruent with the conceptual framework of Orem. Life became complicated for these researchers, however, when they constructed three patient profiles based upon these three dependency categories and tried to get agreement from a sample of nurses regarding the care that these hypothetical patients needed.

A total of 113 staff nurses and sisters responded to these patient profiles (57% of the sample chosen) but while it was possible to find some consensus about the goals of care, absolutely none existed regarding the interventions that were required. As Procter and Hunt commented, their findings illustrate the ambiguity and uncertainty that surround nursing care with many interventions being mutually contradictory. These findings also dismiss the fallacy that 'basic nursing' is unskilled and unproblematic. This is a particularly important point as there are NHS managers who see nursing only as a collection of simple tasks that anybody with a bit of common sense can do. The findings of Procter and Hunt clearly illustrate the difficulties involved in deciding upon the correct course of care for patients. It is naïve in the extreme to assume anybody can plan and carry out 'basic nursing care'. The authors go on to question seriously whether it is possible to develop theories about nursing purely out of practice when that practice is so diverse and contradictory and they also question the use of paper exercises as a means of understanding what nurses actually do.

This study demonstrated a complete lack of agreement about nursing interventions in caring for three patients of different dependency levels. The consensus about goals that Procter and Hunt wrote about was only a relative consensus. There were a total of 327 goals for these three patients that over 80% of the subjects thought were essential! One interpretation of this picture sees the phrase 'evidence-based practice' cleaving through this disarray. If the interventions proposed were based upon research evidence then we would expect some degree of consensus to emerge while if nurses used a range of conceptual frameworks or models to guide their care then we might be able to have less than an average of 109 goals per patient! If a group of practitioners cannot arrive at more of a consensus than this, their claim to accountability is in question. This work suggests something of the complexity of carrying out the correct nursing interventions. It is certainly too complex to be delegated *en masse* to health care assistants. However, the performance of qualified nurses on this exercise falls short of what would be expected if evidence-based practice were the norm as then there should be much more consensus about action.

Again we have to enter the caveat that this was one study only and, presented with real patients, perhaps more of a consensus would have emerged. This study suggests that either paper exercises are unhelpful or too much nursing is based upon individual preferences which lack evidence to support them, thereby undermining claims to accountability. The more widespread use of models or conceptual frameworks might introduce some order and pattern into this apparent chaos with a group of nurses being able perhaps to agree on say 10–12 goals for each patient rather than insist on over 100!

The importance of co-operation and patient compliance with nursing interventions cannot be over-emphasized. If the patient refuses to carry out nurse-suggested interventions, then, whatever model of nursing is in use, nursing care will be of little value. The importance of this for nursing is shown in the fact that according to Connelly (1987) one-half of chronically ill patients fail to achieve maximum health benefit because they fail to follow health-related recommendations. As an example, Harris and Linn (1985) have concluded that four out of five hospital days among diabetic patients were directly related to failure to follow recommended treatment, as were 50% of cases of diabetic coma. Other workers have come to similar conclusions; for example, Levy *et al.* (1982) found that non-compliance with treatment among chronically ill, ambulatory patients brought about more complex and expensive hospital treatment than would have been expected as well as precipitating premature hospitalization.

Nurses and nursing models must therefore address the issue of compliance with nursing (and medical) care. It must first of all be stated that in a free society the patient always has the right to say no and refuse treatment, although it is to be hoped that the decision would be an informed one with all the facts of the situation and risks available to the patient. This underlines the importance of good communication with the patient and of the nurses being prepared where necessary to be the patient's advocate.

By incorporating the elements of patient, environment, health and nursing, a valid model should also help address the problem of compliance as it is related to the patient's perception of health and the way the surrounding environment affects the patient. Non-compliance with nursing advice to give up smoking may be understood not only in terms of nicotine addiction but also the patient's view of their health and the effect they think smoking has on that health. For example one patient the author encountered was adamant smoking was good for him because 'smoking makes me cough and clears my chest'. Other factors may also affect smoking such as whether the patient is surrounded by other smokers at home and work, and also the messages conveyed at great expense by the advertising industry that smoking is a good thing.

The problem of compliance shows that the nurse needs to add an interactionist dimension to any model being used. The nurse must try to understand how the patient constructs any situation if they are to have the best chance of persuading the patient to comply with treatment and care which research evidence suggests will be beneficial to the patient. The patient's developmental status will also affect their ability to co-operate in treatment, whether it be the young child who simply does not understand why they have to take their medicine or the elderly widow who has given up wanting to carry on living as part of a bereavement reaction.

Any discussion of compliance brings in its train the issue of advocacy. This is not a simple concept for it draws the nurse into a conflicting sense of loyalties. The UKCC rightly points out that the nurse:

must not practice in a way which assumes that only they know what is best for the patient. UKCC (1996, p. 13)

If the interactionist perspective that is encouraged by some models of nursing is applied consistently, the nurse should always be trying to see things from the patient's point of view which should ensure practice adheres to the UKCC principle outlined above. The problem comes with the sort of situation where the patient fails to co-operate with or actively refuses treatment. Again we find the UKCC stating:

Advocacy also involves providing support if the patient refuses treatment/care or withdraws their consent. UKCC (1996, p. 13)

This sets up potential conflict within the care team for if the nurse is seen as defending the patient's refusal to accept treatment there will be conflict with the doctor, dietician, physiotherapist or whoever. They may lose confidence in the nurse as a therapeutic agent. We have already argued against relativistic stances, stating that there is right and wrong. The diabetic patient who refuses to control their diet is acting in such a manner as to harm their health. If the nurse follows the UKCC guidelines and supports the patient in their refusal to accept treatment he or she will also be contravening the Code of Professional Conduct as his or her actions are clearly not in the patient's best interests. The only possible way out of this very difficult position might be to argue that by keeping in contact with the patient in a supportive and non-judgemental way now, it might be possible in the future to persuade them to accept treatment. This of course assumes that the nurse does know better than the patient what is best for them. The nurse now contradicts the first of the above guidelines – in short you are damned if you do and you are damned if you do not!

The ability of the nurse to act as the patient's advocate is therefore open to question. As health care advances and nursing roles expand and develop greater accountability *for the delivery of care* (e.g. the nurse practitioner role), so it becomes harder to defend supporting the patient in the non-delivery of care. There are real limits on how far the patient advocate role can be taken. Giving patients information to ensure consent is truly informed and trying to see things from their individual point of view is consistent with a models-based approach to care and the requirements of the UKCC. The problem comes when advocacy is pushed to the extent that it is in the UKCC 1996 guidelines, as in the current state of health care, this can put the nurse in a situation where they are wrong whatever course of action is taken.

Compliance is particularly relevant in considering the care of patients with chronic illness, and in a review of these problems Connelly (1987) emphasizes the importance of self-care in compliance, going on to discuss predisposing factors such as self-concept, family and support networks and psychological status. These are key notions in the work of Orem and Roy respectively, indicating that nursing care derived from these models can tackle problems of compliance.

It will be apparent from the previous sections that use of a model will lead nursing into some new and unfamiliar territory that will involve seeing the patient in a more holistic fashion. One major change that will be noticed in using most models is that the nurse needs to spend more time talking to the patient and this must be recognized as direct nursing care, not just 'having a chat'. Managers and sisters therefore should accept that time spent in conversation, particularly listening to a patient, is very much a part of nursing intervention just as time spent bathing or dressing the patient.

The nurse may find that models start to identify environmental problems whose solutions lie beyond the boundaries of nursing at present. This is particularly true of the community nurse. This is no reason to reject models, although this may be a very frustrating situation for the community nurse to be in. Rather, we must look at ways in which nursing can tackle these new problem areas and not just walk away from them. It may be that closer links with social services are needed. The nurse as patient's advocate is a role that nursing spends more time talking about than practising; perhaps models may force nurses to confront the reality of that role. In this way models can serve as a stimulus to nursing development.

On a larger scale still, perhaps some patient's problems have their origins in political decisions made by national government or perhaps it is the factory down the road producing unacceptable levels of pollution. If nursing models make us recognize the political and environmental causes of some patient problems, there should be no logical reason why nursing should not go forward into these arenas as a legitimate part of nursing intervention.

Models may also lead nurses to place greater emphasis on patients learning to do things for themselves. Not only do nurses need to learn what is involved in allowing and encouraging a patient self-care, but so do patients and their families. The danger is that what to the nurse appears as interventions designed to promote indepen-dence in activities of daily living (Roper) or to improve self-care ability (Orem) may look to the patient like neglect.

This underlines the need for good communication between nur-sing staff, patient and family in order that the patient knows what the nurse is trying to achieve. Misunderstandings which could lead to complaints can be avoided in this way.

Evaluation

Evaluation of care is perhaps the most important aspect of all. As Thomas and Bond (1995) observe, demonstrating the value of nur-sing has never been more important than it is today in the cash-squeezed NHS. There are senior NHS managers and health aca-demics in so-called 'policy think tanks' who simply do not recognize the value of nursing and see only a collection of simple tasks which anybody with an NVQ level 2 can perform. Nursing therefore has to demonstrate its worth; it has to evaluate what it is doing for patients.

Here it is important to remember that the care given may be very different from what is written down. Consequently, how a nurse evaluates care mentally may be very different from how this evalua-tion is recorded in nursing process documentation. It is a dangerous assumption that documentation reflects the quality of care despite the fact that as Christie (1993) observed, the WHO regard documen-tation as essential to ensure good communication, to be a measure of quality and to ensure accountability for care given. The evaluation section of the nursing process is therefore potentially a valuable tool and should be consistent with the conceptual framework or model in use. If care was based upon Orem's model, for example, criteria to evaluate care against might include questions such as how effective have we been in promoting self-care?

The use of criteria to measure the success or otherwise of care is essential and brings us back to the issue of goal setting. It is only possible to measure the effectiveness of care if goals have been set which can be measured. If goal setting is carried out incorrectly, then meaningful evaluation of care will not be possible.

The evidence concerning evaluation as revealed by nursing pro-cess documentation is not re-assuring. The work of Davis *et al.* (1994) referred to earlier found little attempt had been made to evaluate interventions and also that there were few legible signatures for care given. This latter point calls into question the notion of individual accountability.

Other research looking at the overall value of care plans is little better. A study by Bellman (1993) focused on a sample of 43 nurses working on a group of five surgical wards. She found that 83% of the nurses believed that patient care plans bore little resemblance to what nurses actually did, 85% hardly ever referred to care plans throughout the day and 75% thought they were a complete waste of time. This view is supported by Fonteyn and Cooper (1994) who assert that in their experience most nurses thought the written nursing process care plan was only a paper exercise and was of little value. A much larger study carried out by Martin *et al.* (1994) reported that in a sample of 1096 nurses drawn from nine North American hospitals in one urban area, fewer than 30% were happy with the way their care plans were documented and 66.4% stated that care plans were not valued by RNs. Given this degree of hostility towards the nursing process care plan in practice, the whole validity of this approach is called into question. Martin *et al.* conclude by remarking that a supportive organizational culture plus a positive attitude and knowledge are essential requirements to elicit individualized planned care within a nursing process framework. The traditional nursing process care plan clearly did not have that support within their hospitals which suggests that possibly individualized care may be jeopardized by the need to write care plans that staff do not have any faith in. The possibility that, paradoxically, the traditional care plan may be an obstacle to individualized care is explored in Chapter 4.

In recognition of these weaknesses, some nurses have instigated audit projects aimed at using a series of criteria against which the quality of the nursing process documentation may be checked. It is hoped that this will improve the quality of the documented nursing process care plan. One such piece of work was carried out by Roberts and Smith (1993) who developed a check list of 46 items or criteria to measure the quality of the nursing process documentation being written by staff in their hospital. The development of the tool as a bottom-up approach involving clinical staff is welcome; however, the tool was not administered in a standardized way which undermines the reliability of the findings. Wards could either audit their own documentation or invite other wards to do so. The authors claim improvement in the audit scores, indicating that the audit has increased the quality of the documentation and as a result the quality of patient care has improved. There are two flaws in this argument. First, no statistical significance testing has been carried out on the scores, therefore the improvement may not be of any significance. Second, there is no evidence to support the assertion that the quality of documentation and care are related. The evidence cited above suggests that there is little relationship at all. This is not therefore a particularly rigorous or useful piece of research and the same comment could apply to work by Teggart (1993) who also describes developing a nursing process documentation audit tool which it is claimed provided a lot of useful information. Again there are serious doubts about reliability and validity and a lack of statistical analysis which invalidate this paper.

The research evidence is scant and indicates that, in practice, studies using the nursing process documentation to evaluate the quality of care given have been of dubious reliability and validity, whatever model is used. What limited research there is suggests that this is because either the evaluation section of the care plan is poorly filled in, the overall care plan is not valued by staff or there are serious weaknesses in the research which aims to audit care plans and improve quality as a result.

If use of the formal care plan to evaluate care has failed to be effective, what evidence is there that nurses have evaluated the effectiveness of care by other means such as studies of specific interventions? A major review of recently published research into the effectiveness of nursing care was undertaken by Bond and Thomas (1995). Their findings were not encouraging as they commented upon the paucity of replication as no two studies were ever alike. This point has already been made in this chapter; even the best pieces of research tend to be isolated and lack the replication which would increase confidence in their findings. Only a moderate number of studies claim to be able to show the effectiveness of nursing interventions while there are multiple problems with poor study design. Consequently,

Stronger study designs which are able to provide sound evidence of the relationship between nursing inputs and the effects on patients are required. Bond and Thomas (1995)

The cost as well as the effectiveness of nursing interventions must also be considered for as these authors point out, if a new nursing intervention increases costs overall then it is unlikely to be adopted. New interventions must have their costs as well as their effectiveness evaluated. This can of course be turned to nursing's advantage because if nurses can show that nursing care saves money, for example in the prevention of pressure sores, earlier discharges and fewer re-admissions, then nursing has a very strong argument which management will take seriously. Research into the effectiveness of nursing interventions therefore, according to Bond and Thomas, needs to:

- be much more rigorous than at present, particularly with regard to reliability and validity testing and statistical analysis;
- focus more on the evaluation of nursing interventions, including the economic impact;
- place more emphasis on empirical testing and the development of theory from such data;
- involve more replication and multi-centre studies in order that results may be generalized with more confidence;
- concentrate in a consistent fashion upon clinical practice.

This agenda for research into the effectiveness of nursing interventions addresses many of the weaknesses encountered in this chapter. However, it is not a substitute for evaluation by each individual nurse of the nursing care he or she has delivered. There is a lack of convincing evidence that this evaluation is finding its way into the formally written care plan, even if nurses are mentally evaluating their care in practice. There is a case for saying that a conceptual framework or nursing model should facilitate that evaluation process by setting up a consistent structure within which care can be evaluated and goals can be set that are measurable.

Care planning and quality assurance

In this chapter so far we have examined the various stages in what is essentially a linear problem-solving method – the nursing process. It is called linear because the nurse moves in a straight line from one stage to the next finishing on evaluation of care delivered, a crucial step which should feed back into care planning by making evident the success or otherwise of the care provided by the nurse. This approach is consistent with nursing models and is actually facilitated by their use. The nursing process is a problem-solving technique, it is a mental exercise only. Writing out nursing process care plans is a separate issue which, as we have begun to see, has major difficulties.

Some writers, however, consider the nursing process was much more than an attempt at developing individualized care. Latimer (1995) summarizes these alternative views as either seeking to make nursing more professional and accountable on the one hand or trying to make it more cost effective and involved with the developing field of quality assurance in health care. This latter point is crucial for as we have seen in the preceding section, evaluating the effectiveness of nursing intervention has not been done with any conviction in standard nursing process documentation nor by separate research projects. Yet nursing is under increasing pressure to justify itself as pressure on resources in a market-driven health-care system become tighter year on year. There has been a growth in management techniques aimed at controlling expenditure and improving quality to deliver value for money. Resource management, performance indicators, clinical audit, quality assurance; the phrases trip off the tongue and the men in grey suits seem ever more powerful while clinical practitioners in all the professions, not just nursing, become increasingly alarmed.

The quality of nursing care is therefore a crucial issue. Many research projects have foundered upon this difficulty whether they are studies looking at the impact of the nursing process or primary nursing. By the same token, any attempt at introducing a model of nursing or moving towards a more multidisciplinary model of care and attempting to look at the impact upon quality has the same difficulty. If the agenda outlined above by Thomas and Bond (1995) is to be followed, rigorous methods of determining the quality of care will have to be used if the effectiveness of nursing is to be unambiguously demonstrated. Whatever the situation, nurses are held accountable for their care, therefore measures of quality are everybody's business.

It is beyond the scope of this book to launch into a major discussion of quality assurance in health care. However, there are some key points which are of relevance to evaluating the quality of delivered care, whether a models-based framework has been used or not. A useful framework for considering quality has been suggested by Ovretveit (1992) and this involves seeing quality from three perspectives: patient, management and professional. The validity of this approach should be apparent from a moment's reflection. What the patient considers quality care may not be what the nurse thinks of as good care while management have a different agenda again which is much more to do with value for money and cost effectiveness. Simply asking the patient whether they are satisfied with care is unreliable and lacks validity as a measure of the professional and managerial quality of that care. It also lacks the power to discriminate between good and bad as it usually results in 95% of patients saying that they are satisfied. Although asking the patient to state their level of satisfaction has a common-sense appeal, it is fraught with weaknesses such as the fact that it means different things to different people, it is a loosely defined and ambiguous notion, and can be influenced by a whole host of things that are nothing to do with nursing (Bond and Thomas, 1992). It is likely, for example, that many patients will not know what constitutes good care (professional quality) therefore they cannot form a valid judgement, while a great many elderly patients who remember life before the NHS may just be grateful for any care at all.

Workers such as Bell *et al.* (1993) have taken this critique further, working in focus groups to try and discover things that are important to patients. As they point out, unless audit addresses areas of concern to patients, it may result in a waste of valuable resources and fail to deliver improvements that the patient recognizes as such. The patient dimension of quality may therefore be missed altogether while wasting resources is a management quality issue.

Marr and Giebing (1994) offer a useful division of nursing quality-assurance systems into those which have been developed elsewhere (which they call centrally devised) and intended to be bought, ready made, off the shelf for use and those which have been developed internally by staff for their own use (locally devised). Both these approaches to nursing quality are largely what Ovretveit (1992) would call professional quality assurance although it is possible to bring in the patient and management dimensions of quality, particularly with locally devised tools. Examples of the former include Monitor, Qualpacs and the Phaneuf Audit which may be thought of as centrally designed tools while the RCN DySSSy approach is a good example of the latter. The results that are obtained with any method depend upon the tool that is selected, therefore nurses need to be aware of what these methods entail if they are to evaluate the quality of their care.

Reference has already been made to papers by Teggart (1993) and Roberts and Smith (1993) who spent a great deal of time developing an audit tool to assess the quality of nursing process documentation. These papers may be criticized on several grounds, including the lack of evidence of reliability and validity testing and the established gap between documentation and actual care delivered. Therefore, it is worth pointing out that a rigorously tested audit tool has existed for some 20 years to measure the quality of documentation, the Phaneuf Audit tool (Phaneuf, 1976). This gives a score for the quality of the documentation and as its author Phaneuf freely admits, this is not the same as a measure of actual care given. She therefore recommends the use of another audit tool at the same time which looks at the care delivered. If staff wish to audit documentation, before developing their own tool they should ask whether they can justify large amounts of time being devoted to developing a documentation audit tool when a rigorously tested one already exists. That would be poor quality from a management perspective! Christie (1993) offers an example of using Phaneuf's tool in such a UK study aimed at improving patient assessment in A&E.

The other approach taken by centrally devised audit tools involves looking at samples of nursing care and scoring them against pre-set criteria. This characterizes Monitor and Qualpacs and leads to a complex and time-consuming exercise which will produce scores related to the quality of care delivered. There are problems, however, in that both systems are derived from a nursing process approach and therefore have an in-built bias in favour of areas using a strictly orthodox nursing process method of documenting care. We have stated that the nursing process is only one problem-solving approach to care; there are others as we see in the next chapter, therefore nurses using other more flexible methods to deliver care may score badly. In addition, a clinical area implementing a particular model of nursing may have specific types of intervention which go unrecognized by one of these centrally designed tools which were not designed to take into account different nursing models and the range of approaches to care that may flow from their use. Credit may therefore not be gained for good nursing care because it simply is not recognized and therefore scored by the tool. The tool may be blind to some aspects of a model and consequently scores may be distorted.

These criticisms suggest the need for a more sensitive approach to quality, particularly where care is delivered across a wide range of settings other than the traditional general hospital ward or where different conceptual frameworks are used to underpin care. This locally determined approach is characterized by the RCN Dynamic

Standard Setting System (DySSSy). The key ideas involve the staff setting agreed standards of care, then stating benchmarks that can be used to measure whether these standards have been met. These benchmarks are known as criteria and have to be measurable. Criteria can be subdivided into structure (physical aspects of the care environment), process (care delivery) and outcome (i.e. the outcomes of care). This sounds similar to goal setting; the difference is that these criteria (and hence standards) are set for all patients but goals are set on an individual basis. The staff can then audit their performance by measuring how successful they have been in meeting the criteria they have set.

This approach allows staff to develop a quality framework that is sensitive to local needs and which they can feel a sense of ownership in. The DySSSy method allows the differing concepts and ideas in various models to be accommodated within the quality-assurance work. It is a system which allows nurses to look at the quality of care actually delivered but can also incorporate documentation if staff so desire. Crucially, it is free from the nursing process bias that distorts scores from methods such as Monitor and can be adapted to suit whatever form of care planning and documentation is employed. This local method of evaluating the effectiveness of nursing care involves a great deal of work and should focus on a small number of key standards rather than becoming bogged down in trivia. It does have the potential, however, to be a powerful tool in the hands of nurses seeking to demonstrate the effectiveness and value of the care they deliver.

This brief discussion of quality assurance approaches should alert the nurse to the importance of this area. No clinical area can ignore quality assurance and the need to evaluate the quality of care delivered. It is a complicated area, however, and the choice of tool can significantly affect the results. Nurses should not therefore allow management to impose a tool upon them but rather be proactive, selecting an approach which they feel best suits their needs. The DySSSy method meets many of the requirements of a sensitive tool which can demonstrate quality and effectiveness when used with different models of nursing and methods of care delivery other than the standard nursing process. Crucially, it can be customized to fit local needs and whatever nursing models are in use can be reflected in the standards and criteria that are set.

Primary nursing and the organization of care delivery

Recent years have seen the growth in popularity of primary nursing and the named nurse concept, which is not quite the same thing. Primary nursing may greatly help the delivery of care planned within a conceptual framework or nursing model, but it is not the only means of care delivery, just as the nursing process is not the only means of planning care. Various other modes of care delivery exist including the original, traditional task-centred method referred to already. The work-book system which preceded the nursing process documentation illustrates the concern of traditional nursing organization with physical tasks.

The traditional system was based around tasks with each nurse assigned a task to perform for all patients that shift. As we know, this led to fragmentation and depersonalization of care as patients found a bewildering array of nurses coming and going performing separate tasks with no sense of continuity or order. Psychological and social aspects of care never had much chance of developing in this task-centred system. The next development came with the advent of patient allocation. The idea was that, by allocating a group of patients to a team of nurses, or a smaller group to a single nurse, care would become more holistic. Walsh and Ford (1989) have argued that in practice this tends to resemble a small-scale version of task allocation, while the single nurse who has a small group of patients allocated to them for a shift finds it very difficult to practise holistic care because there is no continuity beyond that shift. Come the following day, responsibility has been passed on to somebody else while the nurse is given a new set of patients, again for the duration of only a shift before this game of musical chairs is repeated again and again. Team nursing, which involves allocating the same patients to a group of nurses for their entire stay, was a welcome step forward aimed at eliminating the problem of discontinuity caused by the musical chairs approach. Team nursing does require a ward to have adequate staffing to ensure teams are able to give care consistently to their patients. Unfortunately, this is proving increasingly difficult to provide.

This lack of continuity of care is compounded by the low standard of care planning and documentation that may be due to a lack of time or knowledge of care-planning techniques. The nurse may also have a strongly negative attitude towards the subject, which inhibits good care planning. To take over responsibility for a batch of eight new patients in the morning is a daunting prospect, but when there is only a very scant written record of their problems and care, and that may be several days or even weeks out of date, then the chances of the nurse being able to practise professional individualized care start to become very slim indeed.

A model of nursing can give the nurse a framework and a philosophy to work with, but there has to be a system of nursing that permits a nurse to implement care consistently and in a way that meets the patient's individual needs as well as the need for professional accountability on the part of the nurse. This system is primary nursing.

Primary nursing is another import from the USA, but has a major contribution to make if nursing models and individualized care are to be made to work. The notion is simply that each patient has a nurse who retains overall responsibility for their care in the same way that a doctor does. This nurse, the primary nurse, should assess and plan care, delegating responsibility for the patient to colleagues or associate nurses when off duty.

However, this is a very simple picture of primary nursing for, as Mead (1991) showed, there is a lengthy list of key characteristics which should be present for primary nursing to really function including some very significant changes in the roles of all the nurses on the ward, increased levels of authority and accountability for care delivered which should also be much more patient centred with a substantial element of patient choice in care. Good communications which show the primary nurse to be the key organizer of care are also essential. Mead also highlighted the need for a visible value system and ward philosophy. Such characteristics are also essential if any clinical area is to use nursing models to guide care delivery.

The consistency of care and the involvement with the patient, which are characteristics of models-based nursing, are also essential components of primary nursing. The two therefore go together very well and a primary nursing system will greatly facilitate the introduction and operation of a model(s). Team nursing, however, may also achieve a stable environment within which models-based care may flourish, providing the resources are available to ensure that the teams (usually two on any ward) can operate consistently and are not disrupted by staff shortages and reliance upon bank nurses as stop-gaps. As long as the nurse responsible for the patient's care gets to know the patient well then it is possible to carry out the in-depth assessment referred to earlier and plan care that follows on logically from the assessment and is sensitive to the individual's needs. This can happen within either a primary or team nursing system. There is considerable debate about primary nursing compared to team nursing and in discussing these areas, Ford and Walsh (1994) have pointed out that however appealing primary nursing may appear, there are few studies that have evaluated its effectiveness and convincingly shown improvements in the quality of care that can be attributed exclusively to its introduction. Indeed, there is considerable debate about just what constitutes primary nursing leading to questions such as how will we recognize it when we see it? The views of Thomas and Bond (1995) discussed earlier about nursing's failure to evaluate the effectiveness of nursing interventions should be recalled here together with the in-depth analysis of primary nursing systems of Mead (1991). A final note of caution comes from Mead and Bryar (1992) who remind us of the potential for the introduction of primary nursing to follow the same rocky road as the nursing process. In particular, they point out that both involved nursing giving up time-honoured ways of working and therefore the difficulties in making changes may be partly understood within a framework of loss and bereavement.

The named nurse should not be confused with the primary nurse. The former is a very narrow role and often ends up as little more than a name on a piece of card stuck over the patient's bed with little actual impact upon care. The primary nurse is part of a much bigger and radical change in nursing care delivery. According to Wright and Khadim (1989), it redefines the nurse–patient relationship by bringing both parties together in a completely new way, changing the whole way we think about nursing. That is true, but it is not the only way this new way of thinking can be achieved. Nursing models also have this potential, so does effectively resourced team nursing and, as we see in the next chapter, there are other ways of achieving this goal, particularly in the growing area of short stay and day care.

Summary

In this chapter we have followed through the various stages involved in one method of planning individualized care, the nursing process. As we have seen, it is one method only – just as the nursing care plan is one method only of documenting care. There is considerable criticism of the nursing care plan which is conventionally derived from the nursing process approach and there is evidence to suggest care plans are poorly written, often having minimal impact upon care delivered. This indicates that there is a need to look at alternative approaches to the planning and documentation of individualized patient care, although the notion that a model of care may be helpful in planning and delivering that care still stands. The need to evaluate the effectiveness of care cannot be over emphasized and while primary nursing promises a great deal, especially for models-based care, there is a lack of convincing evidence that it has had a major impact upon patient outcomes so far.

References

Bell L, Morriss B & Brown B (1993) Devising a multidisciplinary audit tool. *International Journal of Health Care Quality Assurance*, **6**(4), 16–21.

Bellman L (1993) The use of nursing care plans in surgical wards. *Journal of Clinical Nursing*, **2**(4), 258–259.

Bliss M (1981) Prescribing for the elderly. *British Medical Journal*, **283**, 203–204.

Bond S & Thomas L (1992) Measuring patient satisfaction with nursing care. *Journal of Advanced Nursing*, **17**, 52–63.

Chapman GE (1983) Ritual and rational action in hospitals. *Journal of Advanced Nursing*, **8**, 13–20.

Christie J (1993) Does the use of an assessment tool in the A&E department improve the quality of care? *Journal of Advanced Nursing*, **18**, 1758–1771.

Clark E (1992) Psychological perspectives. In Robinson K & Vaughan B (eds) *Knowledge for Nursing Practice*, pp. 89–109. Oxford: Butterworth Heinemann.

Connelly CE (1987) Self-care and the chronically ill patient. *Nursing Clinics of North America*, **22**(3), 621–629.

Davis B, Billings J & Ryland R (1994) Evaluation of nursing process documentation. *Journal of Advanced Nursing*, **19**, 960–968.

Faucett J, Ellis V, Underwood P, Naqvi A & Wilson D (1990) The effect of Orem's self care model in a nursing home setting. *Journal of Advanced Nursing*, **15**, 659–666.

Fonteyn M & Cooper F (1994) The written nursing process: is it still useful to nursing education? *Journal of Advanced Nursing*, **19**, 313–319.

Ford P & Walsh M (1994) *New Rituals for Old*. Oxford: Butterworth Heinemann.

Harris R & Linn MW (1985) Health beliefs, compliance and control of diabetes mellitus. *Southern Medical Journal*, **78**(2).

Hilgard E, Atkinson R & Smith E (1987) *Introduction to Psychology*. New York: Harcourt Brace Jovanovich.

Hurst K (1993) *Problem Solving in Nursing Practice*. London: Scutari.

King I (1981) *A Theory for Nursing*. New York: Wiley.

Latimer J (1995) The nursing process re-examined: enrolment and translation. *Journal of Advanced Nursing*, **22**, 213–220.

Levy M, Mermelstein L & Hemo D (1982) Medical admissions due to non-compliance with drug therapy. *International Journal of Clinical Pharacology, Therapeutics and Toxicology*, **20**(12).

Marr H & Giebing H (1994) *Quality Assurance in Nursing*. Edinburgh: Campion Press.

Marriner A (1979) *The Nursing Process*. St Louis: CV Mosby.

Martin P, Dugan J, Freundl M, Miller S, Phillips R & Sharrittes L (1994) Nurse's attitude towards nursing process as measured by the Dayton Attitude Scale. *Journal of Continuing Education in Nursing*, **25**(1), 35–40.

Maslow A (1968) *Toward a Psychology of Being*, 2nd edn. New York: Van Nostrand Reinhold.

McFarlane J & Castledine G (1982) *The Practice of Nursing*. London: CV Mosby.

Mead D (1991) An evaluation tool for primary nursing. *Nursing Standard*, **6**(1), 37–39.

Mead D & Bryar R (1992) An analysis of the changes involved in the introduction of the nursing process and primary nursing using a theoretical framework of loss and attachment. *Journal of Clinical Nursing*, **1**, 95–99.

Ovretveit J (1992) *Health Service Quality*. Oxford: Blackwell Scientific Publications.

Phaneuf M (1976) *The Nursing Audit: Self-regulation in Nursing Practice*. New York: Appleton Century Crofts.

Procter S & Hunt M (1994) Using the Delphi Survey technique to develop a professional definition of nursing for analysing nursing workload. *Journal of Advanced Nursing*, **19**, 1003–1014.

Roberts C & Smith R (1993) Improving nursing records with audit. *Nursing Standard*, **7**(51), 37–39.

Teggart L (1993) Measurement of care planning. *Journal of Clinical Nursing*, **2**, 63–65.

Thomas L & Bond S (1995) The effectiveness of nursing care. *Journal of Clinical Nursing*, **4**, 143–151.

UKCC (1996) *Guidelines for Professional Practice*. London: UKCC.

Walsh M & Ford P (1989) *Nursing Rituals; Research and Rational Action.* Oxford: Butterworth Heinemann.

Wright S & Khadim A (1989) Primary nursing: your questions answered. *Nursing Standard,* **4**(7).

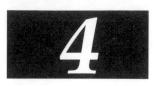

Critical Pathways

Introduction

In Chapter 3 we reviewed the most common method of planning individual care, the nursing process. The documentation that goes with the nursing process, the written care plan, has been the subject of much criticism and complaint. In this chapter we question whether the root of the problem is that nursing is being made to fit the nursing process rather than the other way round. Some nurses in the USA have now rejected the traditional care plan as the norm and moved on to new multidisciplinary approaches to care known as critical pathways (CPs). These form the focus of this chapter as they are now being introduced to the UK and we need to ask whether they can deliver individualized care and, if so, whether nursing models have a place in this brave new world.

Care planning and problem solving

The first three chapters presented two different views of the way nurses work, both of which were described by Benner (1984). On the one hand there is the logical, step by step, rule-bound behaviour of the competent nurse but there is also the expert, at times intuitive, nurse who seems to grasp whole problems at once, often solving them without any visible series of logical steps. Benner argues that these stages lie on a continuum which nurses may traverse as they progress from absolute novices to experts many years later. The nursing process approach discussed in Chapter 3 seems to fit the logical, step-by-step approach to problem solving, but sits ill at ease with the more intuitive approach that is said to characterize experts. This raises the interesting issue of whether one of the major problems with the nursing process is that it simply does not fit with the way that many nurses work. In other words, nursing is being made to fit the nursing process rather than the nursing process having been designed to suit the way nurses work.

In order to gain some insight into this debate, the work of Hurst (1993) is most useful as he summarizes the literature about theories of problem solving and places them within a nursing context. As Hurst observes, there is a great deal written about how nurses ought to solve clinical problems, but very little research done concerning how they actually do in practice.

There are two basic views of how we set about solving problems, the first of which is known as the stages theory. This sees humans as working through a logical set of stages in a linear manner to arrive at a solution to any problem. The most common stages are problem identification, assessment, planning interventions (including goal setting), implementation of plans and evaluation. These stages of course correspond closely with the orthodox view of the nursing process which follows this rigid linear methodology. This identification of the nursing process with problem solving in nursing is so close that Hurst points out that they are synonymous for many people. This insistence that the only way of planning care is with the nursing process has stifled nursing and prevented creative thinking. The adoption of only one method of problem solving by nursing's leaders (e.g. UKCC) may be seen as evidence that nursing is a static profession which has failed to keep pace with change (Hardy and Engel, 1987). Despite the great deal of literature urging the nursing process upon nurses, there is a lack of evidence to show that experienced nurses really do solve problems in this way, to the exclusion of other strategies. To paraphrase Hurst, the stages model (nursing process) is over-supported and under-researched. What research we have uncovered in Chapter 3 indicates that this is an unpopular approach among nurses and the quality of written care documentation produced by the nursing process leaves much to be desired.

There is an alternative problem-solving strategy to the stages model which is known as information-processing theory and it can be summarized as consisting of three components:

- *Task environment*. This is the external representation of a problem to the nurse, for example, a post-operative patient who has had a hip replacement appearing distressed and stating they have pain in their calf.
- *Problem space*. At this level the nurse has internalized the problem. Analysis takes place drawing upon knowledge and previous experience. This places the experienced nurse at a considerable

advantage to the junior. A range of options is explored both mentally and physically, for solving the problem, feedback from trial solutions is digested and the problem re-analysed. An accurate and complete problem space (having access to all the facts) is essential for problem solution. In the above example, the nurse knows about the risk of deep venous thrombosis (DVT) and the presenting signs and symptoms, therefore s/he checks the calf for tenderness, measures calf circumference for comparison with the other leg, checks anti-coagulant medication and ascertains which doctor is on call.

- *Problem-solving strategy.* The solution is arrived at by searching the problem space and a considerable amount of mental effort. It may be arrived at in one attempt or there may be an element of back and forth (iteration) between the problem space and the solution. The solution does not come out of thin air, however. The person does not automatically 'know' the answer as the word 'intuition' may imply, but may have to draw upon considerable knowledge, experience and the ability to recognize patterns and deviations from patterns within the problem space to arrive at a solution. In the example discussed above, the nurse decides the patient may have developed a DVT and knowing the potentially serious consequences if left untreated, decides to bleep the on-call SHO while giving much-needed psychological support to the patient.

This information-processing theory presents a very different picture to the linear, stages (nursing process) model of problem solving. The apparent superiority and intuitive grasp of expert nurses described by Benner (1984) may be attributed to their much greater experience and patterning ability. Perhaps Benner's experts are actually working with an information-processing model of problem solving, which appears invisible because nurses have been brainwashed into recognizing only the stages, nursing process model?

It may be rather like the clock that stops ticking, you only notice it when it stops because you have got so used to its ticking that you are no longer aware of its presence. It may be that expert nurses become so used to certain patterns of patient behaviour that they are not consciously aware of them but are able to recognize subtle deviations before others and arrive at a rapid solution based upon their greater experience and knowledge within the 'problem space' without any explicit problem-solving display. If nurses have only learnt the nursing process and consequently only know a stages model of problem solving, then anything else will appear intuitive.

There is strong support for this alternative explanation of how nurses work from writers such as Tanner *et al.* (1987) and Carnevali *et al.* (1984). They consider that the nursing process is too limiting due to its rigid and linear approach and argue that the nurse's diagnostic reasoning skills are in practice much wider and more akin to the information-processing theory. North American writers such as those cited above are concerned with diagnostic reasoning; that is, how nurses decide what the patient's problem is, which is then expressed as a nursing diagnosis. A nursing diagnosis is a standardized statement of a problem or a label which may be applied to any patient and this has led Hurst to criticize North American writers and researchers who have only concentrated upon diagnostic reasoning for only looking at half the picture. This is because they have not gone on to look at how the nurse decides what to actually do once a diagnosis has been arrived at.

The views of Kim *et al.* (1991) are important here, however, for in describing what a nursing diagnosis consists of they point out that the nursing diagnosis is tied to a meaningful course of action and required nursing interventions. This implies that once the nursing diagnosis has been arrived at, the nursing interventions will be fairly standardized and tend to follow automatically. Kim *et al.* (1991) engage in a dialogue with a leading Scandinavian nurse, Randi Mortensen, who raises the worry that this may become nursing on auto-pilot with no attention paid to individual needs at all. The North American response to these Nordic doubts is that a standardized system of nursing diagnoses will lead to research programmes targeted on specific diagnoses which will provide clear guidelines for evidence-based practice.

This response is not very re-assuring. The use of the future tense raises the issue of what do we do now, before such research programmes are instituted? It sounds a very idealistic solution but given the lack of resources available for nursing research and the difficulties of researching many of the diagnoses it will be many years before it is possible to come to some conclusions. In addition, a characteristic of research is that it tends to raise as many new questions as it answers, therefore the idea that it is possible to have a research programme that can give us all the answers to the patient problems posed by nursing diagnoses is simply unreal, even if the resources and time were available. There are, however, advantages in developing a common nursing language, such as nursing diagnoses, to permit nurses from different countries to communicate better. However, the notion that a nursing diagnosis leads automatically to a pre-set nursing intervention ignores the individuality of the patient. There is no substitute for the nurse using their judgement to deal with patient problems in an evidence-based, accountable but individualized way.

Leaving this short discourse on the question of nursing diagnoses, we now return to the main issue of how nurses work in practice. The linear nursing process approach has been consistently unpopular ever since its introduction and has little research-based evidence to support it. In 1991, the requirement that North American hospitals use formally written nursing process care plans was dropped by the Joint Commission on Accreditation of Health Care Organizations (JCAHCO), a powerful body responsible for setting standards in health care. Fonteyn and Cooper (1994) have argued that it is time to dispose of the orthodox nursing process care plan, citing a series of studies which seriously question the assumption that nurses do work in a linear four- to five-stage problem-solving method. In their view, the nursing process has use as a teaching tool to help junior students understand the complex world of care. This is consistent with the views of Benner (1984) discussed extensively earlier. However, Fonteyn and Cooper go on to point out that the formal nursing process is an over-simplification of the way experienced nurses work and imposes rigid constraints upon practice. Health care has become far more complex over the past 20 years while the nursing process has not changed; it is therefore becoming cumbersome and outdated. In short, it does not fit the real world of health care and is more of a hindrance than a help to RNs.

The following points are seen by Fonteyn and Cooper (1994) as undermining the validity of the nursing process:

- The main accrediting body (JCAHCO) in the home of the nursing process (USA) no longer considers the formal written care plan necessary.
- The increasing complexity of patient problems in modern health care has outstripped the nursing process.
- Patients want more involvement with their care. Perhaps it is possible to find quicker and more flexible ways of documenting care that are more 'patient friendly' than the nursing process care plan which many nurses still do not seem to understand. If the quality of the care plan is as poor as research suggests, how can we share it with patients? In addition, even a well-written nursing process care plan can easily lead to the exclusion of patients from their care if it is rigidly adhered to.
- The increasing number of day cases and 24-h admissions makes writing out the full nursing process care plan an even more time-consuming exercise for little, if any, perceived benefit. It is in danger of being seen as irrelevant by nurses.
- The explosion in the amount of data available about patients has swamped the nursing process. To document all this information in the care plan leads to increasing amounts of duplication and consumes more and more precious time.

In view of these criticisms – the general perception that the nursing process is unpopular with clinical staff and the fact that research shows it is poorly understood and implemented – perhaps it is time to relegate the nursing process from its present pre-eminence. If we see it only as a useful tool for teaching junior students, but move away towards a more problem-based learning strategy involving case studies and selection/prioritization of actions, perhaps we might be giving students an education that is more appropriate for the real world? By the same token, clinical areas can then be freed of the constraints of having to 'do the nursing process' and can develop alternative, more creative strategies that also reflect the increasingly multidisciplinary emphasis on care that is being sought from health service managers. However, we must beware throwing out the baby with the bathwater and reintroducing the old task-centred approach, the needs of the *whole* individual must be paramount to the nurse.

Critical pathways: an alternative approach

In Chapter 3 the notion of standard setting was introduced in terms of the RCN DySSSy system. Nursing staff agree standards for care, set criteria which will demonstrate whether the standards are being met and check performance against those criteria (audit) to evaluate care. This sensible way of approaching the quality issue should be borne in mind when getting to grips with the critical pathways concept as there are striking echoes of DySSSy within this notion.

Critical pathways (CPs) started life in the New England Medical Center's Hospitals in the mid-1980s. The idea brings together all the professional groups involved in patient care to arrive at a consensus about standards of care and expected outcomes for selected patient groups. It is self-evident that patients with a common condition will have a large proportion of their care common to other patients with the same condition. In short, much care is predictable and routine (Layton, 1993) and perhaps nurses' desire to individualize care has gone too far with the result that we try to treat each patient as the exception rather than the norm. This is certainly the view of McNicol (1992) who argues that pre-planning routine care frees up time to deal with individual problems as they occur. The CP therefore recognizes that there will be some degree of individual variation, depending upon factors such as age, pscyhosocial status and other health problems (co-morbidity). It should therefore be possible to plan out a pathway of care for patients with the same medical problem, setting out stages they should reach with the passage of time and defining outcomes which can be measured to assess progress. This can be undertaken as a *multidisciplinary* exercise and providing allowance is made for individual variation within the pathway, the result could be an agreed plan of care which achieves the standards set by all the staff for patient care. The orthodox nursing process documentation is therefore redundant as are other forms of paper notes kept separately by groups such as doctors and therapists. All the information is in one document which does not need writing out anew for each fresh patient.

This then is the CP concept explained simply. A more formal definition is:

The combination of clinical practices that results in the most resource efficient, clinically appropriate and shortest length of stay for a specific medical procedure or condition. Franc and Meyer (1991)

This definition highlights the multidisciplinary nature of CPs as it talks of clinical practices, not medical or nursing interventions. The idea of clinically appropriate practices gives a built-in professional quality dimension while the option of writing a pathway for a 'condition' as well as a medical procedure widens the scope far beyond a patient admitted to hospital for a specific operation, for example. This opens the door to the management of patients in the community or nursing home environment as well as patients in a general medical or elderly care ward and also embraces the field of mental health.

The phrase 'resource efficient' is highly significant because all health services are concerned about the costs of care and this imme-diately gets nurses talking language which managers understand; a key point if support for new ideas is to be forthcoming. CPs actually originated in the concept of managed care, which according to Laxade and Haile (1995) aims to provide care that is cost effective, patient focused, multidisciplinary and collaborative. The managed care concept attempts to ensure that the patient receives the right care at the right time within an appropriate cost–quality balance. This is to be achieved by establishing desired patient outcomes within an agreed time frame and utilizing known resources for each patient group that is identified. A patient-centred approach is essential at all times to achieve these aims. This most useful sum-mary by Laxade and Haile (1995) of the thinking behind CPs shows the importance of multidisciplinary collaboration in ensuring that quality is built into the care that is to be delivered within the CP and the outcomes that the CP seeks to deliver. Health care purchasers in today's NHS are under pressure to buy the best health care they can for the limited amount of money they have at their disposal. Man-aged care therefore is an attractive option and offers health care professionals the opportunity to build quality standards into that care, through CPs. They are therefore potentially a far more power-ful tool than the traditional nursing care plan. Tallon (1995) consid-ers CPs to be *de facto* standards of care which permit staff to validate care they deliver. In the process they demonstrate professional accountability and constitute a significant aid in any legal battle over care.

The baseline for a CP is time and this runs along the horizontal

Table 1 Blank critical pathway. The time scale can be in minutes, hours, days or weeks depending upon the clinical area.

Area of care	Day 1	Day 2	Day 3
Assessments and consultations			
Tests			
Treatments			
Medications			
Diet			
Activity			
Teaching			
Discharge plans			

axis. On the vertical axis care is divided up into various areas. Table 1 shows how such a chart would look using the areas of care which, according to Laxade and Haile (1995), are most commonly used.

The multidisciplinary team agrees in advance what should be happening for each area of care at each day on the pathway and that care is plotted in rather like a graph. Care can be plotted not only in terms of what should be done when (process), but also in terms of what the patient should achieve at set times (outcomes). This corresponds closely with the notion of process and outcome criteria found in the RCN DySSSy standard-setting system. A key step in writing a pathway is to decide the length of the pathway first and then work backwards in time from the end-point. This might be only 30 min for patients admitted to A&E with acute chest pain (Walsh, 1996). Wieczorek (1995) has shown how it is possible to write CPs for patients in theatres on a 6-h time scale with the primary nurse held accountable for the achievement of the CP targets. The time scale may be in days as shown in some case studies presented below but there is no reason why the CP could not run to weeks and months in the case of community or mental health patients.

When a multidisciplinary team sits down to write a CP, Zander (1992) suggests that there are four key questions that everybody should have in mind:

- What does each discipline require in terms of patient outcomes?
- What is the best way of achieving these outcomes?
- Who should be accountable for seeing that the outcomes are achieved?

• How does care need to be restructured to meet the requirements of the first three questions?

Consensus and compromise have to be the watchwords and no professional group, including nursing, can expect to have things all their own way. Many UK nurses might immediately think that medical intransigence would be a major stumbling block and indeed it might. However, you do not know until you try and with the changes that are afoot in medical staffing as a result of the 'new deal' reductions in junior doctors' hours, senior medical staff are realizing that they have to explore new ways of working. The evidence that we review from the USA below does indicate that for a CP to work *all* staff have to be working together for a successful implementation.

The issue of accountability is crucial for CPs, no matter how well written, will be worthless if there is not agreement about who is responsible for seeing that they are carried through. The 24-h presence provided by nursing in hospital and the close involvement with patients and their families that characterizes nursing in the community led to the view that nurses are the best people to be accountable for care delivery in the role of care manager. This is aided by a primary nursing system.

A multidisciplinary team beginning work on a CP focuses on only one agreed condition and aims to produce a CP which applies to patients with that condition *who meet the agreed entry criteria for the CP* (e.g. age). Assessment of the patient to ensure they are appropriate for the CP is essential as no CP can be written that will cover 100% of patients with any one presenting condition. At best, a CP will only be suitable for the majority of patients, never all, and it is crucial that a patient is not forced on to a pathway that is inappropriate for the individual's needs. In starting work on CPs it is best to pick common conditions that account for a high proportion of patients and which have a fairly predictable course. Staff should learn to walk before they can run and therefore gain experience with fairly straightforward conditions before moving on to the more complex. For example, writing a CP for elderly patients with fractures of the upper third of the femur should only be tackled after gaining experience with other less complicated conditions.

The CP forms a guide to care delivery and expected outcomes. It does not, however, replace individualized care required to deal with specific problems unique to any individual which do not fit the pathway. The clinician still has to think and solve problems, but can now do so in a creative way freed from the constraints of the nursing process. When there is a discrepancy between expected and actual events on a CP this is known as variance and the necessary individualized care is recorded as a variance from the pathway. This is the only care documentation that should be carried out with a consequent substantial saving in time. The time thus freed up from writing down routine material for every patient can then be devoted to dealing with individual problems or 'variances'. The documentation of these variances then provides a powerful audit tool to monitor the quality of care and also to allow modification of the CP in the light of experience. A simple procedure is to underline or circle the relevant piece of the CP and mark it 'V1' 'V2', etc. while maintaining a record on a separate sheet of what happened in each case.

It is crucial that a CP is rooted in sound research findings if all staff are to sign up for its implementation; this is particulary important in these days of evidence-based practice. Having such sound rationales for action allows staff to share the CP with the patient with confidence and to justify the interventions and expected outcomes which are clearly identified to the patient. The CP is also tangible evidence to health purchasers that the provider is giving high-quality care and it communicates to all members of the health care team a clear message about the treatment and care the patient should receive together with expected outcomes. This latter point is called normalcy and is defined by Tallon (1995) as a description of the expected course of events for the average patient. In Tallon's view this should cover 95% of patients for each condition although other authorities set lower figures of 70–75% of patients.

A clear view of what should happen is essential if there is to be rapid identification of patients where things are not going according to plan. Co-morbidity is likely to be a major culprit in explaining why some patients do not follow the expected recovery pathway, but psychosocial factors are also possible causes. For example, wound healing may be hindered by diabetes or mobilization delayed by fear of falling. Variance can only be recognized if the original CP sets out expected outcomes at various stages in clear, measurable and unambiguous terms. The importance of these aspects of goal setting was stressed on p. 56 and these points are just as valid in CPs. When a deviation is recognized the explanation has to be found and steps taken to rectify the problem. Problem-solving skills are therefore required on an individual basis and the variance has to be carefully documented. It must be emphasized that the early recognition of variance is vital so that the problem is dealt with when it is only a small problem rather than later when it has become much bigger.

If a patient deviates from the CP in their recovery, this does not necessarily mean there is an error in the CP. Tallon (1995) considers this to be a major misunderstanding about CPs. It may be that an individual factor is responsible or that the CP needs fine tuning in the light of experience. This latter point is particularly true in the early stages of CP usage.

The steps to follow in developing and implementing CPs might be best demonstrated by examining some case studies. Rudisill *et al.* (1994) have discussed CP development on a cardiothoracic surgical unit performing 700 major cardiac operations per year. They stress the importance of starting with a multidisciplinary team meeting and getting everybody's agreement, including the medical staff. Without this, the exercise is futile. The team in Rudisill's unit then set a length of stay for their CP of 5 days post-operatively for those under 60, 6 days if aged 60–70 and 7 days if aged over 70. The importance of starting at the end-point and working backwards has already been stressed and their approach immediately built in a key individual factor which could be easily assessed to ensure the patient is assigned to the correct CP; that is, the age of the patient.

The team then listed post-operative care under six headings: treatment, activity, education, consultation, nutrition and lab tests, and plotted this against time. It is important to note this is an example of using a set of headings to plot care which the staff felt were most appropriate to their patients. However, they refer to care given rather than outcomes. If, for each day, outcomes are listed as well as care to be given, this makes the CP a much more powerful tool as it becomes easier to spot variances. This improves individualized care and strengthens the quality audit. It is one thing to know that something was done when it was supposed to be, but that is only part of the story. It is much more important to know the effects or outcomes of actions. This point is returned to later.

The primary nurse had the responsibility of evaluating care against the CP to plot variances. This brings out the point that not only is primary nursing possible with CPs but it is actually highly desirable as it focuses the responsibility for checking all the patient's care against the CP on to one accountable professional who has the authority to instigate variances in care according to individual need. A patient version of the CP was developed, stripped of jargon, which was presented to the patient on admission. This mapped out care for the patient on each day and formed an invaluable patient teaching tool. Intensive in-service training was given to all staff on the use of the CP before implementation. The involvement of all staff in the original decision to implement a CP and the subsequent writing of the pathway, together with the in-service training, contrasts starkly with the way the nursing process was introduced in the UK.

CPs need to be evaluated after a suitable number of patients have been treated to measure their impact on factors such as length of stay and also to examine the variances that have occurred. The care team needs to see what patterns there may be in the variances as this could indicate weaknesses where care may be improved. In the Rudisill *et al.* study, evaluation took place after 6 months when 168 patients had been admitted on the CP for either coronary artery bypass grafting or valve surgery. It was found that 53% of them were discharged on or before the target date set in the CP, 27% within 2 days of the target date while the remaining patients had much longer stays as a result of serious complications. The group to be targeted for improvements were the 27% of patients who did not have serious complications but who stayed up to 2 days longer than planned, as corrective action here looked easiest to achieve.

The variances charted by the primary nurses among this group could be analysed into three categories: patient, doctor or institution related. The study found that 24% of the variances related to post-operative respiratory difficulties were caused by either pre-existing lung disease, atelectasis or inadequate pulmonary toilet (suction, breathing exercises, etc.). This analysis led to collaborative work between the physiotherapists and the nursing staff to tackle the post-operative problems while pre-operative arterial blood gases were instituted with patients who had known lung disease, to improve pre-operative assessment and preparation for surgery. A surprising variance finding was that 29% of the group of patients with lengthened stays developed atrial fibrillation, which set in train research to investigate this problem and its delaying effect on discharge. Finally, the third major variance related to 17% of the patients being unable to carry out the post-operative mobilization programme as quickly as intended due to low haemoglobin levels leading to fatigue and breathlessness. After discussion, it was felt that the risks of blood transfusions outweighed any potential gain, therefore it was felt best to just recognize that for a significant number of these patients the activity goals were not going to be achieved. This links back to the warning (Tallon, 1995) that staff should not assume the CP is incorrect when a variance occurs, rather it may be that other existing health problems may make some patients lag behind others in their recovery. Analysis of the variances recorded by the primary nurse therefore led to modifications and improvements in care and also sparked off a new research project.

After their experience in introducing the CP for cardiac surgery Rudisill *et al.* felt that the following benefits accrued to their unit:

- Improved nurse/doctor collaboration and practice.
- Quality improvement from a multidisciplinary perspective. However, they did not elaborate on how this had been measured.
- Increased patient and family involvement in care through patients holding their own version of the CP.
- Enhanced nursing accountability.
- Decreased costs and reduced length of stay. Patients on the CP had an average length of stay reduced by 1.12 days at a saving of $1893 per patient.

The unit had a full primary nursing system in place and this was instrumental in the success of the CP. Nurses were given increased knowledge about what was happening by the CP and also increased authority as it allowed them to take the initiative, particularly in areas such as discharge planning. As we have already seen, knowledge and authority are key components of accountability and the CP approach undoubtedly enhanced professional accountability for the nurses in this unit.

An important point concerning the development of a CP comes from the work of Heacock and Brobst (1994) who developed a CP for patients undergoing prostatectomy. We have already stressed the need for CPs to be research based: they must also be based in the realities of current practice so that staff perceive them as realistic. Heacock and Brobst (1994) describe the first stage, once multidisciplinary agreement had been reached, as consisting of examining a sample of patient documentation to describe accurately the current situation. This involves medical, nursing and PAMS (professions allied to medicine) documents being examined together using a data collection form to record the same pieces of information on each patient, for example, patient activity, intravenous infusions, catheter removal. This produced consistent information about the steps in treatment and care with the passage of time during the patient's hospitalization. It also permitted the team to set an agreed length of stay for treatment which fixed the end-point of the time line. The team could then work backwards from the end-point placing various stages on the pathway appropriately. This data-gathering work reviews the current state of affairs and sets the framework against which the CP can be developed. It also prevents enthusiastic staff proposing stages that are unrealistic from a time point of view.

The advantages of the CP approach are summarized below by Heacock and Brobst (1994) after they developed a CP for prostatectomy patients:

- The display of interventions and expected patient outcomes across time is a *visible* guide to care for all staff and the patient.
- Collaboration in care was greatly aided by all the staff working together to develop the CP and everybody became much more aware of each other's roles as the CP was implemented. This was not achieved without substantial differences of opinion emerging from the various professional groups in the planning stage which had to be resolved before progress could be achieved. However, once consensus had emerged, the CP was much stronger as a result of this group ownership.
- Continual evaluation of care against the CP allowed for it to be customized to the individual's needs and any corrective action needed to deal with variances from the CP could be taken promptly as the desired care was so clearly visible to *all* the staff.
- The CP is a powerful patient education tool.
- It greatly helps with the continuity of care if the patient is transferred. (This latter point only holds if the new ward, nursing home or community staff agree with the CP. This emphasizes the importance of involving community staff in CP development if there is likely to be a long-term community follow-up programme of care

such as in the field of mental health or a patient who has had a stroke or suffers from asthma.)

The importance of devising a CP only after careful examination of a sample of recent patient documents is stressed by Grant *et al.* (1995) who developed a CP for patients undergoing mastectomy (Table 2). The multidisciplinary team involved in this work included representatives of community support staff and a patient self-help group. This illustrates the potential for CPs to enhance continuity of care between the hospital and primary health care settings. It also demonstrates how CPs may increase patient involvement as a patient self-help group may contribute to the CP. This builds in the patient dimension of quality referred to earlier (p. 68).

Consideration of Table 2 shows the 10 areas of care used by the staff in developing the CP. They have added a very important extra aspect of care missing from the example shown in Table 1: psycho-social and emotional needs which shows the importance of flexibility in developing CPs according to the needs of different patient groups. A problem with this CP, however, is that it is mostly process based. The CP sets out actions that should be performed by staff rather than patient outcomes that are expected. If the full value of CPs is to be realized they must include outcomes. This point is argued strongly by Woodyard and Sheetz (1993) who point out that just because patient teaching has occurred, the nurse should not assume that the patient has learnt anything. It is an old adage in teaching that it is not what is taught that matters, but what is learnt! It is only half the battle to plan pain control on the day of surgery or therapeutic emotional care on the first post-operative day (see Table 2), what really matters is whether the patient is free from pain and how distressed they feel about the surgery, both of which are about the outcome, rather than the process of care. The CP developed by Grant *et al.* could therefore be improved by the addition of outcome-focused stages stating what the patient should achieve on each day of the pathway.

Woodyard and Sheetz (1993) discuss this problem in relation to their own CPs and point out one of the dangers of CPs; that is, that they may become too task focused. These authors felt the emphasis on process had led to their CPs falling into that trap and losing sight of the whole patient. They therefore felt that the CPs had to become more patient focused and saw that introducing clear statements about patient outcomes would achieve this by shifting the emphasis back on to what the whole patient is doing and away from separate tasks (the process of care).

A problem they found with the process-focused CP was that there was a lack of clarity among staff about what counted as acceptable progress on the pathway as there were no clear milestones against which to measure progress. As an analogy, imagine yourself on a

Table 2 Critical pathway for a total mastectomy

Area of care	Day 1 (day of surgery)	Day 2 (Post-op Day 1)
Assessment and monitoring	Vital signs 4 hrly Fluid balance Pain levels Dressing/drain patency and drainage Ability to pass urine Lab results Emotional response and family coping	Vital signs 8 hrly if satisfactory Fluid balance Pain levels Dressing/drain patency and drainage Passes urine without difficulty Lab results Emotional response and family coping
Consultations	Specialist nurse breast care Pt self-help group	Specialist nurse breast care
Procedure/test		
Treatment	Vacuum drainage system Incentive spirometer Coughing/deep breathing Turn 2 hrly Avoid trauma to arm	Vacuum drainage system Uses incentive spirometer independently Coughing/deep breathing Avoid trauma to arm
Activity	Assist to bathroom in pm	Increase as tolerated with assistance as required Sit out of bed
Medications and IVs	IVI until tolerates oral fluids Analgesia IV or IM Other medication as prescribed	Discontinue IVI Discontinue IV/IM analgesia Start oral analgesia Pain controlled by oral analgesia Other medication as prescribed
Nutrition	Clear fluids Light diet if tolerated pm	Normal diet
Patient/family education	*Explain* Nursing care Pain control Positioning/mobility Deep breathing/coughing Inspiration spirometer Diet/fluid intake IVI and drains	*Explain* Nursing care Arm protection Signs and symptoms of infection Breast awareness Breast care specialist nurse to discuss diagnosis Prosthesis Support groups
Discharge planning	Pt/family discuss and show understanding of CP Plan of care agreed with pt/family	Breast care specialist nurse completes screening for high risk factors
Psychosocial/ emotional needs	Therapeutic emotional care	Breast care specialist nurse to assess counselling needs and initiate support Therapeutic emotional care

Table 2 Continued

Day 3 (Post-op Day 2)	Day 4 (Post-op Day 3)	Desired Outcomes
Vital signs 8 hrly if stable Discontinue fluid balance Pain levels Dressings/drain patency, drainage Lab results Emotional response family coping	Vital signs twice daily Pain levels	Vital signs within normal limits and stable Pain managed by oral analgesia
Breast care specialist nurse Social worker if needed		Seen by breast care specialist nurse
Complete blood cell count haematocrit within 25% of pre-op value		Blood count stable within normal limits
Vacuum drainage, wound and axilla drains Check wound dressing Avoid trauma to limb	Discontinue incentive spirometer Wound drain removed Maintain axilliary drain if present	Drain sites clean No pulmonary complications Wound healing well, no sign of infection
Increase as tolerated		
Explain Nursing care Arm mobility exercises Showering/bathing Activity Follow-up arrangements Counselling Self-help groups	Seen by surgeon Reinforce earlier teaching	*Patient* Identifies support systems and resources Able to discuss/demonstrate arm exercises/protection Breast awareness Signs of wound infection Follow-up arrangements
Community nurse referral Other home help if needed	Plans discussed involving DN. Breast care nurse and outpatients follow up	Pt feels there will be care and support after discharge
Therapeutic emotional care	Therapeutic emotional care	Talks about feelings related to diagnosis/surgery

long motorway journey – the car may be comfortable, your favourite tape playing away in the background, you can make convenient stops whenever you want to at service stations and there are no traffic jams, the process of the journey is fine. However, if somebody has removed all the signposts, including those with mileages to the next town, how will you know whether you are making satisfactory progress towards your destination? Those signposts allow you to measure your journey and inform you on how well you are proceeding; they are in fact measures of the outcome of the last hours' driving.

There are two ways of building outcome measures into a CP. They can either be incorporated under each of the areas of care or listed separately. Woodyard and Sheetz (1993) felt it best to list them separately for the sake of clarity rather than use the main headings on the CP. They developed three broad headings for outcomes as follows:

- Physiological parameters that can be measured such as blood pressure or haemoglobin levels. Pain could also be included here using a simple scale.
- Activity and behaviour such as mobility, continence and psychosocial factors such as mood, orientation, anxiety, etc.
- Knowledge and discharge planning. This focuses on what the patient knows not what has been taught, what the home environment is really like and whether it is suitable for the patient's discharge rather than on whether a date has been set and transport ordered! This focus brings in various cultural and spiritual aspects of care which impact upon how patients learn and what they chose to do with the information they are given. For example, Asian cultures in general have a more fatalistic approach to life than the West which may mean that despite an excellent teaching package being delivered to a diabetic patient (process), little change is made in behaviour (outcome).

To make the quality of care a current reality, it was necessary to set outcome standards for these three areas on a daily basis, which could then be evaluated daily. In making these evaluations the clinician has to draw upon their knowledge base and past experience, accurate observation of the patient and current clinical data. Care is therefore focused on the individual whole patient and the nurse involved is acting in a truly accountable way. Documentation of care now consists of charting by exception, in other words it is only the variances that are recorded. This may be achieved by marking the relevant section of the CP with a 'v' and documenting the problem on a separate sheet kept for variances where the interventions and outcomes may also be recorded. As long as care is taken following the CP and outcomes are achieved, then all that is required is the nurse's signature on the patient's CP in order that accountability is maintained. The savings in nursing staff time are potentially very significant, not only in terms of time spent writing in care plans that nobody reads, but also at handovers which now only focus on variances in the CP. An interesting observation by Woodyard and Sheetz (1993) is that patient teaching has expanded dramatically as staff have realized how ineffective their previous efforts were now they are looking at what the patient has learnt rather than what the nurse has taught.

The value of staff time saved is illustrated by Rasmussen and Gengler (1994) who describe how frustration at increasing workloads and the demands of writing out full care plans for every patient led to the nursing process being seen as a waste of time. (It is doubtful if extra staffing was allocated when the nursing process was introduced into the NHS to allow for the time to be consumed on writing out care plans.) One of the most influential early workers in the CP field, Zander, was of much the same opinion writing that most nurses were dissatisfied with the nursing process, which she saw as totally inadequate and as getting in the way of multidisciplinary care (Zander, 1992).

Development of the CP approach, according to Rasmussen and Gengler (1994) has freed up considerable amounts of time and greatly increased patient involvement as they are presented with their own version of their CP on admission. As an example, Table 3 shows the CP for congestive heart failure with outcomes built into each area of care rather than under separate headings as in the case of Woodyard and Sheetz (1993), while Table 4 shows the patient version. The possible impact upon staff time is revealed by Layton (1993) who claims a 30% reduction in time spent documenting care since the introduction of CPs.

Communication has greatly improved, both with the patient and between the various members of the care team. Primary nurses can advance patients along the CP, making clinically significant decisions without waiting for ward rounds and doctors' permission as the CP is a multidisciplinary document that everybody has agreed to. Rasmussen and Gengler's experience of the introduction of CPs has been that patients appear far happier and have had their mean length of stay reduced while doctors report that they appreciate receiving fewer phone calls for permission to carry out routine procedures. This latter point is very important in the NHS as the reduction in junior doctors' hours means that there will be fewer members of the medical staff available, particularly at weekends and at night. Patient care could be significantly held up by the lack of a doctor to give permission for what is routine care. The CP approach works around that problem by setting out in advance what should happen when, and authorizing the nurse to make sure that it does happen, providing agreed outcomes in terms of the patient's pro-

Table 3 Critical pathway for congestive heart failure (estimated length of stay: 4 days)

Area of care	Day 1	Day 2
Activity	Mobilise as able Meals in bed Commode at bedside Ensure upright position *Expected Outcome* Activity as tolerated	Sit out in chair for meals Walk up to 20m. with assistance ×2 Walk to bathroom with assistance *Expected Outcome* Able to tolerate activity without distress
Nutrition	Low salt diet Refer dietitian if needed Assistance with eating if required	Low salt diet Refer dietitian if needed Assistance with eating if required
Treatments	VS 4 hrly obs Fluid balance chart Weight Heparinised venflon O_2 at 3 l/min Assess lung and heart sounds 6 hrly/prn Assess pedal oedema 6 hrly Waterlow risk score	VS 4 hrly obs Fluid balance chart Weight Heparinised venflon O_2 at 3 l/min Assess lung and heart sounds 6 hrly/prn Assess pedal odema 6 hrly *Expected Outcomes* Pt lost 0.5kg weight or pedal oedema has decreased Breath sound improved
Teaching	Review CP with Pt Give Pt's copy to Pt Explain medications Give info sheet on CHF to pt	*Expected Outcome* Pt can describe and show understanding of present medication
Discharge	Assess for Community Nurse follow up Assess for home O_2	

Area of care	Day 3	Day 4
Activity	Walk 30m ×3 *Expected Outcome* Able to perform ADLs and walking without aid of O_2	As for day 3 *Expected Outcome* Able to tolerate activity without distress
Nutrition	Low salt diet	Low salt diet
Treatment	VS 4 hrly obs Fluid balance chart Daily weight Heparinised venflon O_2 prn Assess lung and heart sounds 6 hrly and prn Assess pedal oedema 6 hrly	VS 4 hrly obs Fluid balance chart Daily weight Remove venflon Discontinue O_2 Assess lung and heart sounds 6 hrly Assess pedal oedema 6 hrly *Expected Outcomes* Foot/ankle oedema resolved Unlaboured respirations

Table 3 Continued

Area of care	Day 3	Day 4
Teaching	Reinforce teaching re medication/diet	*Expected Outcomes* Pt can describe and show understanding of medications
Discharge	DN visit arranged if needed Home O_2 service arranged if needed	Discharge letter to GP
		Expected Outcomes Pt can discuss and show understanding of medication, diet, other health education info., follow up visit by DN and when to contact GP

Table 4 Critical pathway: Congestive heart failure (patient's copy)

Area of care	Day 1	Day 2
Activity	You can move around as able. Avoid becoming overtired or short of breath Meals can be taken in bed	You should increase your activity slowly. Sit out of bed for meals and walk short distances with the help of nurses twice daily
Nutrition	You will be on a low salt diet. The dietitian can come and talk to you about this later if you like. Salt causes your body to hold in fluid which makes your heart work harder and causes the swelling around your feet	Low salt diet
Treatments	Your intake and output of fluid will be measured every day	As for day 1
	Your heart and lungs will be listened to every day to see if they are getting better	
	You may have to use oxygen for the first day or two to help you breathe	
	You will be weighed daily so we can see if you are getting rid of excess fluid	
	You will have a needle placed in an arm vein this can be used to give you medication	
Teaching	It will help if you understand what is going on in your body. Please ask questions if you do not understand what is happening	Now you are a little better we can check how much you know about your medication and heart failure. We will give you a fact sheet on heart failure and talk it through with you
Discharge		We will begin checking what arrangements will be needed for your discharge

Table 4 Continued

Area of care	Day 3	Day 4
Activity	You should be feeling better and able to do mild activities without oxygen. If you can't tolerate this the doctor may suggest using oxygen at home	You should be able to walk the length of the ward without trouble breathing and have a bath unaided
Nutrition	Low salt diet	Low salt diet. Check if you should continue this at home
Treatments	Most treatments will continue but you should use oxygen only when you feel you need it	Your oxygen should not be needed now If you are fit to go home the needle in your arm will be removed
Teaching	You will be given information sheets about the medication you will be on after discharge. A nurse will talk about this with you and s/he will also discuss your diet (as some foods are best avoided) and other useful information about your health	Check you are happy with your medication and knowledge about when to see your GP in future
Discharge		A follow up visit at home by the District Nurse may be arranged. Your GP will be notified of your stay in hospital and may also want to see you

Tables 3 and 4 were adapted from Rasmusen and Gengler (1994).

gress have been met. The nurse is accountable for ensuring that is the case.

We have already stressed the importance of beginning CP work with relatively uncomplicated patient groups. It may be that the complexity of certain health problems limits the applicability of CPs to some groups, particularly the elderly where co-morbidity becomes even more of a problem or emergency admissions where events may follow a much less predictable course. Laxade and Haile (1995) point out, however, that it is possible to write 'mini-CPs' which could be added on to the main CP for problems such as pressure sores or diabetes. Alternatively, the CP could branch into a fast or slower track depending upon the presence or absence of such complicating factors. The outcomes are the same but the time scale is lengthened or shortened according to the patient.

Tallon (1995), in writing about CPs in wound care, is opposed to writing branching CPs or mini-CPs as he considers this will become very complex. He urges staff to look at the core problems in relation to wound care, such as arterial vascular insufficiency, and write a CP for that condition rather than a different CP for each *cause* of that condition such as diabetes, localized tissue ischaemia due to immobility or femoral/popliteal atherosclerosis. The CP then sets outcomes relating to revascularization, increased tissue oxygenation and optimizing pain relief. This is a radical way of thinking that requires writing CPs without thinking in conventional medical diagnostic terms. Tallon does not advance any evidence to show this technique has been used or even how feasible it is. The point about a multiplicity of CPs around the same problem is well made and it may represent one of the main limitations to their usage; that is, some patient conditions are just too complicated to manage this way.

The final case study to be presented therefore looks at how one team set about tackling the problem of developing a CP for stroke patients, an emergency condition mainly affecting older people with a less predictable course of recovery and the potential for many complicating factors.

This work was carried out at a large 900-bed North American teaching hospital which had 170 medical beds and a mean length of stay of 11 days for patients after a cerebrovascular accident (CVA), before discharge or transfer (Hydo, 1995). The initial response to the proposal was negative, partly because it was felt that stroke patients were too variable to be able to have any common pathway and also there was a great deal of territoriality among the various professional groups.

The first barrier was overcome by an analysis of documentation relating to a sample of 30 patients admitted with a diagnosis of CVA which revealed there was actually a substantial body of common problems and associated treatment and care. This emphasizes the importance of looking at all the documentation for a sample of patients as a starting point for pathway planning as the recorded evidence of what is actually happening may be very different from each member of staff's subjective perceptions of what they think happens. The view that there was too much variability in CVA patients did not stand up to scrutiny.

The problem of territoriality was overcome with a stick and carrot approach. The carrot was urging staff to step back from their own point of view and try to see the big picture in terms of total patient care involving all members of the multidisciplinary team. Nurses need to do this as much as doctors or anybody else. The stick was financial pressure on the hospital to reduce length of stay as under the USA Medicare system CVA patients were only funded for a 7-day period of care.

The importance of data analysis on past patients and multidisciplinary discussions is underlined by the fact that after such work it was decided to omit patients with haemorrhagic strokes from the CP as the 7-day target was unrealistic for such patients. The CP was developed after intensive multidisciplinary work and its implementation was accompanied not only by in-service training but also by a booklet explaining how to use the CP which ensured all staff had the same information to start off with. A first evaluation was held after

30 patients had completed the pathway. This highlighted two problems:

- There were difficulties in selecting the right patients to put on the pathway as the diagnosis was sometimes not clear on admission. This highlights the importance of agreed criteria for entering patients on a CP which can be assessed at the outset. This is a lot easier where routine planned surgery is involved rather than emergency admissions.
- There were significant delays in moving patients along the CP. These variances were analysed using the categories of patient, doctor and institution as likely causes. Co-morbidity was the main patient problem. Some 20% of patients initially entered on the CP fell into this category as they had severe musculoskeletal and cognitive deficits and clearly would not be fit for discharge within 7 days. Such patients had to be taken off the CP altogether due to these health problems which complicated their care too much. This was always recognized as a likely problem when dealing with older patients suffering from a medical emergency condition. The degree of doctor variability was less than feared and reduced even further once they got used to working with the common set of outcomes as laid down in the CP. The institutional problems highlighted resulted in delays caused by inefficiencies in the hospital system such as non-availability of PAMS staff and lack of X-ray facilities out of hours. This work led to the setting up of a dedicated stroke unit within the hospital to remove these inefficiencies caused by having a large hospital offering a range of general services scattered throughout the institution and not focused on any particular patient group. Hydo (1995) reports that as a result of this work they have largely achieved their goal of reducing the mean length of stay for stroke patients to 7 days although she does not give any more specific information than that.

Summary of key steps in introducing a CP

1. Identify a group of patients with a common health problem or who are to undergo a specific medical intervention. There should be a reasonably predictable series of events for the majority of patients in this group.
2. Convene a multidisciplinary meeting to secure the agreement of all parties to CP development. The multidisciplinary team should then undertake the following steps.
3. Audit all documentation for a recent sample of such patients to set the framework of what happens at present.
4. Set the time line by agreeing the length of the CP and work backwards from the agreed end-point.

5. Write in the necessary interventions and desired outcomes for each hour/day/week of the CP.
6. Agree clear guidelines as to how patients are assessed for suitability to start a CP and agree who makes the decision that a patient will commence or leave the CP.
7. Decide how variances will be monitored, recorded and actioned together with who will have accountability for the management of variances (ideally the primary nurse).
8. Prepare a version of the CP to be given to the patient on commencement of the CP.
9. Organize in-service training for all staff involved and write a booklet explaining how the CP is to be used.
10. Set up an audit of variances after an agreed period of time so that the CP can be amended in the light of experience. Helpful changes to care delivery may also be identified by the audit. The impact of the CP on care in terms of parameters such as length of stay and cost should also be evaluated.
11. Make changes to care and amend CP in light of step 10.

Critical pathways: the case for and against

The obvious criticism to be made of CPs is that they conflict with the principle of individualized care. However, is care individualized at present? All the research evidence points to a discredited system of care planning based on the nursing process which makes it very difficult to demonstrate individualized care actually takes place. If nursing care plans are to be believed, any individualized care that does occur takes place despite the nursing process rather than because of it! There is a major question mark against the present system therefore, especially as one method is advocated to the exclusion of all others (nursing process) and there is little evidence to show that this is actually how experienced nurses operate in practice anyway. The *nursing* process does little to support multidisciplinary care, another powerful reason to look at new ways of working and documenting care.

The key argument about CPs is that they are a guide to care for the majority of patients but by no means all. They represent agreed statements about what the patient should be achieving at various stages and as such are about standards of care and quality. The interventions necessary to achieve those outcomes still represent a problem-solving challenge to each member of the health care team and therefore the nurse, along with everybody else, has to be able to individualize care to meet the outcomes. The interventions may have much in common but the patients are different and therefore the skill of the clinician is in adapting interventions to the individual patient, varying the order of interventions, persuading the patient to collaborate in care and recognizing early variations from the expected pathway and outcomes. This latter point is crucial to customizing the CP to meet the needs of each individual patient.

As long as CPs are introduced properly and the lessons of the nursing process implementation disaster are learnt, then CPs should lead to more individualized care as staff spend less time writing meaningless routine documentation and have more time to work with the patients on their problems. The idea of a patient version of the CP has great potential in terms of patient empowerment and perhaps one of the most effective ways of individualizing care is to increase patient involvement in that care. The patient's own copy of the CP certainly offers that potential.

If CPs just focus upon tasks to be done, there is a real possibility that they will represent a step backwards towards task-centred care and we will lose the holistic view of the patient. This is a real danger and it emphasizes the needs for patient outcomes to be written into the CP at each stage if for no other reason than to get staff asking what is the *whole* patient doing today? The central role of the nurse as care manager is crucial here for in monitoring variance they have the overview of what the patient is doing. Primary nursing would seem to facilitate CPs and the introduction of CPs may well *de facto* lead to a primary nursing system as nurses are held accountable for the overall management of specific patient's care.

This issue of nursing accountability opens up a potential problem area because, as we have seen, accountability requires knowledge and authority. The CP gives the nurse a great deal of information about what is happening; they need to have the knowledge and ability to be able to interpret that information meaningfully to make the correct decisions about progress along the pathway. Much of that information is coming from the biomedical sciences and we have already discussed the need for nursing to retain at least one foot firmly in the world of science (Chapter 1) if the individual is to have the credibility to make decisions within the CP protocols. Professional updating and continual education become even more important, especially in the more technical and scientific areas. This links into the even more important issue of authority for if the nurse is to be held accountable as the care manager for pathway implementation and variance monitoring, they must have the authority to implement stages on the pathway such as removing IVIs or starting discharge arrangements, subject to the agreed outcomes in the CP being met at the previous stage.

The Royal College of Nursing (RCN, 1993) has raised the issue that clinical protocols, which are similar to CPs, may have more to do with utilizing fewer qualified staff and cost containment than improving the quality of care. Registered nurses are essential in the use of CPs as they are the cement that holds the whole thing together. Without their skills and knowledge it is difficult to see how variance monitoring and individualization of care could be achieved. Cost containment is not in itself a bad thing as increased efficiency means more patients can be treated with the same resources. This permits real efficiency savings rather than using the term to provide a smokescreen for the service cuts that have been forced upon NHS Trusts in recent years. The CP has quality safeguards built into it as it really consists of a statement by the staff about the standards of care they expect patients to receive, as measured by specific outcome measures they have written into the CP. The RCN (1993) recognizes the benefits of consensus and consistency between health care professionals working together that CPs can bring about.

Perhaps the most important criticism concerning CPs is the quality of the evidence which supports their use. In Chapter 3, Bond and Thomas (1995) were very critical of studies in the UK looking at the effectiveness of implementing new ideas in care (p. 66). One of their main criticisms focused on weak research designs and lack of rigorous statistical analysis of data. The case studies cited in this chapter do not present a convincingly rigorous analysis of data to support the claims that CPs have greatly improved care and reduced costs. This analysis may have taken place, but unfortunately hard data are only presented in one paper by Rudisill *et al.* (1994) with the claim of a cost reduction of $1893 per cardiac surgery patient. They do not elaborate as to whether this figure is arrived at after a comparison with a similar group of patients to those on the CP. This is a crucial point as you can only compare like with like; or, in research jargon, there must be an equivalent control group.

The evidence presented in the North American literature is interesting, but largely anecdotal. Health care providers in the UK are right to be very interested in CPs as they offer many potential benefits to both patient, provider and purchasing health authority as well as to nurses. Implementation of CPs should use the lessons learnt in the USA and the UK, particularly with reference to the nursing process implementation. Further, there must be rigorous evaluation of the effects of CP introduction involving the management (costs and length of stay), professional (standard setting) and patient dimensions of quality.

Nurses should not think of CPs as being the answer for all patients, as they are not. For any condition it seems likely that a significant minority of patients will not fit the CP due to complicating factors. The CP concept also stresses recovery; however, many patients will not recover and this is most obviously true in the field of palliative care. This does not invalidate the idea, it merely makes writing the expected outcomes more difficult. A pain-free and dignified death may not be the sort of statement that staff feel happy writing down as the expected outcome for their patients, but that is often the reality. A great deal of sensitivity is required in writing outcomes but the idea of a multidisciplinary approach to planned care which has built-in quality standards makes the CP idea worthy of serious investigation in this field.

If nursing only focused on CP development, it would be doing those patients who do not neatly fit into a pathway a disservice. It is important to explore new ways of planning and documenting care for patients but this time working closely with clinicians so that any new approaches are based on reality rather than being imposed on nurses from above. CPs may be a very useful tool, but they are only *one* tool and just as a jack is very useful for changing a flat tyre, you also need something to remove the wheel nuts. One tool on its own is rarely enough to complete any job!

On balance, the potential advantages of CP introduction suggest that it is a worthwhile initiative that may lead to significant benefits for some patients, but by no means all. It is one way of planning care, but not the only way, and we should not rush to a blanket implementation like nursing did with the nursing process or the Roper, Logan and Tierney model of nursing. This is, of course, an appropriate time to look at how CPs might sit alongside nursing models, which we shall now do.

Nursing models and CPs

Consideration of the CPs in the earlier part of this chapter shows that there is no specific area of care shown that is labelled 'nursing care'. This presents a challenge to nursing as it would be very easy to forget about the holistic nursing approach to care as it became subsumed under a dominant medical focus. In writing CPs nurses face a dilemma; they have to step away from the familiar safe haven of an area labelled nursing in the interests of a truly multiprofessional approach to care. On the other hand, however, we have to keep the essentially nursing dimensions of care available to the patient.

We have to realize that the traditional nursing process care plan has failed as a tool for planning and documenting care and therefore we have to move on to try something better and in the process be brave and confident enough in our own professionalism to work with documents that do not carry a specifically nursing label. The trick is to make sure that the essential qualities that we recognize as nursing are written into the CP documentation and that the holistic view of the patient that nurses hold is best utilized within the CP operation. This of course means that the nurse not only provides direct care but acts as the overall manager of care, responsible for spotting any variances early and subsequent variance problem solving. This can occur directly or by bringing in the appropriate member of the multidisciplinary team, such as the doctor or physiotherapist, for example.

As a group of expert staff sit writing a CP, it is easy to forget the patient's point of view, a point made by Hampton (1994). It is essential that any CP be individualized to the patient's own needs and nursing models which emphasize working with the patient and trying to discover the meanings which they place on various care situations are therefore to be commended to any team engaged in CP production. These are, of course, the interactionist models (p. 30) and Hampton is a powerful advocate of King's principles of mutual goal setting in working with CPs (Hampton, 1994). This also underlines the need to produce a patient's version of the CP which patient and nurse work with together. As King (1981) stresses, when patient and nurse work towards the same agreed goals, there is a much greater likelihood that they will be achieved. Hampton argues, therefore, that working towards achieving mutually agreed goals with patients as partners, will allow the nursing profession to meet the many challenges it faces in today's harsh and difficult health service climate by demonstrating the real value of nursing.

There is a strong ring of truth about this observation as the health service is increasingly a results-and-outcomes driven organization governed by market forces rather than patient needs. If nursing focuses only on demonstrating that it can meet patient needs, however professionally correct that may be, the danger is that we are backing the wrong horse. The horse to have our money on is called 'achieve your goals and get results'; in other words we have to show that nursing makes a difference to patient outcomes while still functioning within an ethically and professionally sound environment. King's approach to mutual goal setting is in tune with the increasing reality of health care in the late 1990s and while the brief account of her work in Chapter 8 presents her model as predominantly mental health focused, the key principle embedded within her work, mutually agreed goal setting, can be applied to many situations, including CP development in general nursing settings. The emphasis on outcomes which is increasingly driving health care requires that for moral reasons if no others, we must ensure that outcomes (goals) are mutually agreed with patients, if we are to steer this juggernaut along an ethically correct route.

The first stage in contributing to the writing of a CP is therefore to ensure that the nursing model is not lost, before looking at the influence of any specific model. If the holistic patient-focused perspective of nursing (the nursing model) is to be written into the CP, the nursing staff must have an agreed philosophy of care to give a cohesive approach to their work. This could be enhanced if they were also working with a nursing model that was appropriate for the kind of CP being written.

A key issue revolves around the initial nursing assessment. The CP requires on-going assessment and monitoring as part of the pathway (e.g. vital signs, pressure areas, anxiety, mood); however, there is also a need for an initial assessment before the patient is entered upon the pathway. This should determine whether the patient is appropriate for the pathway as a major mistake would be to try and force patients into pathways that are not suited for them. It will also determine whether even though the patient is suitable for the pathway, there are any significant individual problems which have to be taken into account, such as English not being the person's first language or the presence of a physical problem such as diabetes. There needs to be a rational framework for such an assessment and this of course is provided by a model of nursing which takes on board a holistic view of the patient. This holistic assessment needs to be carried out and recorded within the documentation that contains the CP. The North American practice commonly involves statements of nursing diagnoses within the CP derived from the assessment although they can be replaced with patient problem statements as shown in Table 3.

Ensuring that the assessment is compatible with a holistic philosophy that consistently underpins the CP will greatly facilitate care. For example, on a surgical ward writing CPs for patients undergoing mastectomy or stoma surgery could reflect on the importance of ensuring that their patients adapt successfully to surgery and therefore examine the key areas that are outlined in Roy's adaptation model such as self-concept and role function. Are these concepts assessed and written into the CP? The mastectomy CP in Table 2 could have been improved if the heading 'psychosocial/emotional needs' had been more focused by the inclusion of outcomes written for self-concept and role function. It would be helpful to have dates by when the patient would be expected to look at her wound in the mirror (physical self-concept) and to begin to talk about her feelings as a woman/wife/mother after surgery (personal self-concept and role function).

In a medical or elderly care ward it might be possible to build

Table 5 Key nursing points in building Orem's self-care model into a CP for stroke patients

Area of care	Specific self-care considerations
Consults and assessment	Assess self-care requisites (see p. 115)
Tests	Nil specific
Treatment	Nil specific
Medication	Ability to take responsibility for self-medication
Diet	Ability to drink and feed self unaided or with assistance
Activity	Ability to control elimination and mobilize unaided or with assistance
Teaching	Understanding of patient/family about cause of illness, future preventative actions and possible complications such as pressure sores or urinary/chest infections
Discharge planning	Will patient be able to meet universal self-care requisites after discharge, e.g. prevention of hazards, balance between solitude/socialization, feeding, elimination, activity?

Orem's self-care model (1990) into a CP written for stroke patients. Table 5 lists the eight areas of care described by Laxade and Haile (1995) as commonly used in CP construction and shows how Orem's self-care model might assist in ensuring that a strong and relevant nursing perspective is built into the CP (see p. 115 for more detail concerning Orem's model).

There are some key areas of Orem's model not touched upon here such as developmental self-care which requires the nurse to consider where the patient lies on the life continuum, in this case probably an elderly patient with problems such as fear of losing their independence and becoming a burden on their family. Using an Orem-based nursing assessment form will ensure this key is assessed before the CP is implemented. Orem also requires us to look at the effects of what she calls 'health deviance' or illness on self-care, in this case what are the possible cognitive and communication problems resulting from the stroke, such as confusion and loss of speech. These are key areas that require assessment before commencing a CP to ensure the patient is appropriate for the CP.

Orem's concept of normalcy refers to how the individual sees themselves in relation to others and the effects this may have. A patient with disability after a stroke is probably going to see themself as abnormal as they may have become incontinent and lost the use of half their body (hemiparesis). The result is possibly to make the patient depressed, angry or withdrawn. Reflection upon Orem's self-care model therefore highlights a range of psychosocial factors that are not included in the eight commonly used headings of a CP and assessment of which will benefit patient care.

There is therefore a strong case for adding a psychological or mental functioning area which considers factors such as orientation and mood, while the area of communication must also be added to the CP. This can either be as part of a heading such as Activity or Teaching (as it is an activity and it is necessary part of teaching; however, this feels rather artificial) but given the importance of communication, it probably deserves a heading of its own although it may be subsumed under the extra heading of Psychology or Mental Functioning already proposed.

In this example, we have shown that drawing upon Orem's self-care model we can ensure important holistic aspects of patient care are built into the CP under the commonly used headings and also that there are important areas not covered which deserve new headings of their own. Having set up the right framework for the CP, the nurse should now try and ensure that the self-care philosophy is built into care both in terms of interventions which should be directed to helping the patient/family practice self-care but also in terms of outcomes. The development of a patient version of this CP then makes the approach clear to family and patient from the beginning, avoiding possible misunderstanding. What to the nurse is encouraging the patient to care for themselves in readiness for discharge may look to the family like the staff are too busy to do things for the patient or even do not care. This potentially damaging misunderstanding can be largely avoided by having a patient version of the CP available at the outset which clearly sets out the philosophy of care.

The use of the Roper, Logan and Tierney model alongside CPs is potentially unhelpful as this model focuses very much on the physiological side of the patient, to the neglect of the psychosocial dimensions. It is precisely these psychosocial aspects that tend to be overlooked in writing CPs and the use of the Roper model is therefore likely only to reinforce this vital omission.

As we have seen, one of the main aims of the CP is to make care consistent. The use of a model as a framework to help shape the nursing input to a CP enhances this consistency and also means that observed variances will be approached from a point of view that is consistent with the nursing input to the rest of the CP. Further examples of the application of nursing models to CP development are presented in Chapter 5.

This section suggests that the use of nursing models with CPs is both possible and desirable if the necessary holistic and individual nursing input to care is not to be lost and to help enhance the consistency of approach that is one of the CPs main aims. A models-based nursing input to the multidisciplinary CP means that while the nursing label may be lost, the care remains.

Multi-professional care and the patient-focused hospital

There is one other aspect of the multidisciplinary approach to care that is finding increased favour with managers which should be briefly considered in this context: the patient-focused hospital (PFH). This idea also originated in the USA and is finding favour in a modified form in some areas of the NHS. One of its operational features is the development of clinical protocols, an idea closely related to critical pathways except that they lack the outcome focus of a CP (Laxade and Haile, 1995). Unfortunately, the terms are sometimes used loosely and interchangeably, which causes confusion.

The PFH concept originated in the work of Booz-Allen and Hamilton (1990) and is based on the view that large modern hospitals are inefficient because there are too many specialist staff who will only perform a very limited range of tasks. This inefficiency is compounded by the fact that there are too many centralized specialist departments (e.g. X-ray, pathology) which means patients or clinical samples are continually having to be transported around the hospital at great expense both in terms of time and money. The solution is therefore to break down the large hospital into smaller units of around 100 beds which will be self-sufficient for many of the previously centralized functions which will now be delivered at the bedside and to go for multiskilled staff rather than professional specialists. Booz-Allen and Hamilton (1990) claim that the same member of staff can perform routine X-rays, ECGs, routine physiotherapy, phlebotomy and simple lab tests without the patient leaving the ward and that the efficiency savings will more than pay for extra equipment that has to be purchased. Tempting claims of potential savings of around 30–40% on staffing costs were made by Booz-Allen and Hamilton in their proposals as they argue for a change in emphasis away from the process of care (e.g. who carries out care) to the care itself. The result according to Manthey and Watson (1994) is that care is delivered by fewer people who can do more things.

Writers such as Hanrahan (1991) have developed the theme further dwelling on the structural inefficiencies built into hospitals where the famine or feast syndrome is widespread. There are therefore times of day when staff cannot cope with the volume of work leading to a possible reduction in standards and yet there are other times when staff are idle as there is insufficient for them to do. Hanrahan argues this is an inevitable result of the traditional and largely *ad hoc* way hospitals evolved with a large number of specialist professions and no integrated organizational structure. The goal therefore is to:

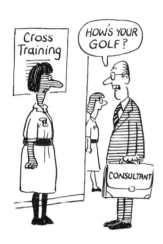

. . . shrink the number of job categories and management layers by cross-training to reduce the specialised infrastructure. Hanrahan (1991)

Hanrahan goes on to argue that nurses in partnership with doctors should manage this brave new world with significant enhancement of nursing accountability, autonomy and recognition. Nurses should then become engineers of care, freed from a lot of things they currently do which are not nursing, such as going to pharmacy for drugs, performing domestic tasks and unnecessary paperwork. Weber (1991) presents a series of case studies of early pilot PFH schemes in which the common factor seems to be the development of teams of multiskilled care workers led by nurses. Weber is an enthusiastic proponent of the PFH idea and while his case studies are all very positive, there is a lack of hard evaluative data which makes his paper little more than anecdotal evidence. It certainly does not meet the rigorous criteria that Bond and Thomas (1995) have argued for in evaluating the cost effectiveness of changes in practice before full-scale implementation.

There are immense implications in this radical approach to care. Whatever the professional arguments, there are some major practical problems inherent in the NHS which mitigate against a full-scale PFH. It seems unlikely that British hospitals will be able to provide the physical conditions needed by the PFH concept as newly designed and built 100-bedded operating units are required. The

NHS simply does not have the money to undertake this kind of building programme and as the delay between starting planning for a major new hospital building and its final opening is regularly the order of 15–20 years, it seems likely that a PFH-designed hospital is unlikely to open its doors in the UK before the year 2010. Cynics might mutter that it would probably have to close within a year anyway if the experience of the new Royal Derby Children's Hospital is any guide, opened by the Trust in 1996 amid talk of its possible closure within 5 years as part of a rationalization programme.

The promised savings, however, mean that NHS managers are looking seriously at utilizing some of the ideas in the PFH concept, even if full-scale implication would be many years away for the sort of practical reasons mentioned above. Black and Garside (1994) argue that NHS managers are actually interested in the PFH concept not from a cost-savings point of view but rather that it will be cost neutral but deliver higher quality care. It is very early days in the UK and there is little evidence to show that the pilot schemes have had any significant effect. However, the sort of inefficiencies highlighted by Hanrahan (1991) will be familiar to many nurses and clearly we should be looking at new ways of running hospitals to reduce such problems.

Black and Garside argue that it only takes 12 weeks to effectively cross-train care team members to perform a wide range of tasks normally carried out by other professions. The benefits are said to include a greater continuity of care by a team of staff sharing the same goals and objectives while each individual member of the team spends more time on direct patient care. In one of the earliest sites to trial the PFH concept, the Central Middlesex Hospital, Layton (1993) reports that cross-training has worked well, allowing staff to cross professional boundaries and deliver care when it is needed rather than the patient have to wait for a specialist to attend. This includes tasks previously carried out by junior doctors and if the purpose of the exercise is to deliver care promptly to patients, then avoiding lengthy delays while another member of staff attends is clearly beneficial. However, the patient will not benefit if the care is not carried out to an acceptable standard, which underlines the importance of quality education in new roles and careful monitoring of the outcomes of interventions rather than just whether the interventions were performed.

Three levels of work are identified in these early projects for the care team:

- care giver/clerical officer/housekeeping tasks;
- care giver/team assistant;
- care programme manager/assistant.

There are many implications for skill mix as such schemes are developed and the professions allied to medicine such as physiotherapists, radiographers, etc. are understandably very concerned about what will happen to their professional identity. Nurses too are anxious about being merely 'multiskilled care givers' while the RCN is very concerned about the danger that these moves focus only upon tasks and consequently fragment patient care leading to the PFH initiative being dubbed the task-focused hospital (RCN, 1992).

Manthey and Watson (1994) have discussed this issue of staff losing their professional identity but feel it is a red herring. They argue that the purpose of PFH is not to dilute the professions but rather to draw upon the different educational backgrounds and bring together the separate professional identities in order to focus on the single purpose of delivering patient care. Cross-training is seen as a way of sharing skills to the patient's advantage and they argue further that a profession is not solely defined by a set of skills, therefore a nurse taking an X-ray does not become a radiographer or any less a nurse.

It is true that professions are not defined by skills alone; there are a range of ethical, educational and philosophical issues which set the context within which the skills are practised. Some writers would argue that nursing is not even a profession. Porter (1992) launched a scathing attack on nursing's pursuit of professionalization arguing that it was all rhetoric and nursing should abandon the ideology of professionalization. Support for Porter's view is limited, therefore we will stay with the argument that nursing is a profession for now and therefore we must recognize that skills are practised in a professional context.

If skills are seen as independent of the practitioner's professional background, an assumption inherent in the PFH concept, then a radiographer or a physiotherapist will perform a bed bath in exactly the same way as a nurse. Many nurses will feel uncomfortable with that deduction and there is a lack of evidence to test that hypothesis. Radiographers spend less time communicating with patients than nurses, while physiotherapists probably communicate with patients in different, more directive, ways than nurses. The problem is that the interpersonal communication skills involved will be different and so will the professional ethos. The nurse is therefore more likely to notice that the patient is withdrawn or anxious and follow this up; communication becomes a therapeutic tool in a way it cannot with other professionals.

It therefore seems prudent to recognize that the differing backgrounds of practitioners means that not all skills can be performed with equal benefit to the patient by members of different professional groups. Cross-training needs to concentrate on more than just the mechanical skills and explore also the ethical, philosophical and educational differences between the differing professional backgrounds. As a further example, the concept of self-care is not likely to figure prominently in radiography but the nurse may be working hard to increase a patient's independence prior to discharge with the result that two practitioners may approach the same task from very different points of view leading to inconsistencies and contradictions in care. This also highlights the problems that arise from a focus on tasks at the expense of the whole patient.

In order that patient care may be delivered in a consistent fashion within a PFH environment, it is essential that there is an overall conceptual framework guiding care to which all members of the team subscribe, whatever their professional background. Clearly, a conceptual model of nursing provides that sort of framework although it may need adapting in the interests of multiprofessional agreement. In setting up PFH approaches to care, therefore, it is essential to have all the team openly discuss their own professional approaches to care and explore the differences as well as the similarities that exist. This paves the way for agreement on a philosophy and a model of care. In this way the problem of skills being divorced from the individual's professional background can be largely avoided and with it the inconsistency and confusion that may develop. Such work leads naturally on to the development of clinical protocols and CPs (see below) which reflect the agreed model of care that staff are working with.

The notion that team members who are basically involved in domestic housekeeping duties and have no nursing background might start to expand their areas of function into direct patient care involving monitoring vital signs, for example, fills most nurses with alarm and should be opposed at all times. The UKCC (1992) have made it clear that the RN will always be held accountable for delegated care; therefore, whatever may happen, the RN will be held accountable for the consequences of a person who is basically a domestic taking a patient's vital sign observations incorrectly.

The PFH initiative is underpinned by the development of clinical protocols which as we have seen are very similar to CPs, except they tend to be more task and process focused. They may therefore easily lack the holistic approach that characterizes an outcome-led CP (p. 89). The nurse developing CPs should be aware therefore of PFH initiatives and not confuse a CP containing clear statements of outcome for the whole patient with a clinical protocol which is a more task-focused plan of interventions by time. If the idea of developing clinical protocols is suggested the nurse should try and upgrade the suggestion to the more powerful CP which could still be used in a PFH initiative. The CP is actually a superior tool because of its greater potential for enhancing quality and the picture which it paints of the whole patient.

The PFH principles of greater multiprofessional teamworking to deliver more efficient higher quality care at the same cost are ones that nurses cannot really argue with. They need, however, to be aware of the potential dangers that this may lead to as a greater proportion of care could be taken on by staff who lack the necessary expertise and education. The danger of moving back to a task-focused rather than a holistic approach must be kept firmly in mind and finally the differing professional backgrounds of staff may mean they bring a very different approach to the same task. There is, therefore, a need for an agreed conceptual framework to guide care and a nursing model is a very good place to start developing such a multiprofessional model. It is imperative that professional considerations should be put forward to counter an NHS management point of view that at times is more concerned with the cost side of the quality equation and which fails to value and recognize the contribution that professional, specialist carers can make, be they nurses, physiotherapists, occupational therapists, radiographers or any other members of the professions allied to medicine.

Summary

This chapter started with the problems of using the Nursing Process style care plan as a means of planning and delivering nursing care. This approach is a useful tool for students beginning to try and understand the complexities of care, but has served registered nurses in the clinical environment very poorly and is increasingly becoming discredited. The use of critical pathways (CPs) as an alternative was explored and while there are dangers and problems of losing the individuality of the patient, they seem to have much to offer as a potential new tool for care planning. The use of a nursing model to help shape areas of the CP could potentially strengthen the concept a great deal, particularly with reference to the more individualistic needs of the patient. There is a significant move afoot towards a more multiprofessional approach to care and CPs look to have the potential to assist in delivering an integrated and more efficient approach to care. The patient-focused hospital (PFH) concept was explored finally and elements of this approach to care are being tried out in the UK. Again, there are potential benefits to care and potential dangers; the use of a conceptual framework to help overcome the very different professional backgrounds that PFH teams are drawn from is seen as essential in order that care is delivered in a consistent manner. Care delivery cannot be isolated from the professional context of the individual practitioner and must be harmonized around the holistic needs of the patient.

There is a vital role therefore for models or conceptual frameworks in pulling together the wide range of individual practitioners if a truly multidisciplinary *team* is to be assembled to work with patients whether with CPs or within a patient-focused context. Nursing models offer a good starting point for such team building, but nurses will have to accept that the models will require adaptation to make them multiprofessional.

References

Benner P (1984) *From Novice to Expert*. Menloe Park, CA: Addison Wesley.

Black A & Garside P (1994) Patient focused care. *Health Service Journal Supplement*.

Bond S & Thomas L (1995) The effectiveness of nursing; a review. *Journal of Clinical Nursing*, **4**, 143–151.

Booz-Allen and Hamilton (1990) Operational restructuring; the patient focused hospital. London: Booz-Allen and Hamilton Management Consultants.

Carnevali D, Mitchell P, Woods N & Tanner C (1984) *Diagnostic Reasoning in Nursing*. Philadelphia: Lippincott.

Fonteyn M & Cooper L (1994) The written nursing process; is it still useful to nursing education? *Journal of Advanced Nursing*, **19**, 315–319.

Franc C & Meyer J (1991) Facing the challenge of providing cardiac care in the 1990s, Pt II. *Journal of Cardiovascular Management*, **November–December**, 15–27.

Grant E, Newton M & Moore S (1995) Keeping patients on the right track. *Nursing* **95**, 57–59.

Hampton D (1994) Kings theory of goal attainment as a framework for managed care in a hospital setting. *Nursing Science Quarterly*, **7**, 170–173.

Hanrahan T (1991) New approaches to care giving. *Healthcare Forum Journal*, **July/August**, 33–38.

Hardy L & Engel J (1987) The search for professionalisation. *Nursing Times*, **83**(15), 37–39.

Heacock D & Brabst R (1994) A multidisciplinary approach to critical path development; a valuable CQI tool. *Journal of Nursing Care Quality*, **8**(4) 38–41.

Hurst K (1993) *Problem Solving in Nursing Practice*. London: Scutari.

Hydo B (1995) Designing an effective clinical pathway for stroke. *American Journal of Nursing*, **95**(3), 44–50.

Kim M, Camillert D & Mortensen R (1991) Nursing diagnosis and nursing practice: dialog with Nordic nurses. *Vard I Norden*, **21**(11), 30–33.

King I (1981) *A Theory for Nursing: Systems Concepts Process*. New York: Wiley.

Laxade S & Haile C (1995) Managed care; an opportunity for nursing. *British Journal of Nursing*, **4**(5) 290–294.

Layton A (1993) Planning individual care with protocols. *Nursing Standard* **8**(10), 32–34.

Manthey M & Watson P (1994) The patient focused approach; professional identity and the multiskilled approach. *Journal of Nursing Administration*, **24**(1), 9–14.

McNicol M (1992) Achieving quality improvement by structured patient management. *Quality in Health Care* Suppl. 1, 40–41.

Porter S (1992) The poverty of professionalisation; a critical analysis of strategies for the occupational advancement of nursing. *Journal of Advanced Nursing*, **17**, 720–726.

Rasmussen N & Gengler T (1994) The route to better communication. *Nursing 94*, **February**, 47–49.

Royal College of Nursing (1992) *Task Focused Hospitals or Patient Focused Care?* London: RCN.

Royal College of Nursing (1993) Protocols; guidance for good practice. *Nursing Standard*, **8**(8), 29.

Rudisill P, Phillips M & Payne C (1994) Clinical paths for cardiac surgery patients; a multidisciplinary approach to quality improvement outcomes. *Journal of Nursing Care Quality*, **8**(3), 27–33.

Tallon R (1995) Critical paths for wound care. *Advances in Wound Care*, **8**(1) 26–34.

Tanner C, Padrick K, Westfall V & Patzner D (1987) Diagnostic reasoning strategies of nurses and nursing students. *Nursing Research*, **36**(3), 358–363.

UKCC (1992) *Scope of Professional Practice*. London: UKCC.

Walsh M (1996) *A&E Nursing: A New Approach*, 3rd edn. Oxford: Butterworth Heinemann.

Weber O (1991) Six models of patient focused care. *Healthcare Forum Journal*, **July/August**, 23–31.

Wieczorek P (1995) Developing critical pathways in the operating room. *AORN Journal*, **62**(6), 925–929.

Woodyard L & Sheetz J (1993) Critical pathway patient outcomes; the missing standard. *Journal of Nursing Care Quality*, **8**(1), 51–57.

Zander K (1992) Critical pathways. In Melum M & Sinior M (eds) *Total Quality Management: The Health Care Pioneers*, pp. American Hospital Publishing.

5 Some Models Used in this Book

In the next section of the book, models are critically evaluated in various fields of nursing by the process of attempting to devise assessments, care plans and critical pathways (CPs) based upon the work of Orem (1990), Roy (1984), King (1981), Roper, Logan and Tierney (1996) and the FANCAP assessment scheme of Abbey. The application of these models to general adult nursing, both hospital and community, and mental health nursing is explored.

In this chapter, a very brief outline of the salient features of the respective models is given for reference. However, the reader is strongly recommended to use the reading list given at the end of the chapter to explore in detail both the original writings of the authors, and the various interpretations of their work that are available. It is only by reference to the original sources that the reader will come to understand the full philosophy of the model and the stance that the authors have taken in expressing their ideas. All models contain assumptions which are always open to question; again these will become apparent only by reference to the original sources.

The selection of models reflects those which are most commonly used and also those which seem most relevant to practical nursing. In developing the care plans, jargon has been avoided as far as possible and the documentation has been freely adapted from the author's ideas in a way that seems easiest to work with. Given the immature state of model development, the nurse is encouraged to consider further modifications beyond those that have been used here. Such work should be undertaken in the light of practical experience and also with reference to the literature in order that the nurse does not lose touch with the author's ideas.

Orem's self-care model

Orem's basic philosophy is that people strive to achieve self-care either by their own efforts or by the efforts of significant others such as friends or family. When they are unable to achieve self-care, a self-care deficit exists, which is defined as a patient problem requiring nursing intervention. The basic philosophy of nursing in this model is therefore to help the patient and family achieve self-care.

The ability to carry out self-care is referred to as the self-care agency of the person and this depends upon factors such as the resources the person has to provide a healthy diet and a home for themselves. Knowledge coupled with the person's attitudes and beliefs towards health make up another key component of self-care agency. Social factors such as the home and family circumstances and the person's role in society will also influence the ability to practise self-care as will their age and developmental status. Illness and disability will arise as a result of the person's self-care agency being unable to meet their self-care demands which may then further reduce their self-care agency. In this way, a downward spiral may arise with the person's health steadily deteriorating as their inability to practice self-care causes further health problems which reduces even more their self-care ability. The notion of self-care agency therefore brings in a holistic view of the person, requiring the integration of biological, psychological and sociological insights if the person is to be returned to an improved health status.

A further key principle is the notion of dependent care agency. This refers to the resources, knowledge, etc. available to a person to care for another. Orem's model does not just focus on the self but also sees care for others as an integral part of human behaviour whether they be family members or next-door neighbours. Evidence to support these assertions has been presented by Hart (1995) who showed that in a sample of 127 pregnant women, measures of self-care agency significantly correlated with pre-natal care actions. Hart also explored the notion of dependent care agency with these women, which at this stage relates to the ability to accept the role of mother and form a relationship with the foetus. These may be seen as the necessary foundations for any woman to develop a dependent care agency; that is, the ability to successfully care for her child. In Hart's study, her measures of self-care agency correlated with dependent care agency and subsequently with infant birth weight which may be seen as an objective measure of the mother's ability to practise self-care. Hart concludes by pointing out that these findings lend support to the ideas which make up Orem's conceptual framework. This is indeed so; however, this is only one study carried out in South Georgia, USA, and a great deal more evidence would need to be assembled before it would be possible to claim a solid foundation for Orem's model.

Patients may be envisaged as lying on a spectrum of self-care demand stretching from, for example, an unconscious patient being ventilated on ITU through to a diabetic person who needs advice about their injection technique. The former patient is unable to meet any of their self-care needs and requires total nursing intervention, which Orem calls a wholly compensatory nursing system. The latter patient requires only some advice from the nurse to provide for all their self-care needs; this is known as an educative supportive nursing system. Between these two extremes, nursing is said to be partially compensatory, implying that the patient can meet some but not all of their self-care needs.

Orem's model may analyse the nursing care for goals using the above framework and some writers insert a column on the care plan in which the nurse notes whether the nursing care for any goal is wholly or partly compensatory, or educative/consultative. This practice has not been followed in this book in the interest of simplifying the paperwork.

This model of nursing therefore acknowledges that patients can have a wide range of dependency and emphasizes the role of the nurse not only as a provider of care but also as an educator about health. The aim of the nurse is to help patients to move along this continuum of self-care need until they can achieve the maximum possible self-care with the nursing role ideally limited to support and advice.

The model emphasizes that self-care should be therapeutic; that is, beneficial to health, hence the phrase 'therapeutic self-care demand' which means the challenges the person faces in order to practise self-care which results in health. The patient's perception of self-care may not actually improve their health status, for example, smoking may be seen as reducing stress and therefore to the patient may appear self-care. This dilemma of whose point of view is correct, the patient's or the nurse's, recurs in other models and requires the nurse to adopt an interactionist point of view in applying systems or developmental models.

Many health problems can be seen as originating in lack of knowledge or in self-neglect. The Orem model seeks to highlight these causes of ill health, and by stressing the importance of the educative supportive nursing system offers a way of tackling these problems. Hartweg (1990) has analysed Orem's model from the point of view of health promotion, defining this to mean positive action taken by a person to benefit health. This is congruent with Orem's ideas about self-care and Hartweg has shown that these ideas can be incorporated within the universal and developmental self-care aspects of Orem's model, making the model suitable for health promotion work.

Assessment involves two approaches. The obvious aim of assessment is to establish the person's self-care agency and the therapeutic self-care demand that they face. This gives the nurse a picture of what the patient can do for themselves (self-care agency) and the demands being made upon them in order to remain healthy (therapeutic self-care demand). Where a gap occurs between these two aspects, Orem refers to this as a self-care deficit and a problem is said to occur. These self-care deficits may be actual or potential.

For example, a patient who has had a hemiplegia after a stroke is immobile. The therapeutic self-care demand required for healthy tissue over bony prominences is such that there should be a normal capilliary circulation to ensure well-oxygenated cells. As the tissue interface pressure between the average person and the average hospital bed over a bony prominence is well in excess of capilliary pressure, unless the patient's position is changed frequently to relieve pressure, ischaemia will develop leading to tissue death and pressure sore formation. The person's self-care agency is probably so impaired by the stroke, however, that they cannot change position, therefore a self-care deficit exists with the potential for the development of pressure sores. Nursing assessment should reveal the existence of this self-care deficit and the use of nursing theory will predict the probability of pressure sore formation. The reader should recall the discussion of theory given on p. 3 which links theory to prediction but only within limits of probability.

There is, however, another area in which self-care assessment should be carried out. Consider the example of the 19-year-old insulin-dependent diabetic patient who has poorly controlled blood sugar levels. Assessment reveals that they know how they should balance their insulin injections and diet to keep blood sugar within normal limits. They therefore appear to have the self-care agency necessary for good self-management of their diabetes. However, questioning reveals that they periodically miss injections and rarely adhere to their diet, therefore are not practising therapeutic self-care. There are a range of internal and outside influences at work. They may be coping with their diabetes by denial or they may feel under pressure to conform. Peer group pressures (real or imagined) lead to them wanting to be like everybody else by consuming several pints of lager in the pub on a Friday night while eating what everybody else eats during the day. This example shows how a range of internal and external factors influences a person's ability to practise self-care (self-care agency) or to care for another (dependency care agency).

This analysis opens up the issue that there may be areas of self-care deficit which are beyond the individual's control. Social and environmental factors such as unemployment, poverty, poor housing and atmospheric pollution are not factors which the individual can do a great deal about. This places the nurse in something of a dilemma as they may unearth several likely causes of the patient's health problems upon which nursing can have little impact, or can it? Nurses have traditionally fought shy of politics and macro-issues such as these are the responsibility of government. Perhaps it is therefore time that nurses heed the call of Casey (1996) and did engage the political process in a meaningful way. The nurse might not be able to do anything for the individual patient today, but by actively campaigning for better social conditions, it may be possible to improve the health of a great many people tomorrow.

Assessment should therefore try to discover what internal or external factors affect the self-care agency as well as what the self-care agency consists of. It is not just the obvious outside physical ability to practise self-care that matters, it is also what the patient is feeling and thinking in response to their current life situation and previous upbringing, expectations *and* experiences that matters. Only by looking in both these areas can the nurse really discover the extent of the person's self-care agency. After all you would not buy a car without looking under the bonnet!

Assessment is required under three broad areas, which are known as the universal, developmental and health deviancy self-care demands:

- *Universal self-care* is primarily concerned with normal functioning and involves the required intake of air, water and nutrients to maintain health, and also their excretion. There has to be effective prevention of hazards to life and also there has to be a balance between rest and activity, social interaction and solitude. Finally, this social theme is developed into the concept of normalcy, meaning the human ability to function in groups and the desire to be accepted and seen as normal. The importance of the normalcy concept has already been seen in the above example of the diabetic patient. Many patient's apparent lack of co-operation or non-compliance may be traced to their desire to conform with others or with their own perception of themselves as different. How such perceptions and desires affect their self-care agency is a key insight into assessing the person's health status.
- *Developmental self-care* partly reflects the way a person's developmental status affects their universal self-care ability. However, adult life also has various developmental milestones in the same way as childhood. These adult milestones may be seen as positive events such as marriage and childbirth or negative events such as divorce, redundancy at work or bereavement. The nurse needs to assess the person's ability to cope with these events and take into account how they will affect self-care ability in other areas.
- *Health deviancy self-care* looks at the actions required by the person to cope specifically with illness and/or disability. They may be seen as a logical sequence starting with the ability to recognize that there is an illness problem and that medical attention is needed. The next steps involve the ability to recognize the likely effects of illness, being able to carry out medically prescribed treatments and being aware of possible side-effects of such treatments (e.g. drugs or diet). Finally, patients need to be able to adapt

their self-concept in line with their illness, learning to live with its effects while maximizing personal achievement and quality of life.

Orem's model therefore offers a comprehensive assessment of the person seen from a self-care perspective. This must then follow through into the care that is planned and delivered. Goals must be set as things that the patient will achieve and care should be directed towards the patient doing things for themselves. As we saw on the previous page, patients exist on a continuum of self-care abilities and nursing's role is to move the patient towards the increasingly self-care end of that continuum. The notion of dependency care is equally important as health care moves towards an increasingly community focus. Increasingly, children experience short periods of hospitalization with as much care as possible carried out at home by parents while adults with chronic health problems are also seen as best cared for in the community. This leads to many people with deteriorating health due to conditions such as multiple sclerosis or Alzheimer's disease being cared for by relatives supported by primary health care nurses.

A simplistic view of self-care, which takes the phrase literally, suggests this is an inappropriate model for such patients as they will never be able to care for themselves and their overall health will deteriorate to the point of death. Orem has never written in such simplistic terms; however, she sees nursing as incorporating the family and significant others in caring, hence the term dependent care which is seen as a key component of the wider concept of self-care. Self really means the individual, their family and significant others in their life. Therapeutic self-care aims to maximize the person's health status but also acknowledges that in absolute terms this may deteriorate in certain disease conditions. The point is that the nurse should assist the patient to make the best of what they can while they can. A useful analogy might be to imagine a person falling from an aeroplane, the descent to the ground is inevitable but it can be slowed down, the experience greatly improved and the landing made a lot softer with the use of a parachute. Nursing is the parachute which allows a person with a chronic deteriorating health condition to have a soft landing, even if that condition ultimately is responsible for their death.

The increasing move towards community-based care therefore makes a model such as Orem's very useful as it tackles the reality of care for many patients, short episodes of hospital care in between lengthy periods of care by self, family and significant others.

It is important that the nurse wishing to learn more about Orem's model should go to the original source material and study it in depth. It may serve as nothing more than a useful way of thinking about nursing and encourage nurses to develop a philosophy for their practice which is about maximizing self and family care. It is possible to take the conceptual framework a little further and structure nursing around Orem's three concepts of universal, developmental and health deviancy self-care demand. Assessment looks at how well the patient copes with everyday living activities, where they are in their life span and how well they can cope with the specific effects of illness. Care is directed towards ensuring that the patient and family/significant others can manage the maximum self-care in everyday living and in dealing with the effects of illness, given the age and developmental status of the patient. These two positions represent different stages of integration of Orem's model into practice and are well short of a full-blown implementation of the model. They both, however, offer potentially beneficial contributions to patient care, particularly in areas which have a strong rehabilitation and discharge focus such as units caring for the older person, medical wards and staff working in the community.

The nurse could take some of Orem's ideas further and utilize a concept such as normalcy to obtain insights into the psychosocial dimensions of the person, particularly in conditions where non-compliance is such a major problem (e.g. diabetes, asthma). The concept of health deviancy could be used as a framework to help build a patient teaching package. In a condition such as asthma the nurse might construct a patient teaching leaflet in response to the following questions which are readily derived from Orem's health deviancy concept (see p. 118).

- What are the signs and symptoms that suggest your condition is deteriorating?
- How can you obtain medical help?
- What might happen if you do not seek help at this stage and a full acute exacerbation of your asthma develops?
- Can you use your inhaler properly?
- What the the correct drugs to use and what are their effects?
- What side-effects might there be from these drugs?
- What are the other factors in your life that might make your asthma worse and how can you integrate the requirements of managing your asthma into everyday life in a balanced way?

This approach could be used with a range of medical conditions.

A wide range of useful applications of various parts of Orem's conceptual framework is possible, including integration into CPs. The unit or ward may even chose to implement the whole approach and redesign care plans or CPs accordingly. This of course leads up to the important question of whether there is any evidence to support such a change. Some research-based evidence has been cited in support of Orem's model so far, but it is not a great deal. This presents us with a major problem and it is a problem that all other nursing models face, for despite the great deal of interest shown in models in the 1980s, we have to admit 10 years later that there is a dearth of research evidence to support their use. By the same token there is also a dearth of evidence to contradict their use.

The root of the problem is that very few places have actually implemented models meaningfully and then attempted to evaluate the effect of the changes made. As a result there are few published reports to persuade others to try out a new model, consequently in the highly pressurized conditions that exist in many parts of the NHS, new models are not trialled. It seems as if a vicious circle has become established which means that it is impossible to provide any research evidence on model implementation, therefore nobody will try out models and so there can be no research evidence. At a time when survival has become the main aim of many NHS Trusts, experimentation with new ways of delivering care that does not have an obvious financial benefit has been relegated to the bottom of the pile in terms of priority. Thus evidence to support, or otherwise, models such as Orem's or Roy's is lacking. We return to this theme later in this chapter.

The Roy adaptation model

Roy considers health to be a function of adaptation to stressors which may be physiological, psychological or social in origin. Successful adaptation may be equated with health and therefore the nurse's role becomes one of assisting the patient to adapt to the stressors to which they are exposed. The model is behaviourist in nature since at its core lies the question of how the patient behaves in response to the various stressors of life. These stressors are known as stimuli in the Roy model and nursing care is seen wherever possible as being directed at the stimuli; that is, the causes of the patient's problems.

If a person is exposed to pathogenic micro-organisms but their body defence systems successfully prevent an infection developing, we may say they are healthy because they have adapted to the stressor. The stressor lay within the person's adaptation range, they were capable of dealing with it as the body had the appropriate antibodies, etc. If the micro-organism was one which the body could not deal with, for example a strain of influenza virus to which immunity had not developed, it could be said to lie outside the adaptation range of the body and illness, that is, flu, results.

This principle of adaptation can be applied to psychosocial situations as well. Thus, a woman undergoing mastectomy will be exposed to many stressors in addition to the obvious physical stresses of surgery and cancer. She faces a major challenge to her self-concept of her body and worth as a person, along with her role function as a woman and as a sexual partner. This in turn affects her interdependence with others such as her husband or partner.

To assess a patient using the adaptation model it is necessary to describe the patient's behaviour and pick out those areas which show signs of an inability or failure to adapt which is then defined as a patient problem. The next step is to consider what is causing that behaviour, that is, the stimulus, as this is ideally going to be the target for nursing intervention. The model suggests that the causes of problems can be analysed into three types: focal, contextual and residual stimuli.

The focal stimulus is the immediate cause of a problem, a contextual stimulus is seen as any environmental factor that may contribute to that problem, while a residual stimulus can be either a previous experience or an attitude or belief system which may also be a contributory factor. Thus, for every problem identified there should be a focal stimulus, and there may or may not be a contextual and/or residual stimulus.

Consider a patient who is in pain after surgery. That is a behaviour we have observed within the physiological mode. The next step is to find out what is causing that pain and obviously the immediate answer is the direct effect of the surgery. This then is the focal stimulus or immediate cause of the pain. However, Roy's model urges the nurse to look further to see whether there are other causes.

The patient may be worried about some of the things going on around them in the ward and, as Hayward (1979) has shown, anxiety increases pain. This is an example of a contextual stimulus, an environmental factor contributing to pain. The patient may also have the belief that they should expect pain after surgery and so would not have asked for analgesia that could have relieved the pain. This is a belief or residual stimulus contributing to the patient's pain. The nurse using the Roy model would do more than give post-operative analgesia, they would also find out what the patient was anxious about and by explanation reduce anxiety and pain and also engage in patient teaching about pain relief to encourage the patient to ask for analgesia as soon as pain was felt rather than suffer in silence because of a mistaken belief.

Assessment is therefore a two-stage process. The first stage consists of describing patient behaviour and discovering how the individual is feeling and thinking, then trying to pick out problem areas. This is known as the first-level assessment, while the second stage, or second-level assessment, involves trying to discover the causes of the patient's problems identified in the first stage.

It may be argued that some stimuli are not amenable to nursing intervention; for example in the case above, surgery is seen as the focal cause of the patient's pain yet clearly there is nothing the nurse can do about the fact that the patient has had surgery. The common-sense approach is to acknowledge that sometimes the causes of patient problems (stimuli) are not amenable to nursing intervention. However, the nurse can still do much to alleviate the effects of the stimuli, for example in this case give analgesia.

An alternative, more rigorous approach is that of Logan (1990), who argues that only those stimuli that are amenable to direct and independent nursing action should be included in the assessment. Independent action is defined as actions which nurses perform under their own initiative without needing consent or written instructions from others. According to this definition, giving analgesia is not an independent nursing action since it needs a doctor's written instructions in the form of a prescription on a drug chart.

The problem with Logan's approach may be illustrated by considering a patient who is vomiting after surgery. This could be due to a post-operative ileus or the side-effect of opioid analgesia (the stimuli in Roy's language). As there is nothing the nurse can do to directly resolve the ileus, and as giving analgesia is not an independent nursing action, Logan seems to be suggesting that these should be ignored in the second-stage assessment process. The result is a patient who is vomiting yet, according to Logan's interpretation, we ignore the causes of the vomiting because they are not amenable to what she defines as independent nursing actions! In this book the more practical common-sense approach has been adopted rather than Logan's more extreme view.

To give structure to the assessment, the model suggests four different areas of behaviour that should be assessed: physiology, self-concept, role function and interdependence. Physiology is subdivided into oxygenation and circulation, fluid and electrolyte balance, nutrition, elimination, rest and activity and regulation, including body temperature, hormonal control and the nervous system. This latter area includes the crucial area of pain.

Self-concept includes both physical (i.e. the body) and personal self-concept (i.e. self-worth).

Self-concept has two dimensions: the physical self and the personal self. The former is concerned with how the person sees their appearance and their body and their ability to adapt to changes in their physical self. This obviously connects to surgical nursing where major changes in the body may occur. A woman may lose a breast because of surgery for cancer, an individual may lose a leg due to PVD while stoma formation may drastically alter a person's abdominal wall and excretory functions. The patient's perception of their body may of course be very different from the nurse's and this distorted self-image is seen most strikingly in young women suffering from anorexia. The personal self concerns the moral and ethical view that the person holds of themselves, it is about self-esteem. The tearful and distressed elderly woman who has sustained a fractured upper femur may be convinced that she will be a burden to her family, the 60-year-old man who has had a stroke and lost bladder control, the ability to speak properly or feed himself may lash out in anger and frustration before sliding into a deep depression as he sees himself reduced to the level of an infant, while the mother of the child who has had a serious accident is consumed with guilt as she blames herself for not preventing the incident. All these and many other examples illustrate the devastating consequences of a diminished personal self-concept in response to some outside event or stimuli.

Role function describes the various roles that we have in life and Roy suggests that they may be considered as primary, secondary and tertiary. Primary roles are enduring characteristics over which we have no control and typically include age, gender and the role expectations that society has accordingly. Being a son or a daughter falls into this category also. Comments such as 'That is no way for a grown man to behave' or 'But she is only a child' and 'At his age what do you expect?' testify to the power of such primary roles and the expectations that society places upon us. If the individual sees him or herself, in response to the challenge of illness, as failing to behave in the approved way, then this may well cause serious psychological distress. Others may also interpret behaviour which does not conform to a primary role as evidence of illness or at least as cause for disapproval. Nurses are potentially as likely as anyone else to disapprove of a patient in a same sex relationship for example. Secondary roles are those which we have a degree of choice over but which are fairly permanent such as occupation or marital status, while tertiary roles concern less important and more transient roles associated with leisure activities such as being a member of a football team supporters club or a cricket team. These other roles are also constrained by various expectations and norms and the patient may experience a great deal of distress as a result of fear that illness may impair their ability to fulfil these roles. A major area of concern involves roles as sexual partners which may be affected by a range of medical conditions. Other non-medical causes may have significant effects upon health however, such as redundancy which may seriously undermine a man's traditional role as breadwinner. It is obvious from these two examples that role function and self-concept are closely interlinked.

The final area of adaptation that Roy explores involves interdependence, the amount of dependence that we have on other people. The examples cited above in connection with self-concept and role function clearly impact upon interdependence and these three aspects of adaptation form a complex triad which cannot be ignored. A great deal of patient distress and unhappiness, not to mention non-compliance, may be understood in these terms.

In order to explore these areas with a patient it is necessary to get to know them, making Roy's model inappropriate for clinical areas such as A&E or day surgery. However, where longer interaction with the patient is possible, Roy's model opens up a sophisticated and insightful way of planning and carrying out nursing care that is particularly relevant to areas such as surgery where the patient often has to adapt to major changes in their body.

As with Orem the nurse can integrate Roy's model into practice at several different levels. The basic concept of adaptation may simply be used in building a philosophy of care or the nurse may go further and adopt the two-level assessment concept. Patient assessment in future may seek not only to describe the problem but also to try and explain the causes of the problem. In trying to understand these causes the nurse may also look beyond the obvious direct cause and wonder what contributing factors there may be in the patient's home environment (contextual stimuli) or what previous experiences and beliefs they bring with them (residual stimuli). The nurse may chose to pick up on concepts such as self-concept and role function and build them into care to give a broader, more holistic approach. Roy's ideas can also be incorporated into CP construction. These are all examples of the potential value of Roy's conceptual framework, even if the clinical area does not wish to take on board the full model, although it would be an exciting development if some UK clinical areas were prepared to tackle the challenge of Roy's model.

In the preceding section, the lack of research evidence to support nursing models was referred to. It was suggested this was caused simply by the lack of areas implementing models and subsequent evaluation studies. One such evaluation has been carried out however by Weiss *et al.* (1994) and this produced very interesting results. The Women's Center and the Acute Division of Sharpe Memorial Hospital, San Diego, California had both implemented Roy's model by 1988 and after several years felt it time for an in-depth asessment of the model.

As Weiss *et al.* point out, evaluation of nursing models by empirical methods has not yet occurred and while these authors cite many case studies advocating the benefits of switching to a models-based approach to care, hard research evidence is thin on the ground. Given the immense complexity of empirical research into the quality of nursing care, these authors opted for a qualitative approach relying on semi-structured interviews with a sample of 20 RNs chosen from a sampling grid to ensure all areas of the hospital were covered. Their aim was to explore and describe the perceptions held by nurses of the Roy model after several years of implementation with an orthodox nursing process documentation. The methods adopted were therefore appropriate to this research goal.

When the degree of integration into practice was explored, the researchers found it was possible to describe four levels:

- *Conscious:* nurses identified Roy as the framework for their care and talked about their care with Roy's model in a very explicit fashion.
- *Unconscious:* aspects of Roy's model were discernible in the way

these nurses talked about care even though they did not overtly refer to Roy.

- *Directed:* these nurses were aware of Roy's model but gave the impression that their use of it was document driven, rather than having any great understanding of or support for the model. (The assessment forms and care plans were written in a format derived from Roy.)
- *Lacking:* here there was a complete lack of awareness of Roy's model.

At a general level, the researchers felt that the nurses integrated the ideas and concepts inherent in Roy's model into their practice although they did not use the specific terms and jargon that Roy uses. Those nurses who had studied Roy as part of their training or in subsequent continuing education work showed the greatest utilization of her ideas.

When the advantages and disadvantages of using Roy's model were explored, there was a great deal of support for the idea that it gave nurses a clear structure that everybody used. This structure was valuable for assessing patients, planning care and most interestingly, actually doing the work. This latter point is important when arguments such as 'nursing models have nothing to offer in practice' are deployed! Staff commented that using Roy gave a much more thorough psychosocial assessment of the patient and also that the depth of the model required them to develop new skills (presumably in areas such as communication skills and counselling although frustratingly this point is not expanded upon in Weiss *et al.*'s paper). Nurses also commented that the use of such a framework advanced the professional status of nursing. The disadvantage was that the nursing process documentation was very time consuming and often contained irrelevant sections that wasted even more time. This seems more a familiar criticism of the nursing process rather than Roy's model. The other main point raised was that the language of the model was very difficult to follow, a comment that has been made many times in the UK. While it is reassuring that Californian nurses also found this problem, it does point to the need to simplify the language which after all should express ideas and elucidate meaning rather than hide them behind a smokescreen of jargon.

Weiss *et al.* (1994) conclude that the Roy model had become well integrated into practice and was seen as having made a very beneficial contribution to care. Education about the model was the greatest facilitator and the use of the nursing process was the biggest drawback.

Again we should beware the trap of reading too much into a single study, but this study was carried out with rigour and lets the nursing voice speak clearly about Roy's model. Unless models are given a chance to work and then carefully evaluated there will never be the research data that will allow other units to give them a try. Evidence-based practice cannot occur without the evidence, but there has to be some practice to gather the evidence in the first place!

The FANCAP
assessment
scheme

Strictly speaking, this is not a model of nursing but rather a quick and comprehensive guide to assessment (Abbey, 1980) that can be bolted on to the nurse's own philosophy of care or used on its own in very acute situations such as A&E or ITU. The FANCAP scheme, therefore, is potentially a very useful building block for nurses constructing their own model, hence its inclusion.

The six letters in FANCAP are the initials of the key words Fluids, Aeration, Nutrition, Communication, Activity, Pain. The order has no significance, it is simply to make an easily remembered word. As an aid to assessment it is suggested that some of the headings are readily broken down into notions of in and out, for example fluids or nutrition.

A key idea in using the scheme is that the six headings should be interpreted in ways other than their literal meanings; this lateral thinking gives the scheme greater flexibility and scope. The sorts of parameters that should be assessed may be summarized as follows:

- *Fluids*
  - In: Oral hydration, IVI.
  - Out: Urine, vomit, wound drainage, sweat (temperature).
  - Lateral: Fluidity means flowing along without friction, how well therefore does the person relate to others? Is he or she isolated, difficult to get along with or socially integrated and easy to get along with?

- *Aeration*
  - In: Airway patency, breathing, (rate, effort, rhythm) skin colour if Caucasian, evidence of cyanosis.
  - Out: Expiratory wheeze, cough, sputum production, cardiac output (BP, P).
  - Lateral: Aeration implies ventilation of feelings, 'getting it off your chest'. Is the patient expressing/supressing emotions?

- *Nutrition*
  - In: Dietary intake.
  - Out: Bowel habit.
  - Lateral: The mind needs feeding as well as the stomach. What is the quality and quantity of mental stimulation reaching the patient?

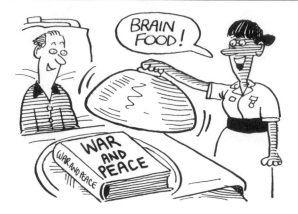

- *Communication*   In: Sensory nervous system, central nervous system, ability to understand language, orientation in time and space, other neurological signs, endorine system as an internal communication system.

    Out: Language use, ideas expressed, non-verbal communication.

    Lateral: Communication means a route between two separate locations, thus a wound is communication between the outside world and inside the body. Assess wounds under communication.

The last two headings do not lend themselves to the structures suggested above as it is not possible to distinguish between in and out nor is there any obvious benefit from a looser more lateral interpretation of the key words.

- *Activity*   Rest and activity, sleep and mobility, social activity (recreation, family, etc.) and work activity should be assessed here.

- *Pain*   Physical pain is obvious, but a looser interpretation leads to a consideration of psychological pain, i.e. fear and anxiety.

The sequence in which a patient may be assessed will vary according to the patient and their condition. Thus, in an A&E unit or ITU, aeration would be the first priority followed by pain, while in a renal care unit fluids would be the logical starting point. The nurse should make use of the various assessment tools that are available in assessing the different areas such as a pressure sore risk calculator or a pain rating scale.

The lateral thinking aspects of the scheme are often greeted initially with some scepticism, but after usage it is usually acknowledged that the scheme is made more comprehensive and sensitive by such an approach. This has been the author's experience in teaching third-year students to use FANCAP in a variety of settings.

The FANCAP scheme is deliberately left loose for nurses to adapt to their own clinical areas so that it can be used in conjunction with any philosophy of care to build a nursing model suitable to that clinical area. It is a challenge to the nurse's creativity and powers of independent thinking.

The Roper activities of living model

This model is derived from the notion that humans carry out a series of everyday activities which are essential to normal functioning. The model claims that 12 such activities of living may be identified and structures nursing around this framework as follows:

- maintaining a safe environment;
- communicating with others, both verbally and non-verbally;
- breathing;
- eating and drinking;
- elimination of body wastes;
- personal cleansing and dressing;
- controlling body temperature;
- mobilizing, both locomotion and manipulation;
- working and playing;
- expressing sexuality (appearance, relationships, etc.);
- sleeping;
- dying.

The model considers that humans exist on an independence–dependence continuum and this is reflected in each of these 12 activities of living (ALs). Thus, a person can be positioned somewhere between the two extremes for each of these 12 ALs with factors such as age and illness playing a major role in determining their exact location.

The function of nursing is seen as trying to promote maximum independence for each AL and meet the patient's needs that arise due to increasing dependence. It is important to maintain the patient's normal routine as far as possible. Where this is identified as having contributed to the patient's illness, the nurse is seen as being responsible for trying to change the patient's attitudes to be more compatible with health. The nursing role can vary from giving information to the patient through to actually carrying out an AL if the patient is unable to do it for him or herself.

The model identifies three other components of nursing besides those carried out directly in relation to these 12 ALs. These are the preventing, comforting and dependent components of nursing.

Clearly, prevention of harm to the patient is a nursing responsibility which extends to encompass health education. Comforting, as its name implies, is directed at improving the physical comfort of the patient, while the dependent component of nursing involves performing tasks for the patient which they cannot carry out unaided. There seems a lack of clarity in separating out these three components from the AL component and the authors admit that they overlap and interrelate very closely.

The use of the Roper model involves a checklist assessment of the patient's normal level of functioning under these 12 headings followed by an assessment of the patient's current levels of independence. The goal of nursing care is to restore the patient to their previous level of independence, or where this is not possible to help the patient cope with a reduced level of independence.

The reader may question the absence of any psychological or social dimension to this model and may also wonder whether human behaviour can be broken down into these 12 components. Rourke (1990) is very critical of the model for the way it falls into the trap of reductionism, leading to a dehumanizing process. The whole person dissolves into these 12 fragments, each of which is viewed from the negative point of view of a failure to achieve.

Why 12? Why not 10 or 15? What evidence is there to support the claim that these 12 headings represent a comprehensive and definitive view of human behaviour? Self-concept and self-worth, the patient's view of things, attitudes and beliefs spring to mind as topics not covered in this rather simplistic approach to assessment. Questions can be raised about how emotions and fears, anxiety and stress can be assessed and the problems arising from these psychological components of the human condition accounted for. There are also the effects of family, environment, housing conditions, poverty and unemployment to be accounted for.

Although the philosphy of promoting independence is one which many nurses can agree with, the above analysis suggests that the Roper model is open to significant criticism.

The Roper Logan Tierney (RLT) model has its advocates also and, in defending the model, Bellman (1996) argues that its simplicity is a major strength. While agreeing that simplicity is always desirable, over-simplification can lead to distortion and inaccuracy. Models such as Orem's and Roy's are complex because people and nursing are complex, their complexity is a reflection of reality. A nursing model that over-simplifies is not helpful and the reductionist approach inherent in RLT tends to predispose to the loss of the psychosocial areas of care. Bellman asserts that these areas are well represented in the RLT model, it is just the way it has been implemented that has led to their loss.

If Bellman's assertion is correct, that still leaves the issue of why has the implementation been so flawed. Could that not have something to do with the way the model is written and presented in this fragmented, check-list style? Other factors have probably contributed to this state of affairs, such as British nursing's traditional reluctance to embrace the psychosocial dimensions of care and the blanket implementation of the RLT model without due time to consider whether it was appropriate to get to grips with understanding it. It was almost as if nurse managers decided to imitate Tommy Cooper 'Pick a model, go on, pick a model, any model, as long as it's Roper!'.

Bellman (1996) set out to study whether action research with the RLT model could be used as a means of enhancing care on a surgical ward that was using the model already. It is interesting to note therefore that she found a major problem area in need of attention on this ward using the RLT model was psychological care. Patients reported that they shared their fears and anxieties with the ward physiotherapist as the nurses seemed too busy with physical care. Bellman notes the comments of Fraser (1990) that there is no empirical evidence to support the RLT model (none has appeared since) and therefore sets out on a different research route using qualitative techniques to try and understand the nursing staff's perspective on care and the model. In this way her work is similar to Weiss *et al.* (1994) who used such an approach to evaluate Roy's model. There is a key difference though as Bellman used an action research methodology which involved her in the work as an on-going participant.

Bellman identified three areas where the RLT concept of moving patients towards greater independence could lead to innovations that the staff agreed were worth trying: the introduction of patient-controlled analgesia (PCA), patient self-medication and the development of operation-specific information leaflets for patients. This is a good example of how the basic philosophy underlying a model can be a catalyst for change even if the detail of the model is not pursued.

The action research approach that aimed to introduce these changes, however, struggled because of the ambivalence of the nursing staff towards the medical staff. While agreeing that the proposed changes were worthwhile, they also felt that the doctors would provide such an unassailable barrier to change there was little point in trying. At the end of the 15-month study, it is worth noting that when the 12 ward nursing staff involved in the project were interviewed about the RLT model, very few displayed any knowledge of it. Attempts at getting them to keep a reflective diary had also failed. The nurses did seem more aware of their individual practice as a result of the project, however, even if they remained largely in the dark concerning the model that the ward espoused to practice.

There are several valuable lessons to learn from Bellman's brave attempt to use a nursing model to get to grips with practice:

- On a ward which espoused the use of the RLT model, patients felt they gained more psychological support from the physiotherapist than the nursing staff.
- At the end of a 15-month study, few nurses on this ward displayed any understanding of the model, suggesting that the RLT model was superficial and had no real roots in the ward culture. Was it merely cosmetic?
- Staff were unwilling to engage in meaningful dialogue with doctors because of the perceived power imbalance, nor were they prepared to engage in dialogue with themselves through the medium of a reflective diary.
- The philosophy behind the RLT model provided a means to engage staff in a serious attempt to change practice, though not within the psychosocial domain, which met with a limited degree of success. Bellman is not very specific about exactly what change was achieved, however.
- Staff were made more aware of their own practice by the exercise.

This study does little to support the use of the RLT model and helps to confirm one of the main criticisms of it; that is, its lack of attention to the psychosocial area of patient care. It does, however, show that by working with the philosophy behind a nursing model it is possible to push forward change in practice. It also illuminates the difficulty in changing practice if there is no interdisciplinary co-operation. The discussion on CPs in Chapter 4 is very pertinent here.

Alas, this is a single study only and this has been a theme throughout this chapter. Nursing will not be able to advance its thinking about nursing unless ideas can be tried out in practice and evaluated. The only thing worse than a complete absence of new conceptual frameworks being evaluated is one model in place everywhere, the omnipotent RLT model which is *not* being evaluated. But is the omnipotence of the RLT model an illusion as in practice it is merely cosmetic, a fig leaf to cover nursing's conceptual nakedness?

This chapter highlights the need for a range of studies using qualitative as well as quantitive methodologies, to explore how the ideas and concepts inherent in a range of models, including home-grown ones, work in practice. The three dimensions of quality referred to in Chapter 4, patient, professional and managerial should all be utilized in an attempt to get to grips with models and their potential impact. The three studies in this chapter may be thought of as involving patient quality (Hart, 1995 – Orem) and professional quality (Weiss *et al.*, 1994 – Roy; Bellman, 1996 – RLT). There is room for many more such studies but first there has to be the innovation to allow new ideas to be tried out. To the doubting Thomas who questions innovation and all these newfangled models, perhaps the last word belongs to Benjamin Franklin who when asked two centuries ago what was the use of a new invention replied 'What is the use of a new born child?'.

References

Abbey J (1980) The FANCAP assessment scheme. In Riehl JP & Roy C (eds) *Conceptual Models for Nursing Practice,* pp. Norwalk, CT: Appleton Century Crofts.

Bellman L (1996) Changing nursing practice through reflection on the Roper Logan Tierney model: the enhancement approach to action research. *Journal of Advanced Nursing,* **24**, 129–138.

Casey N (1996) Editorial. *Nursing Standard,* **11**(2), 1.

Fraser M (1990) *Using Conceptual Models in Practice: A Research Based Approach.* New York: Harper & Row.

Hart M (1995) Orem's self care deficit theory; research with pregnant women. *Nursing Science Quarterly,* **8**(3), 120–126.

Hartweg DL (1990) Health promotion self-care within Orem's general theory of nursing. *Journal of Advanced Nursing,* **15**, 35–41

Hayward J (1979) *Information: A prescription against pain.* London: Royal College of Nursing.

King I (1981) *A Theory for Nursing.* New York: Wiley.

Logan M (1990) The Roy Adaptation Model: are nursing diagnoses amenable to independent nurse functions? *Journal of Advanced Nursing,* **15**, 468–470.

Rourke Λ (1990) Professional labelling. *Nursing Standard,* **4**(42), 36–39.

Weiss M. Hastings W, Holly W & Craig D (1994) Using Roy's adaptation model in practice. *Nursing Science Quarterly,* **7**(2), 80–86.

Bibliography

Aggleton PJ & Chalmers H (1986) *Nursing Models and the Nursing Process.* Basingstoke: Macmillan.

Vaughan B & Pearson A (1986) *Nursing Models for Practice.* Oxford: Heinemann.

6 Models and Critical Pathways in Adult Hospital-based Care

This chapter aims to explore the requirements and ideal characteristics of a model of nursing suitable for the care of adults in a general hospital setting. These ideals will be tested by using representative patient assessments and care plans based on the Roy (1984), Orem (1990) and Roper, Logan & Tierney models along with the FANCAP assessment scheme. It is hoped that the reader will benefit by seeing how to apply these theoretical models in practice and also it is interesting to see how effectively the models meet the criteria set out at the start of the chapter. Examples are also included of how models may influence critical pathway (CP) development.

Ideal model characteristics

This section is not meant as a definitive list of characteristics essential for a model – it cannot be, as different nurses will have different points of view about nursing and patient priorities. However, the sort of issues raised here might usefully serve as a basis for discussion, or a starting point, when staff are considering models of nursing and what might best fit their own philosophy of care.

The whole thrust of nursing in the last decade has been directed towards seeing the patient as an integrated, individual human being rather than as a piece of malfunctioning anatomy. The patient is a person not 'the mastectomy in bed 3' or 'the man with the leg'. This means that any model of nursing must take into account the patient's psychological and social functioning as well as anatomy and physiology.

Hospitalization is a very stressful event, carrying with it the threats of radical change to the person's body and the way it works or even the possibility of death. The whole network of social roles that have evolved over a lifetime are disrupted, for example roles of worker, parent, spouse or lover, possibly permanently by the hospital experience and its aftermath. The person's very existence may be threatened and their independence removed. In the light of these assaults on a person's psyche, it is evident that nursing care cannot ignore the psychological or closely related social aspects of a patient.

It is possible that the interplay of social and psychological factors was responsible for the patient's illness in the first place. How else can we explain the findings of the by now classic report *Inequalities in Health* (Black *et al.*, 1981)? This major piece of work showed that for most forms of illness and trauma, mortality and morbidity were closely linked to social class – the poorer a person was the more likely they were to suffer or die from any given disease. Much work has been done since the publication of *Inequalities in Health* that suggests this differential persisted throughout the 1980s and into the 1990s (Whitehead, 1987).

Social and environmental factors are a major component of illness and need to be considered not only in relation to causation, but also when planning discharge, for the patient will return to the same sort of environment that contributed to their illness in the first place.

A model of nursing therefore needs to allow the nurse to assess the role played by social and environmental factors in causing the patient's health problems. It should make it possible to explore the patient's anxieties and fears while in hospital and how they feel about the future after discharge. The likely social setting into which the patient will be discharged should feature in the model, together with the effects this may have on the patient's progress both in hospital and subsequently. Insights into the patient's feelings and emotions together with his or her family and social networks must become apparent from the model if the nurse is to achieve the aim of providing integrated, individualized care for the whole patient. The alternative is to resort to the medical model of concentrating only on the malfunctioning piece of anatomy.

Although the psychosocial aspects of care have been emphasized, the nurse must not lose sight of the physiological aspects either. The model should be sensitive to immediate life-threatening problems, to pain, and other essential aspects of bodily function.

The assessment scheme should therefore commence with the 'ABCD of resuscitation' priorities of airway, breathing, circulation and disability. The patient's respiratory and cardiovascular status are normally the highest priority for nursing assessment, followed by pain. The early discharge policy being pursued over the last few years coupled with the changing demographic profile of the general population has meant that the hospital population has become increasingly dependent and frail. The ability to cope or self-care is therefore pivotal to discharge and links to areas such as mobility are essential if a whole host of potential problems are to be avoided. Other key areas such as fluid balance and nutrition, along with personal hygiene and wound care, must also feature prominently in the assessment if problems relating to these areas are to be detected or, better still, prevented. The patient's mental status under-pins all these areas, however, for if they are confused or depressed, this will have a major impact on such aspects of care.

The reality of many hospitals today is a very rapid turnover of patients leading to discharge becoming ever sooner. The hard-pressed community services, however, cannot provide the level of care that the hospital can. This not only requires the nurse to have an increased awareness of social factors (as discussed above) but it also emphasizes the need for hospital nursing care increasingly to pre-pare the patient for self-care at home. Patients need more knowledge about areas such as managing their diet or medication, caring for wounds or carrying out physiotherapy after discharge.

The traditional nursing role of acting for the patient is no longer adequate for the patient's needs. Early-discharge policies require nurses to promote independence and self-care while the patient is in the supervised environment of the ward. Patients should be able to show that they are technically competent to perform whatever tasks are required and have the necessary understanding of what is involved before they can be safely discharged. The model of nursing in use therefore should lay emphasis on the nurse teaching the patient and/or family to be self-caring. A health education, patient teaching approach to nursing should be a major constituent of such a model. This would reflect a greater awareness of nursing being involved in the active promotion of health, rather than an exclusive focus on caring for the ill.

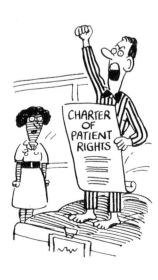

The self-care approach leads the nurse into negotiation with the patient, which in turn results in the realization that the patient also has a point of view. Nurses cannot plan care that ignores the patient's wishes and perceptions. The basic human rights of patients dictate that they must consent to the care being carried out and that consent should be informed consent. Nurses must explain not only what they are doing but why, and seek the patient's approval. In that way patient co-operation is much more likely, leading to the like-lihood that care will be more effective.

It is possible that a patient's apparent lack of co-operation simply stems from a deeply held, but erroneous, belief. Areas such as diet or sexual behaviour abound with such beliefs. Only when the nurse has discovered what the patient believes can his or her behaviour be put in context and more fully understood. Consider the following real example of a 55-year-old male surgical patient who continued to smoke 20 cigarettes a day despite every exhortation to the contrary pre- and post-operatively because he believed this was good for him. The reason he gave was that it allowed him to 'Have a good cough and bring up all that phlegm'. Seen from that point of view there is logic to his actions and, given that insight, the nurse now has a more realistic chance of persuading him to give up or at least reduce the smoking. The nurse might do well to try seeing a situation from the patient's perspective, things may not seem so illogical that way!

The model of nursing chosen therefore needs to be able to recognize the patient's point of view and if possible, explore beliefs and attitudes held about areas relevant to health.

The demographic changes referred to earlier are reflected in the increasing number of elderly hospital patients. The elderly have different needs from the young and middle-aged adult population. The later years of life are marked by substantial physical changes in the body, and also by social changes as families grow away from their elderly parents, who in their turn face increasing dependency upon their adult sons and daughters. Changes such as retirement, moving home and bereavement require great adaptation on the part of the elderly. A model of nursing therefore needs to acknowledge the rapidly changing nature of an elderly person's life. It is easy to think of the elderly as static and unchanging. Once that mistake has been made, the nurse is no longer thinking of an elderly person as a living human being, rather that person has become fossilized. A developmental perspective is therefore essential that acknowledges the dynamic, changing nature of the patient's world, whatever their age.

One final area that has to be discussed is the question of how 'user friendly' the model is. Hospital wards are very busy places and theoreticians should temper their deliberations with a healthy dose of realism. This suggests that a model should be capable of providing a comprehensive assessment, but in a reasonable amount of time, and producing a care plan that is practical. Excessive use of jargon is counterproductive, although there is no reason why nurses should not convert difficult language into more readily understood English whatever the model.

For the successful use of a model, both nurse and patient need to be able to see the practical relevance of its ideas and concepts to the real world.

Summary

The ideal model of nursing for adult general wards should have the following characteristics.

- It needs to show the patient as an integrated, individual human being with psychological and social components. Problems in these fields must be readily identified.
- It should permit immediate identification of physiological problems, particularly relating to life-threatening conditions involving the respiratory and cardiovascular systems, and also pain.
- The model must have a developmental dimension allowing for ageing and its associated changes.
- The ability of the patient to function outside the hospital must be a key element in care; models therefore should ideally be applicable in a community setting as well as in hospital.
- There needs to be emphasis on health education and patient teaching.
- The patient's point of view must be recognized as important and actively fed into the care planning process. Questions such as why the patient holds a point of view need to be explored.
- The model must be realistic and practical to apply.

The four models of nursing that are considered in this chapter are each applied in turn to two different but representative patients. The reader is invited to test the models against the above list, adding ideas of their own as appropriate.

Example 1: **The Orem model in acute medicine;** John Harper

John Harper is a 55-year-old married bus driver with a history of angina and mild hypertension. He awoke this morning feeling unwell and collapsed with severe gripping central chest pain. His wife dialled 999 and he was brought to A&E where a medical diagnosis of acute myocardial infarction was made and he was admitted to CCU after 5 mg IV diamorphine and 12.5 mg IM prochloperazine were given. There follows an assessment and care plan based on Orem's model which could be adapted to suit many patients with an acute medical condition who are largely confined to bed.

Normal self-care ability (prior to admission)	Current self-care ability (after admission)	Self-care deficit (patient problem)
AERATION Breathing normal except on exertion when becomes short of breath (SOB) and develops chest pain which is relieved by rest and GTN. Smokes 20/day, has smokers' cough at times, no sputum at present.	RR 12, shallow. Skin pale. BP 90/60 P86 Unable to cough. ECG sinus rhythm occasional vent ectopics, ST elevation II, III, aVf. No pain at present.	(1) Inadequate ventilation (A). (2) Unstable heart rate, possible arrhythmias (P). (3) Unable to cough (A). (4) Chest pain (P).

Normal self-care ability (prior to admission)	Current self-care ability (after admission)	Self-care deficit (patient problem)
FLUID BALANCE Normal intake of fluid except likes a few pints of beer several times a week. No probs passing urine, gets up once a night to p.u.	Too drowsy to drink, feels nauseous. Cannot walk to toilet.	(5) Unable to drink at present (A). (6) Cannot p.u. in toilet (A). (7) Feels nauseous (A).
NUTRITION Ht 1.72 m Wt 90 kg. Pays little heed to health ed. advice. High saturated fat low roughage diet. Bowels irregular.	Too drowsy to eat. Cannot walk to toilet.	(8) Cannot walk to toilet (A). (9) Poor diet (A,L). (10) Overweight (A,L). (11) Constipation (A,L).
ACTIVITY/REST Works as bus driver. Hobbies: plays darts for pub, watches TV a lot, supports local football team. Sleeps well, 7 h.	Drowsy, sleepy. Bed rest 48 h.	(12) Pressure sores (P). (13) Inadequate exercise (A,L).
SOLITUDE/SOCIALIZATION Married, 2 married sons both live near. Outgoing popular man. Owns own house.	Not saying much as drowsy. Looks anxiously around CCU when eyes open.	(14) Feelings of isolation in unfamiliar surroundings (P).
HAZARDS Has not paid heed to advice re diet, smoking, drinking, etc.	Sleepy and drowsy, though appears oriented at present.	(15) May fall if tries to get out of bed (P).
NORMALCY Happy person, jokes about being overweight and BP/angina problems.	Anxious, has asked 'Am I going to die?' but said later 'Don't feel right here, let me go home.'	(16) Anxious about being in CCU/ diagnosis (A).
DEVELOPMENTAL Recently became grandfather, delighted! No worries re job, bought council house had lived in for many years.	Realizes seriousness of condition, anxious about death.	(17) Anxious about diagnosis (A). (18) May become depressed (P,L).
HEALTH DEVIANCY Reluctant to see GP. Takes GTN for angina, Atenolol for BP. See 'Hazards'.	Occluded coronary artery for which is receiving streptokinase therapy. Diamorphine prescribed for pain IM.	(19) Bleeding disorder (P). (20) Chest pain (P). (21) Non-compliance with health education advice (P,L).

The care plan needs to take the 21 problems identified here and prioritize them. The six long-term problems are unlikely to be of much significance during his 24–28 h on CCU, which leaves 15 short-term problems that need to be ordered in some sort of priority. The reader should consider how many of these could be included in a CP for any patient on CCU, and also how many are relevant when the patient moves to a general ward.

Care plan from 10:00 25/1/97

Problem	Goal	Nursing care
(1) Cardiac arrhythmias (P).	(a) Sinus rhythm. (b) P70–85. BP95/60–130/90.	1. Continual 3-lead ECG monitor. 2. Bed rest. 3. Give medication as prescribed. 4. Record P, BP hourly. 5. Give correct medication.
(2) Unable to maintain normal respiration (A).	RR12–18	1. Monitor RR, inform Dr if < 12. 2. Give O_2 via nasal canulae 40%, 4 l/min.
(3) Chest pain which Pt cannot relieve (P).	No pain will be felt.	1. Reduce anxiety (see (4)). 2. Give analgesia prn. 3. Ensure comfort.
(4) Anxiety (A).	Pt will state understands what is happening.	1. Give explanations about equipment and progress. 2. Encourage Pt to ask and answer questions. 3. Keep family informed of progress, visiting times, etc.
(5) Bleeding due to streptokinase (P).	Pt will not suffer internal haemorrhage.	1. Monitor stools for occult blood, urine for haematuria. 2. Check for headaches.
(6) Unable to maintain fluid balance (A).	Intake of 2.5 l fluid/24 h.	1. Monitor & care for IVI. 2. Offer oral fluids (see 7:2). 3. Give anti-emetics. 4. Fluid balance chart.
(7) Feels nauseous (A).	Pt will not vomit.	1. Give anti-emetics. 2. Small sips of oral fluids.
(8) Cannot walk to toilet (A).	Urine output > 1.5 l/day.	1. Put urinal in convenient place. 2. Monitor urine output. 3. Ensure privacy while in use.
(9) Unable to relieve pressure on bony prominences (A).	Pt will not develop red or broken areas of skin.	1. Turn 2-hrly. 2. Encourage Pt to turn self. 3. Explain need for turning.
(10) Unable to attend to personal hygiene (A).	Pt will state is satisfied with hygiene.	1. Bed bath. 2. Progressively encourage Pt to wash self, etc.

The care plan outlined above sufficed for the first 24 h on CCU. The problems are written from the point of view of self-care and many therefore reflect things that the patient cannot do for himself. Goals are set consequently in terms of outcomes that the patient will achieve (e.g. Nos 3, 8, 9 and 10). The health deviancy aspect of Orem's model has led the nurse to identify problems relating to the immediate disease problem (Nos 1, 3) and to the side-effects of medications which are being administered, such as the risk of respiratory depression (No. 2) or nausea (No. 7) due to opioid analgesia and bleeding due to streptokinase therapy (No. 5).

Assessment of normalcy suggests that the patient feels anything but normal, he is distressed at being in the strange surroundings of a CCU and this anxiety is compounding the anxiety he is experiencing as he realizes he has suffered a potentially fatal medical emergency. This has made him aware of the possibility of death which he raised when the nurse asked him how he felt.

In this first 24 h after admission the nursing staff will be carrying out a large proportion of the care required by Mr Harper as he is unable to care for himself. This is logically described by Orem as a wholly compensatory nursing system and aims to accomplish therapeutic self-care for the patient by compensating for his inability to do so himself. Even so, the following morning the patient will be given a washbowl and encouraged to wash his own hands and face as a step back towards self-care.

Mr Harper fortunately developed no further complications on CCU and was transferred to a general medical ward the day after admission. Several of the problems that characterized the first 24 h now disappear as changes in medication diminish potential side-effects such as nausea and respiratory depression and it is deemed safe to allow the patient to take a more active role in his self-care. For example, he can now be encouraged to wash himself in the bathroom and walk to the toilet. After transfer to the ward, problems such as Nos 2, 6, 7, 8, 9 and 10 drop off the care plan and are replaced by some new concerns as care focuses on psychosocial areas and patient teaching ready for discharge. The following three problems now need to be added to the care plan:

Problem	Goal	Nursing care
(11) Pt anxious and withdrawn (A).	Pt will talk about why he is so anxious.	1. Discuss progress with Pt in privacy. 2. Ask if he wants to ask any questions. 3. Talk with family.
(12) Pt fears he is useless now. Afraid of sex & losing job (A).	Pt understands can continue 'normal' independent life.	1. Allow Pt to talk about worries. 2. Discuss cardiac rehab. programme. 3. Offer health ed. leaflets. 4. Involve family in discussions. 5. Introduce Pt to another who has made good recovery. 6. Emphasize positive action as in prob. (13). 7. Refer for cardiac rehab. programme.

(13) Has shown a lack of motivation to follow health education advice re smoking, diet, alcohol intake & exercise (A).	(a) Pt will discuss these topics and how they affect his condition.	1. Talk to Pt/wife, review Universal S/C demands from health ed. perspective, encourage questions. 2. Give Pt health ed. leaflets. 3. Discuss medication for angina & BP.
	(b) Pt will agree series of goals with wife to (i) stop smoking, (ii) lose 10 kg in 4 months, (iii) reduce alcohol intake by 50%, (iv) change diet to high-fibre low-saturated fat.	1. As above. 2. Negotiate goals that are acceptable to Pt/wife, such as (i)–(iv). 3. Make appointment to see dietitian. 4. Refer cardiac rehab.

The nurse used Orem's concept of developmental self-care to explore with Mr Harper how he saw his life going after discharge and discovered negative perceptions about his future. He is afraid of losing his job and fears problems with his sex life and hence his relationship with his wife and family. These developmental self-care deficits are well described in Orem's model and form a key area of nursing intervention over the next few days prior to discharge. This is a good example of the holistic nature of nursing which is concerned with far more than restoring Mr Harper's myocardium to a healthy state.

The health deviancy aspect of Orem's model also led the nurse to explore the area of health education with Mr Harper to see if he would be more willing to practise self-care in this area. This involves knowing and dealing with the effects of pathology, improving health through active self-care and taking medication with a full understanding of possible side-effects. There is therefore a serious health education agenda opened up by Orem's model that the nurse has to tackle with Mr Harper before discharge. This rehabilitation and health improvement programme continues after discharge, however, and the nursing staff on the ward must ensure that the cardiac rehabilitation services are fully informed about Mr Harper. The notion of dependent care agency must also be explored; that is, the ability of his wife to be involved in care after discharge. It is likely, for example, that she will continue to cook his food and can play a major role in modifying his diet while she too must understand that their sex life can continue normally.

As the patient is transferred from CCU to the ward the nurse withdraws from the wholly compensatory nursing system into a partially compensatory system. In this way he or she may still do some things for the patient but assists him to do others and encourages him to carry out other tasks independently. By discharge the nurse is operating in a supportive–educative nursing system where the patient is carrying out self-care completely and the nurse is providing support, teaching and direction to the patient and family.

Orem's model is very appropriate for patients suffering from a myocardial infarct as the whole aim of care is the speedy return home of a largely self-caring person who has the necessary understanding and motivation to manage their medication and life style in such a way as to maximize their health status. However, this statement highlights a key assumption in Orem's work; that is, that patients want to be self-caring. Self-care implies that patients want power and control over their health which as Smith and Draper (1994) suggest may not be so. Their research suggested that nurses wanted more control over their own personal health than their patients actually did. We should therefore be careful not to judge people by our own standards and automatically assume that patients do want a high degree of control over their own health. This needs to be explored as part of the assessment process as it has clear implications for the willingness of patients to undertake self-care and hence for the appropriateness of Orem's model in some circumstances.

An alternative approach involving the use of a CP is given below. This CP incorporates Orem's model with its emphasis on self-care and patient management of medication. It is, however, a single multidisciplinary document that can be used by all the staff and which gives the nurse extra information such as what tests are due when, what the doctors are planning to do, what referrals have been made and how plans for discharge are proceeding. All staff also know the outcomes that are being sought by other colleagues on different days such as activity levels, pain relief, knowledge of cardiac rehabilitation, etc.

The monitoring of variances against this pathway may show any problems that occur with for example streptokinase therapy or what proportion of patients develop other complications such as arrhythmias and what effect this has on length of stay. Making explicit outcomes, such as patient knowledge about management of future angina attacks or sexual activity, allows monitoring of the effectiveness of patient teaching in such important areas of self-care. Apart from improving the quality of the patient's stay in hospital, this approach also makes it easy to answer queries concerning length of stay from purchasers of health care such as fundholding GPs or health authorities. It may, for example, be possible to show that the development of arrhythmias extends length of stay by an average of 3 days which explains why certain patients are in hospital longer than others and therefore cost more to treat.

Table 1 Critical pathway for uncomplicated myocardial infarction incorporating Orem's self-care conceptual framework

Aspects of care	Day 1: CCU	Day 2: Ward
Assessment	Cardiac monitor Vital signs (VS) 1/2-hrly (if on streptokinase) VS hrly if not on streptokinase Pulse oxymetry S/S bleeding Nausea Pain Height/weight Diaphoresis Anxiety, feelings about being on CCU Orientation, mental status 2 hrly Risk factors such as smoking, family history, diet, exercise Full systems examination Understanding of what has happened and Pt's view of health status	SS bleeding VS hrly if on streptokinase VS 2–4 hrly if not on stpknse. Breath sounds S/S heart failure Feelings/anxiety Pain Ability to learn Motivation to self-care Understanding of health status Domestic circumstances Check fit transfer to ward
	Outcomes Above assessment complete within 2 h On-going assessment carried out as per CP. Vital signs within normal limits Sinus rhythm Clear breath sounds	*Outcomes* Vital signs within normal limits No S/S heart failure Pain free Pt verbalizes feelings Assessment of psychosocial status complete
Referrals		Dietitian
		Outcome Referral made
Tests	Cardiac enzymes Full blood count, U&Es Blood glucose 12-lead ECG Chest X-ray INR	Repeat enzymes INR if on anti-coagulant Rx Repeat 12-lead ECG
	Outcomes Tests complete within 1 h admission	*Outcome* Tests completed Results known where possible
Medications	Thrombolytic therapy if meets criteria Opioid analgesia/anti-emetic Nitrates and/or inotropes as indicated (topical, oral or IV as appropriate) Heparin Anti-hypertensive as indicated	As for Day 1 except for thrombolytic therapy
	Outcomes Thrombolytic therapy started within 30 min if not already begun before admission Pain free, no nausea or vomiting Medication given as per script	*Outcome* Medication given as per script Pain free

Table 1 Continued

Aspects of care	Day 1: CCU	Day 2: Ward

Teaching	Orientate to CCU
	Explain: monitor, IVs, treatment, etc.
	      importance of reporting chest pain
	      MI and how it affects Pt
	Discuss CP with Pt/family
	
	Outcome
	Done within 1 h admission
		Orientate to ward
		Begin cardiac teaching re smoking, diet, exercise
		Explain balance between rest/activity on ward
		
		Outcomes
		Teaching carried out
		Pt shows evidence of understanding

Self-care	Give O_2 2–4 l/min Low fat, low Na diet Monitor fluid balance Urinal/commode at bed side Bed rest Bed bath in am Give nurse call buzzer Offer emotional support, explore feelings *Outcomes* O_2 saturation > 90% Fluid intake > 2 l in 24 h Output > 1.5 l in 24 h > 6 h sleep Self-care achieved Pt talks about feelings	Sit out of bed 3 × 2 h Use commode, urinal Monitor fluid balance Low fat, low Na diet Wash with assistance Offer emotional support, talk about feelings, coping *Outcomes* Fluid intake > 2 l/24 h Output > 1.5 l/24 h > 6 h sleep Pt satisfied with personal hygiene Pt has talked about coping and how he or she feels
Discharge	Talk to family re time to discharge *Outcome* Family visit and discuss progress	Check whether social worker needs to be involved Transfer to med. ward *Outcomes* Social worker contacted if needed Pt settled on med. ward

Aspect of care	Day 3	Day 4
Assessment	As for Day 2	VS 06.00 & 10.00 As for Day 3 otherwise
Referrals	Physio for mobilization Cardiac rehab. programme *Outcomes* Seen by dietitian Mobilizes with physio	 *Outcome* Seen by rehab. nurse
Tests	As for Day 2	12-lead ECG

Table 1 Continued

Aspect of care	Day 3	Day 4
Medication	Oral analgesia Stool softener Nitrates oral or topical Anti-coagulant Other medication as prescribed *Outcomes* Pain free Bowel movement without straining Medication given as prescribed	Stool softener Nitrates oral/topical Anti-coagulant Other medication as prescribed *Outcome* As for Day 3
Teaching	Continue with cardiac teaching programme: how to cope with chest pain, side-effects of medication, sexual activity and work *Outcomes* Pt can state correct action to take if experiences pain, can describe effects and side-effects of medication Pt begins to talk about work/sexual activity	Review knowledge of risk factors, limits of activity, work, sexual activity, how to cope with chest pain, knowledge of medication Explain cardiac rehab. programme *Outcome* Pt demonstrates adequate knowledge of above
Self-care	Uses bathroom/toilet independently Out of bed during day Low fat/low Na diet Discuss feelings/emotions Explore coping mechanisms Mobilize with physio *Outcomes* Can attend to personal hygiene unaided Sits out of bed for 8 h Talks about feelings and coping Can walk 20 m unaided	Continue emotional support Mobilize with physio Low fat/low Na diet Self-caring for personal hygiene *Outcomes* Can climb flight of stairs Cares for own personal hygiene Expresses positive views about coping after discharge
Discharge	Discuss discharge plans with Pt and family, checking suitability of home environment If needed involve DN/GP Discuss with social worker Arrange transport Get medication written up for discharge *Outcomes* Above carried out and family/Pt willing for discharge Prescription ready to take to pharmacy Transport arranged	Arrange follow-up appointment Medicines from pharmacy Letter to GP Check referred to rehab. Decide whether fit for discharge today or tomorrow *Outcomes* Ready for discharge to safe home environment today or tomorrow Follow-up appointments all made Takes medication home Letter sent to GP

NB Discharge will probably take place on Day 5 in which case the CP for Day 4 continues into Day 5. The CP given above is an indicative example and local policies will obviously vary from this CP.

Example 2:	**The Orem model in trauma care;** Mabel Bush

Mabel Bush is an 81-year-old widow who lives alone in her own house. She fell during the night, sustaining an intertrochanteric fracture of her left femur and lay on the floor until a neighbour found her this morning. Her medical notes indicate that she has been treated for atrial fibrillation and heart failure requiring two admissions in the last 3 years, her latest being 6 months ago when she was discharged on a regime of frusemide, digoxin and potassium supplements in the form of effervescent tablets. She was admitted to the ward at 13:30 from A&E and has been scheduled for internal fixation on tomorrow morning's operating list.

Assessment at 14.00 on admission 22/1/97

Normal self-care ability (prior to admission)	*Current self-care ability (after admission)*	*Self-care deficit (patient problem)*
AERATION Breathless if has to walk more than 20 m on flat. Only takes stairs slowly. Non-smoker. 'A bit chesty in winter'.	RR22 sounds 'rattly', no cough, skin pale. BP110/60, P98 irreg. T35.5°C.	(1) Unable to maintain adequate circulation due to heart failure. (2) Chest infection (P).
FLUID BALANCE Complains of going to toilet a lot especially at night so does not drink much in case of accidents. Has little idea of when to take frusemide.	Skin appears very dry. Reluctant to drink. Clothes were wet with urine on admission, passed 80 ml of cloudy urine, protein++, offensive smell.	(3) Appears dehydrated, unable to achieve own rehydration (A). (4) Urine infection is probable (A). (5) Unable to p.u. on her own (A).
NUTRITION Ht 1.52 m Wt 40–45 kg (estimated) looks frail. Does not bother to cook for self often. Snack diet low in roughage, vits, protein. Constipation for which takes liquid paraffin.	Not interested in food. Bowels last open 2 days ago, no urge to defecate at present.	(6) Constipation (A). (7) Poor diet leading to malnourishment (A,L).
ACTIVITY/REST Manages stairs slowly, good manual dexterity. Can only walk 20 m with aid of stick (see aeration). Poor sleeper, catnaps during day. Reads a lot, enjoys needlework, knitting.	#L femur, pain rated 2 on a 5-point scale at rest, 4 if attempts movement. Cannot turn in bed due to #. Norton Score=12. Cannot wash self except hands & face.	(8) Pain which she cannot relieve (A). (9) Cannot prevent pressure sores developing (P). (10) Cannot see to personal hygiene (A).
SOLITUDE/SOCIALIZATION Lives alone. No family in area. Neighbour sees she is OK each day, shops for her once/week. Sees old friends once/twice week. Admits lonely at times.	No family notified yet. Neighbour has locked up house, has been told by A&E of diagnosis.	(11) Family/friends unaware she is in hospital (A). (12) May become lonely (P).

Normal self-care ability (prior to admission)	Current self-care ability (after admission)	Self-care deficit (patient problem)
HAZARDS Worried about living alone in big house, has been afraid of falling.	Confined to bed by injury & traction. Will need surgery and general anaesthetic (GA).	(13) Risks of surgery under GA tomorrow (P).
NORMALCY Feels isolated since husband died 5 years ago, misses him a great deal. Feels the world just passes her by now.	'I want to go home.' Very tearful, does not understand or accept her injury despite pain.	(14) Anxious and distressed (A). (15) Lack of understanding may lead to confusion (P).
DEVELOPMENTAL Widowed 5 years, retired 21 years. Two sons, one lives Australia, other 320 km away with own family. No close family just some old friends.	Very distressed now. 'I don't want to be a burden, I've had a long life, there's nobody left, just let me die.'	(16) Sees no point in living, lacks motivation to carry on (A).
HEALTH DEVIANCY Does not like doctors, rarely sees GP. Is not aware of effects of medication she is on or of correct time/dose.	#L femur. Does not appear to accept injury. ECG = atrial fibrillation.	(17) Will not follow prescribed medication (P,L). (18) Does not accept or understand injury (A).

Care plan 14:00 22/1/97 to surgery 11:00 (approx) 23/1/97

Problem	Goal	Nursing care
(1) Pain which Pt cannot relieve (A).	Pt will be pain free.	1. Give prn analgesia as needed. 2. Try to reduce anxiety. 3. Ensure comfort.
(2) Pt appears very distressed and anxious (A).	Pt will appear calm and talk about her fears.	1. Listen to what Pt is saying. 2. Try to see things from her point of view. 3. Offer explanations and answer questions. 4. Contact son. 5. See prob. (1).
(3) Pt unable to prevent pressure sores (P).	Skin will be unbroken, no red areas.	1. 2-h pressure care. 2. Ripple mattress. 3. Check traction 2-hrly. 4. Sheepskin for R heel/sacrum.
(4) Pt unable to maintain hydration (A).	Fluid intake 2.5 l by 11:00, 23.1.97.	1. Explain importance of oral hydration to Pt. 2. Provide drinks she likes. 3. Encourage drinking. 4. Fluid balance chart. 5. Discuss IVI with Dr if 1–3 not successful.
(5) Urinary infection.	Pt will have no UTI in 5/7.	1. Take MSU. 2. See prob. (4). 3. Administer antibiotics.

Problem	Goal	Nursing care
(6) Unable to maintain continence (P).	No incontinence of urine.	1. Use slipper bedpan. 2. Offer to Pt hourly. 3. Give Pt nurse call buzzer. 4. Ensure privacy when on bedpan.
(7) Unable to maintain good circulation (A).	Good cardiac output as shown by P60–80, reg. BP120/60–150/90, RR< 22.	1. Monitor BP, RR, P 2–4-hrly. 2. Support back with pillows in sitting position. 3. Give medication as prescribed.
(8) May lose orientation, confusion (P).	Will be oriented in time & space.	1. Give detailed explanations. 2. Ensure spectacles available. 3. Keep informed of time.
(9) Hazards of surgery under GA on 23.1.97	Pt will have no complications from surgery.	1. NBM from 05:00. 2. IVI overnight (see prob. (4)). 3. Follow standard pre-op prep. 4. Discuss surgery with Pt.
(10) Pt unable to maintain own hygiene (A).	Will state she is satisfied with hygiene.	1. Give bed bath. 2. Encourage maximum self-care during bed bath.

The above care plan saw Mrs Bush through to surgery 24 h after admission. The assessment highlighted her pain and the potential for several problems, especially confusion and disorientation associated with several factors. The disruption in her normal living and her enforced move to a strange and highly stressful situation may be compounded by the side-effects of opioid analgesia, dehydration, urinary tract infection and cerebral hypoxia associated with heart failure. Clouding of consciousness will impair her ability to self-care across all of Orem's key areas and seriously disrupt her recovery from surgery. This is therefore a key area for nursing care in addition to the obvious requirement of pain relief. The nursing staff were working largely in a wholly compensatory nursing system in this first 24 h as Mrs Bush could do little for herself and the main aim was to deliver her to theatre in the best possible condition for surgery.

A re-assessment carried out after surgery saw several changes in priority as problems associated with preparation for theatre had obviously been dealt with while new problems had arisen in the health deviancy area as a result of the surgery (described by Orem as the deleterious effects of medical treatment). These are summarized in the care plan below and relate to factors such as the wound and a post-operative chest infection. Her lack of knowledge concerning medication was another aspect of health deviancy self-care that was important in progressing to discharge.

Problem	Goal	Nursing care
(11) Wound over L hip.	Wound will heal by 3.2.97 with no infection.	1. Care of wound drains. 2. Remove drains if drainage <25 ml/12 h. 3. Monitor wound dressing for signs of infection, change only if needs changing. 4. Remove sutures when Dr instructs.
(12) Pt has chest infection.	RR & T will be normal in 5/7.	1. Monitor vital signs 4-hrly. 2. Encourage coughing, deep breathing between physio visits. 3. Sit upright. 4. Give medication as prescribed.
(13) Pt reluctant to mobilize.	Pt will walk 20 m with zimmer by 29.1.97.	1. Explain advantages of mobility. 2. Offer encouragement. 3. Ensure analgesia given 1 h before exercise. 4. Set limited goals day by day.
(14) Pt reluctant to drink.	Fluid intake 2.5 l oral/day.	1. Explain importance of drinking. 2. Ensure ready access to toilet. 3. Fluid balance chart. 4. Ensure drinks are what she likes. 5. Give frequent encouragement.
(15) Pt is eating very little.	Dietary intake of 2000 kcal/day by 29.1.97.	1. Discuss importance of eating. 2. Offer small meals more often. 3. Find out preferred foods. 4. Provide dietary supplements in form of drinks. 5. Consult dietitian.
(16) Pt is tearful at times and withdrawn.	Pt will talk of future plans in positive way.	1. Spend time finding out her point of view & listening to her. 2. Encourage son to visit. 3. Enquire if she wishes to see a minister of religion. 4. Talk positively of the future but realistically. 5. Contact social worker to see what support is needed/ available. 6. Encourage maximum independence while in ward. 7. Try and give Pt sense of control over what is happening, involve in all decisions.
(17) Pt has poor knowledge of medication.	Pt will state purpose, dose & time of different drugs by discharge.	1. Tell Pt about drugs as given. 2. On 30.1.97 give teaching session.

Problem	Goal	Nursing care
		3. On 31.1.97 check how much remembered.
		4. Reinforce teaching on subsequent days.
		5. Provide written instructions.

Her frail condition made progress towards self-care a slow affair. Nursing staff were unable to move beyond a partially compensatory system of nursing care and Mrs Bush's view that 'nurses were there to care for her, after all they were supposed to know what was best', suggested that she did not want to take control of her care in the way that some nurses might wish. However, if she was to be fit for discharge she had to achieve a certain level of self-care. Final discharge plans would depend upon how much self-care ability could be recovered. A range of options was discussed with her ranging from going back to her large house on her own to selling the house and getting a small bungalow or moving into a residential home. Aspects such as the balance between solitude and socialization were important while the developmental self-care area made the nurse aware of issues such as the effects of change of residence to an unfamiliar environment, loss of neighbours and friends, problems of social adaptation and the effects of long-term disability.

It was possible to work through these problems sympathetically with Mrs Bush and help her come to terms with the fact that she would not be able to manage in her old house on her own and that a sheltered housing development might offer her the best balance between maintaining her status as an independent person yet having aspects of life she could no longer cope with taken care of. It also offered her an acceptable balance between solitude (privacy) and socialization that would not be found in a residential home. Eventually, a co-ordinated self-care policy between nurses and therapists succeeded in returning Mrs Bush to the community, ambulant with the aid of a stick, living in her own ground floor flat within a sheltered housing project.

In examples 1 and 2, the Orem assessment headings have been adapted so that the four universal self-care needs of intake of air, water, food and excretion have been amended to the three headings of aeration, fluid balance and nutrition. This has been done to give a more integrated approach to each of the three basic physiological parameters of air, food and water. The concept of aeration more accurately describes what the body is actually doing, as simply taking air into the body is only the beginning of a complex process involving both the cardiovascular and respiratory systems.

Example 3: **The Roy adaptation model in surgery;** Charlie Hackworth

Charlie Hackworth is a 74-year-old married man who has been admitted for a right below-knee amputation due to peripheral vascular disease. He has been diagnosed diabetic for 8 years, for which he takes glibenclamide and relies on diet for control. This assessment was carried out on 20.2.97 after he had been admitted for surgery the following day. As an area of maladaptive or problem behaviour is described in the first-level assessment it is underlined and numbered[1]. The second-level assessment then focuses on that behaviour and seeks to explain it in accordance with Roy's ideas of immediate cause (focal stimulus), environmental factors (contextual stimulus) and previous experiences, attitudes and beliefs (residual stimulus). As far as possible the nursing care should be designed around the second-level assessment which is attempting to discover the causes of the patient's problems.

First-level assessment	Second-level assessment		
	Focal	*Contextual*	*Residual*
(1) PHYSIOLOGY *Oxygenation*: RR20 BP180/100 P84[1] Smoked 30/day for 60 years.[2] Occasional cough. L foot cold, gangrenous 3–5th toes, R foot cool, pulse weak.[3]	(1) CVD.	Diabetes. Smoker.	Belief smoking does no harm.
	(2) Addiction to nicotine.		See (1).
	(3) See (1).	See (1).	See (1).
Fluid balance: Appears hydrated. Drinks average 12 pts beer/wk,[4] does not like coffee.	(4) Enjoys beer.	Likes pub company.	Belief drinking does no harm.
Nutrition: Ht 1.8 m Wt 92 kg	(5) Poor diet.	Wife does all cooking.	Traditional beliefs about diet.
Looks overweight,[5] admits he eats a lot of sweet food, but protests he eats little bread, only a few chips, no rice or pasta. Has poor knowledge of current thinking on dietary control of diabetes.[6]	(6) Has not bothered to update on current thought.	Does not like GP so reluctant to attend.	See (5).
Elimination: Bowels open every 2 days, no problems. Difficulty in starting passing urine, has to get up every night, some dribbling.[7]	(7) Prostatic enlargement.		
Rest & exercise: Sleeps 7 h a night. Can only walk 50 m[8] when calf pain forces him to stop.	(8) Intermittent claudication.		
Regulation: Pain on walking[9] in L leg. Non-insulin-dependent diabetes[10] since 1988. Good hearing, glasses worn for reading. T 37.3°C[11].	(9) See (8). (10) Failure of pancreas to make enough insulin.	Overweight.	See (5).

First-level assessment	Second-level assessment		
	Focal	Contextual	Residual
	(11) Infection of gangrenous toes.		
(2) SELF-CONCEPT *Physical*: Understands will have below-knee amputation. Very <u>worried how he will manage</u>[12] to get about, especially stairs. <u>Anxious</u>[13] in case other leg goes the same way. <u>Sickened by sight</u>[13] of L foot. *Personal*: Feels he just will not be the same person, <u>very anxious</u>[13] will wake up in op.	(12) Loss of leg. (13) Fears spread of disease. (14) Gangrene. (15) Fear of anaesthetic.	Large 3-storey house. Has seen another Pt with bilateral amputation.	Fear 'I am rotting away'. Heard of Pts waking up during ops.
(3) INTERDEPENDENCY Always been self-reliant, does not want to cause any bother to people. Feels his wife depends on him a lot, <u>anxious</u>[13] how she will cope while he is in hospital.	(16) Hospitaliza-tion for surgery.	Wife lives 32 km away, no car.	Believes it is his job to look after her.
(4) ROLE FUNCTION Retired engineer though very active still as odd job man. Father of 3 children who all live nearby, enjoys being granddad. <u>Worried how they will think of him now.</u>[1]	(17) Surgery.		Fears he may become a burden on family.

There are three components in writing a care plan for Charlie: the need to prepare him safely for surgery tomorrow, the need to plan care that will deal with the effects of surgery, and finally the need to tackle the long-term health problems that will remain after discharge.

The assessment allows the intial stage of the care plan to focus on the key physiological areas of care necessary to prepare Mr Hackworth for surgery but it also discloses that the area of anxiety goes deeper than losing a leg. It shows a man very concerned about his role within the family and therefore indicates to the nurse that in talking to the patient, he or she needs to focus on a range of things to try and deal with his fear and anxiety. Talking optimistically about how effective a prosthesis can be and how many other patients have successfully adapted to amputation is not enough. It is necessary to begin to explore how the patient sees himself in the family and how he sees his wife and the relationship between them. Such issues cannot be resolved in one talk on the eve of surgery, but they can be put on the agenda and returned to later post-operatively as part of the preparation for discharge.

Pre-operative care plan

Problem	Goal	Nursing care
(1) Abnormal blood sugar levels (P).	Capillary blood glucose (CBG) 4–9 mmol/l.	1. Give medication. 2. Check CBG level 4-hrly. 3. Ensure correct diet. 4. Care of insulin/glucose IVI when NBM.
(2) Anxiety and fear (A).	Pt will talk of his fears.	1. Encourage Pt to talk. 2. Discuss how wife will manage without him. 3. Discuss his role in the family. 4. Talk positively about artificial leg and the advantages of increased mobility and less pain. 5. Teach about what to expect pre- and post-op. 6. Cover L foot with dressing.
(3) Poor circulation to lower limbs (A).	R foot still shows no signs of gangrene.	1. Avoid trauma to foot. 2. Discuss measures that can be taken by Pt after discharge to care for foot.
(4) Difficulty passing urine (P).	Pt will pass 1 l urine by 08:00 21.2.97.	1. Encourage upright position when using bottle. 2. Show where toilets are. 3. Fluid intake >1 l by 24:00.
(5) Hazards of going for surgery (P).	Pt will suffer no avoidable complications.	1. Follow standard pre-op preparation. 2. See probs. (1) & (2).

When a patient has had surgery, it is essential that there should be a thorough reassessment on return to the ward. In Charlie's case this led to the following new data being fed into his assessment sheet.

First-level assessment	Second-level assessment		
	Focal	Contextual	Residual
PHYSIOLOGY *Oxygenation*: BP135/75, P84, <u>RR12</u>[1]. Looks pale. *Fluid balance*: <u>NBM</u>[2] IVI 1 l/8 h. *Nutrition*: <u>NBM.</u>[3] *Elimination*: <u>Catheterized, therefore access for bacteria to urinary tract.</u>[4]	(1) Opioid analgesia. (2) Post-op nausea. (3) See (2). (4) To facilitate surgery.	Very drowsy. Cross infection from other sources on ward.	
Good output 50–75 ml/h. *Rest & exercise*: <u>Very drowsy</u>[5] <u>L below knee amputation, stump dressing, 2 drains.</u>[6]	(5) Anaesthetic. (6) Surgery.	Pt is diabetic & has peripheral vascular disease.	

First-level assessment	Second-level assessment		
	Focal	Contextual	Residual
Regulation: Omnopon infusion for pain control, drowsy, but agrees when asked if in <u>pain</u>[7] rated 3 on a 5-point scale	(7) Surgery.	Pt is anxious.	
SELF CONCEPT *Physical*: <u>Can still feel leg.</u>[8] *Personal*: 'Glad it's all over'.	(8) Phantom limb.		
ROLE FUNCTION & INTERDEPENDENCE No change, very drowsy.			

The post-operative assessment led to new problems being added to the plan of care (p. 156) while problems Nos 4 and 5 were no longer relevant. Problems No. 6–13 were of greatest importance in the first few days but gradually became less important as the patient was able to adapt by increasing oral fluid intake, performing his deep breathing exercises and working with the physiotherapist to avoid a chest infection. Co-operation in the regime of progressive mobilization also ensured successful adaptation to the loss of the limb and ensured pressure sores and contractures did not develop. This allowed attention to switch to the other problems identified (No. 14–17) after the first few days as meeting these challenges was going to be essential if Mr Hackworth was going to be able to maintain a positive state of adaptation to ensure the best quality of life after discharge.

The use of patient-controlled analgesia (PCA) would have greatly helped this patient adapt to the effects of surgery and would also have given him a great deal more control over the situation as he would have been controlling his own pain. Wards committed to a philosophy that supports patient involvement, whether it be Orem's self-care model or the Roy adaptation model, should be urging their medical staff to implement PCA if they have not already done so.

If this patient is to go home and achieve a high degree of independence with his prosthesis, he needs to adapt positively to his altered role as a husband and the inevitable changes in interdependence that will occur with regard to his wife. He also needs to be able to look in the mirror when he goes to bed or look at himself in the bath and accept the major alteration in his body that accompanies the loss of a limb. All the fears and anxieties raised in problem No. 2 therefore remain post-operatively, intensified by the physical reality of his loss. This then had to be a theme running throughout his post-operative care and it is the sort of issue that requires nursing staff to get to know the patient. The primary nurse was best placed to develop this work with Mr Hackworth and it emphasizes the need for nurses working with Roy's model to have counselling skills and also the time to get to build up a relationship with the patient.

Problem	Goal	Interventions
(6) Post-op shock (P).	BPsyst > 100.	1. Maintain IVI as per chart. 2. Monitor BP, P, RR prn ½–4-hrly. 3. Observe stump bandage, wound drain for excess bleeding.
(7) Respiratory depression (P).	RR> 10.	1. See (6)2. 2. Give O$_2$ as prescribed.
(8) Pain (A).	Pt will state is pain free.	1. Monitor pain levels ½-hrly. 2. Give analgesia as required. 3. Give information, reduce anxiety.
(9) Dehydration (P).	Fluid intake >2.5 l/day.	1. Care of IVI. 2. Fluid balance chart. 3. Encourage oral fluids.
(10) Failure of wound to heal properly (P).	Wound will heal without infection in 14 days.	1. Monitor wound drains. 2. Remove if drainage < 25 ml/ 12 h. 3. Leave dressing untouched as long as possible. 4. Change bandage prn. 5. Monitor Temp 4-hrly. 6. Remove sutures in accordance with surgeon's instructions.
(11) Chest infection (P).	No chest infection.	1. Encourage deep breathing coughing exercises. 2. Nurse in upright position. 3. Encourage mobility, see (12).
(12) Immobility (A).	No pressure sores, DVT/PE, hip contractures will occur.	1. Turn 2-hrly. 2. Explain need for Pt to move self around in bed. 3. Sit out of bed 1 h 1st day post-op. 4. Lie face down twice daily ½ h. 5. Carefully apply TED stocking to R leg. 6. Monitor pressure areas 2-hrly. 7. Use wheelchair when able. 8. Discuss temporary prosthesis.
(13) Urinary tract infection (P).	No urine infection will occur.	1. Catheter care prn. 2. Fluid intake >2.5 l/day after catheter removed.
(14) Smokes 30/day (AL).	Will give up.	1. Discuss & provide health ed. literature.

Problem	Goal	Interventions
(15) Overweight (AL).	Will lose 10 kg from post-op wt in 4 months.	1. Teach about diet. 2. Arrange for dietition to see Pt and wife together. 3. Order correct diet. 4. See (17).
(16) Poor dietary control of diabetes (AL).	Will describe correct diet by discharge.	1. See (15).
(17) Drinks too much alcohol – 25 units/wk (AL).	Will reduce intake by 50% to 12 units per week after discharge.	1. Health ed. advice. 2. Discuss low-alcohol beers.

A CP may also be developed for the management of lower limb amputation utilizing Roy's conceptual framework. This is presented below and incorporates expected outcomes on a multidisciplinary basis covering the first 6 days of care. Monitoring of variances against this CP may indicate areas that need revision or highlight problems that can be tackled to improve the patient's progress. The variance analysis again provides important information for purchasers of health care and the development of a patient version of this CP would be expected to improve the patient's understanding of what was happening to him.

Table 2 Critical pathway for first 6 days: elective amputation of the lower limb incorporating Roy's conceptual framework

Area of care	Day 1 (pre-op)	Day 2 (day of surgery)
Assessment	Systems examination Chest X-ray 12-lead ECG Self-concept Interdependence Role function	Standard pre-op checklist Vital signs 1/2-4 hrly Pain Stump dressing Output from wound drains Fluid balance Systems examination Pressure areas (Waterflow) Orientation/awareness
	Outcome Assessment carried out and documented	*Outcomes* VS within normal limits Pain free Dressing clean and dry Wound drains functioning Breath sounds normal Fluid intake/output balance No evidence of redness on pressure areas Pt is aware of surroundings
Referrals	Physio for chest physio and assessment for post-op mobilization Social worker	

Table 2 Continued

Area of care	Day 1 (pre-op)	Day 2 (day of surgery)
	Outcome Visited by physio, social worker	
Tests	Bloods FBC/U&Es group and cross-match Doppler studies	FBC/U&Es
	Outcome Tests performed, results available before surgery	*Outcome* Within normal limits
Medication	Normal medication administered	Pre-med given if ordered PCA morphine after loading dose opioid given in recovery Antibiotic (cephalosporin) and anti-emetic given as prescribed Other medication given as prescribed
		Outcomes Medication given as ordered Pain free, no nausea
Treatment and care	Discuss how patient sees him/herself adapting to loss of lower limb, effects on family	O_2 post-op if needed Encourage deep breathing and coughing exercises NBM 6 h pre-op Maintain IV Encourage voiding 2-hrly turns Fleece for surviving foot Emotional support
	Outcome Pt will talk of fears/anxieties and how feels about future	*Outcomes* Will p.u. within 6 h of return Restful night's sleep post-op See Assessment for other areas
Teaching	Review patient version of critical path with Pt Explain prep for surgery, operation and post- op care, especially pain management and phantom limb pain, stump care and deep breathing exercises Visit from amputee support volunteer Orient to ward	Reinforce teaching pre-op
	Outcomes Pt will be able to describe main stages of care and plan for pain management Will be visited by volunteer	
Discharge	Discuss with social worker	

Table 2 Continued

Area of care	Day 3 (post-op Day 1)	Day 4 (post-op Day 2)
Assessment	Vital signs 4-hrly Check stump dressing Wound drainage Systems assessment esp. breath and bowel sounds Pressure areas Fluid balance Pain Awareness and orientation Emotional state *Outcome* VS within normal limits Pain free Pressure areas intact, no redness Dressing clean and dry Normal breath sounds Bowel sounds present Fluid intake/output balance Awake and aware of surroundings	Vital signs 4-hrly Check stump dressing Systems assessment esp. breath and bowel sounds Pressure areas Fluid balance Pain *Outcome* As for Day 3
Referrals	Dietitian if Pt is diabetic *Outcome* Seen by dietitian if needed	Nil
Tests	4 h capilliary blood sugar if diabetic *Outcome* Within normal limits	As for Day 3
Medication	Discontinue PCA Oral/IM analgesia Insulin if diabetic (sliding scale) Stool softener Other medication as prescribed *Outcome* Medications given Pain free Blood sugar within normal limits	As for Day 3 plus laxative if needed
Treatment and care	Deep breathing and coughing exercises Blood transfusion if needed Bed bath Bed cradle Turn 2-hrly Encourage oral fluids Discontinue IVI if oral fluids are tolerated Encourage light diet Offer urinal in bed Sit out $\frac{1}{2}$h $\times$ 2 daily Fleece for foot Re-apply stump bandage	Deep breathing and coughing exercises Assisted wash in bed Bed cradle Encourage movement 2 hrly Oral fluids and light diet Range movem't strength exercises Sit out $\frac{1}{2}$h $\times$ 2/day Fleece to foot Support knee Explore feelings re self-concept Offer emotional support Encourage maximum independence

Table 2 Continued

Area of care	Day 3 (post-op Day 1)	Day 4 (post-op Day 2)
	Support knee avoiding knee flexion Offer emotional support Heparinized Venflon if IV antibiotics needed Start range of movement and leg strengthening exercises	Re-apply stump bandage Lie prone 20 min × 3 daily Stand with walking frame/physio Mobilize bed to chair with nurse and walking aid
	Outcomes Above care given Will commence light diet and oral fluids Urine output > 1 l in 24 h Pt will begin to talk about surgery	*Outcomes* Above care given Oral fluids > 2 l/24 h Light diet taken Pt willing to begin to do things for self e.g. wash self, etc. Pt can stand with assistance of physio and walking frame
Teaching	Reinforce Day 1 teaching	Reinforce physio exercises
Discharge	Nil	Begin talking to Pt re discharge

Area of care	Day 5 (post-op Day 3)	Day 6 (post-op Day 4)
Assessment	Vital signs 4-hrly Check stump dressing for signs of infection Systems assessment with particular attention to breath sounds and state of skin over pressure areas Capilliary blood sugars if diabetic	As for Day 5
	Outcomes VS within normal limits No signs of wound infection Normal breath sounds Pressure areas intact and not showing signs of redness Blood sugar within normal limits	
Referrals	Nil	Send referral to rehab. unit
Tests	As for Day 3	As for Day 3
Medication	As for Day 3	As for Day 3
Care and treatment	As for Day 4 except Assisted wash sitting out of bed Physio for ambulation training, strength and range of movement exercises Lie prone 20 min × 3 daily Mobilize bed to chair with nurse and walking aid Offer emotional support and explore feelings about self and family Introduce to wheelchair	Re-appy stump bandage Normal/diabetic diet as appropriate Oral fluids > 2 l/day Commode to encourage bowel movement Assisted wash sitting out of bed Lie prone 30 min × 3 daily Physio for ambulation training, strength and range of movement exercises Will mobilize with walking frame and nurse 10 m × 3 daily Offer emotional support, explore how Pt sees future in terms of principle roles and relationships as well as how sees self

Table 2 Continued

Area of care	Day 5 (post-op Day 3)	Day 6 (Post-op Day 4)
	Outcomes Above care given and goals achieved Pt will be able to look at stump during bandage change Pt will show evidence of motivation to recover, begin to talk positively of the future and of discharge Talks of how he or she will cope at home	*Outcomes* Above care given and goals achieved Stump will have healed with no sign of infection Transfers unaided bed to wheelchair Pt displays motivation to recover, talks positively of the future and discharge Explores coping mechanisms within family/ social life including work/recreation
Teaching	Offer written materials on rehab. after amputation and discuss with Pt Reinforce exercise teaching Explain use of walking frame Discuss prosthesis fitting	As for Day 5 plus explain rehab. work in future
	Outcome Pt will demonstrate understanding of areas covered	*Outcome* As for Day 5
Discharge	Explore provisional arrangements for rehab. & discharge, inform Pt and family	Discuss rehab. and discharge plans with Pt/ family to give indicative date depending upon progress
	Outcome Discussions with Pt/family take place	*Outcome* Pt/family aware of rehab./discharge plans and are involved in the planning process

Example 4:   **The Roy adaptation model in surgery;** Valerie Wilkins

Valerie Wilkins is a 58-year-old woman who has been diagnosed as having cancer of the rectum. She has been admitted for anterior resection of the rectum and temporary formation of a colostomy. In example 3 we saw how the care plan was made up of two components, pre-operative and post-operative, based on two separate assessments; the same approach is used here. The following assessment was therefore carried out on admission the day before surgery.

First-level assessment	Second-level assessment		
	Focal	*Contextual*	*Residual*
PHYSIOLOGICAL *Oxygenation*: RR16 BP165/70 P94;[1] non-smoker, warm dry skin. *Fluid balance*: Looks well hydrated, occasional alcohol. *Nutrition*: Ht 1.67 m Wt 50 kg. Has lost weight recently.[2] Poor diet low in roughage.[3]	(1) Anxiety and fear. (2) Lost appetite. (3) Lack of knowledge.	Ward environment. Suffering from cancer, see (3). Lack of motivation since husband died last year.	Had hysterectomy 9 years ago, very painful. Fears death.

First-level assessment	Second-level assessment		
	Focal	Contextual	Residual
Elimination: No problems with passing urine. Seems <u>embarrassed</u>[4] to talk of bowels. Last 6/12 <u>constipation and diarrhoea</u>[5] with some blood staining. Has <u>always had a tendency to be constipated.</u>[6]	(4) Belief it is not polite. (5) Cancer of rectum. (6) Lack of knowledge about diet.		Traditional beliefs re diet.
Rest & exercise: <u>Sleeps poorly</u>[7] since death of husband. Fully mobile, enjoys reading, TV, knitting. *Regulation:* Had hysterectomy 9 years ago. T36.8°C. Wears glasses for readings.	(7) Death of husband.		
SELF-CONCEPT *Physical*: Feels she got over her hysterectomy, relieved it stopped her menstrual problems. <u>Very worried about stoma</u>[8] formation, 'But if it has to be done, it has to be done'.	(8) Probable stoma formation after resection of rectum.	Afraid people will smell it.	Embarrassed about bowel function.
Personal: <u>Afraid cancer will kill her,</u>[9] worried it has spread already, also afraid it might return elsewhere. A neighbour died in this way.	(9) Cancer.		Experience of seeing a neighbour die of cancer.
ROLE FUNCTION: Widowed 12 months. Has 3 married children who live in the area, close supportive family. Works as part-time shop assistant. <u>Admits to feeling</u>[10] <u>lost without her husband,</u> lets things drift along, still cries over him, visits his grave and 'talks to him'. She became very tearful at this point.	(10) Grieving for husband.		
INTERDEPENDENCE: Tries to be independent. 'I don't want to bother anybody'. Acknowledges children have own lives to live. This was said with some sadness as if she finds it <u>hard to adapt</u>[11] to children's <u>independence.</u>	(11) Children have become independent of her.		Needs to feel wanted as a mother, especially since widowed.

This assessment led to the following pre-operative care plan being written.

Problem	Goal	Nursing care
(1) Anxiety due to fear of: (a) surgery, (b) cancer, (c) effects of stoma, (d) further erosion of her role in the family (A).	(a) Pt will talk of her fears pre- & post-op. (b) Pt will appear positive in talking of these problems by discharge.	1. Give information. 2. Encourage questions. 3. Stoma specialist to see Pt pre-op. 4. Discuss (a)–(d) with sensitivity and in private.
(2) Complications of surgery (P).	Pt will suffer no avoidable problems.	1. Standard pre-op procedure.
(3) Pt may develop peritonitis due to contamination of surgical field by faeces.	Rectum and bowel will be empty of faeces.	1. Bowel washout today × 2 and in morning. 2. Fluids only.

As with the previous model, the assessment, particularly under self-concept, provided the nurse with several different leads to pursue in helping Mrs Wilkins adapt to her surgery. The brief pre-operative period only allows time to set the agenda, there will have to be a lot more work carried out post-operatively to explore the key areas that will help Mrs Wilkins cope with her stoma. The second level assessment has supplied the nurse with a range of factors which need to be worked through if Mrs Wilkins is to be helped to adapt successfully to her stoma.

Mrs Wilkins was then re-assessed on return from theatre the following day after resection of her rectum and stoma formation.

First-level assessment	Second-level assessment		
	Focal	Contextual	Residual
PHYSIOLOGICAL *Oxygenation*: BP95/60 P98 RR18.[1] Breathing shallow.[2]	(1) Hypovolaemia. (2) Pain.	Moderate pain, post-GA.	
Fluids: NBM[3] Blood transfusion running. *Nutrition*: NBM[4]	(3) No bowel sounds.	Nauseated.	
Elimination: Urinary catheter good output. Naso-gastric tube mod drainage.	(4) See (3).		
Colostomy L. lower quadrant.[5] Looks pink, bag empty. Two wound drains from lower abdominal wound, slight oozing.[6]	(5) Surgery for cancer. (6) See (5).		
Rest & activity: Drowsy, reluctant to move in bed.[7]	(7) Pain.	Afraid of 'drips and drains'.	
Regulation: Pain[8] is rated 3 on a 5-point scale. T36.9°C.	(8) Surgery.	Anxiety.	Frightened to ask for analgesia.
SELF-CONCEPT *Physical*: Has refused to look at stoma.[9] *Personal*: Relieved it is all over.	(9) Embarrassed.	Already very distressed 'I've been through enough today'.	
INTERDEPENDENCE Has not asked for help despite pain.[10]	(10) Desire to maintain independence.		
ROLE FUNCTION Family anxious to see her.			

Mrs Wilkins' care plan was therefore added to, reflecting immediate post-operative priorities (problems (4)–(10)) but with long-term problems such as (1), (9) and (11) figuring increasingly in care as she recovers from the immediate effects of surgery.

Problem	Goal	Nursing care
(4) Pain (A).	Pt will state she has no pain.	1. Monitor pain levels with 5-point scale. 2. Give analgesia as needed. 3. Give information and try to reduce anxiety. 4. Make comfortable. 5. Discuss importance of asking for analgesia.
(5) Hypovolaemic shock (P).	BPsyst > 90.	1. Ensure IVI runs to time. 2. Record BP, P, RR ½-hrly. 3. Monitor wound & drains.
(6) Dehydration (P).	Fluid intake > 2.5 l/day.	1. Fluid balance chart.
(7) Nausea and vomiting (A).	Pt will not vomit.	1. Naso-gastric tube free drainage. 2. NBM until bowel sounds return. 3. Give anti-emetics prn.
(8) Pt is not able to eat.	Will start light diet within 4 days.	1. Keep hydrated, see (6). 2. Ask what she likes. 3. Discuss diet and stoma. 4. Avoid nausea, see (7). 5. Offer supplement drinks.
(9) Failure of colostomy to work (P).	Stoma will start to work < 3 days.	1. Check appearance of stoma is normal. 2. Ask Pt if she feels any wind. 3. Listen for bowel sounds.
(10) Pt is unable to accept stoma (A).	(a) Pt will look at stoma < 3 days. (b) Pt will help nurse change bag < 6 days. (c) Pt will change bag alone before discharge.	1. Encourage and discuss stoma with Pt. 2. Make it an ordinary part of care. 3. Stoma specialist to visit. 4. Arrange visit from other stoma patient. 5. Talk to family about stoma at visiting times. 6. Reinforce temporary nature of colostomy.
(11) Surgical wound (A).	Wound will heal without complications 14 days.	1. Remove wound drains when drainage < 25 ml in 12 h. 2. Do not disturb dressing unless necessary. 3. Monitor T 4-hrly if > 37°C. 4. Remove sutures according to surgeon's instructions.
(12) Pt lacks motivation and has tended to neglect self since being widowed.	Pt will express positive views about going home.	1. Allow her to talk of her husband. 2. Discuss her job with her. 3. Reinforce temporary nature of stoma. 4. Encourage visiting by family. 5. Explore new things she could do with her life, new interests.

Mrs Wilkins also had problems surrounding her inability to maintain personal hygiene and potential problems of chest infection, pressure sores, DVT, and urinary tract infection from an indwelling catheter. Reference is made to the previous care plan (Charlie Hackworth) to see how these may be dealt with.

It is worth reflecting on a significant insight into human behaviour that is associated with Roy's model and Mrs Wilkins provides a nice example of this point. The different disciplines of physiology, psychology, sociology, etc. all have strong theoretical strands running through them concerning adaptation, but as Fawcett (1995) points out, Roy has brought these separate themes together into an integrated holistic view of human functioning rather than leaving them in their own professional pigeon holes.

Thus the surgeon knows that the body will adapt to the changes he or she has made in the anatomy providing there are no complicating factors such as infection or anastomotic breakdown. Psychologists have developed theories that explain how we adapt, or fail to adapt, to varying levels of stress and how different types of stimulus produce different responses. Thus the stimulus of seeing bowel protruding from the abdominal wall is likely to produce a response of disgust. Sociologists have described how stressors affect groups of people and how we wish to belong to groups within society. A stoma may therefore make a person feel an outcast. The strength of Roy's approach is to unify these different perspectives under the one banner of nursing for it is only with such an integrated holistic approach that we can help Mrs Wilkins become a functioning, independent person living her own life again as part of her family and social network. The surgeon alone cannot do that, nor can the social worker or a clinical psychologist.

The care plan therefore requires the nurses to address the various physiological issues to make sure that the patient regains normal eating and drinking patterns (Nos 6,7,8) and is pain free (No. 4) while the stoma is functioning successfully (No. 9). However, the nurse is also working with the patient's social networks exploring her role function and interdependence (No. 12) while working through the psychological aspects of adaptation (Nos 1,10,12).

Example 5	The FANCAP assessment scheme in A&E

Assessment in A&E is based on the well-known 'ABCD of resuscitation' protocol which requires airway, breathing, circulation, and dysfunction involving the cervical spine and consciousness to be the first priorities. This is a reliable method for assessing immediate life-threatening problems; however, it does not go beyond the urgent problems. FANCAP can be used to give the same priorities as the ABCD scheme, but has the advantage of exploring other areas. If the assessment begins with 'Aeration', airway, breathing and circulation will be covered; 'Activity' should make the nurse look for any sign of limb weakness or neck injury, while 'Communication' requires an assessment of level of consciousness. Pain should be assessed next, leaving fluids and nutrition until last. Thus, in A&E the FANCAP scheme becomes AACPFN, suggestions are invited for an easy way of remembering this acronym!

Nurses in A&E rarely have the luxury of time in which to write detailed care plans and care planning is frequently done in the nurse's head rather than on paper. CPs offer one solution to this problem, even if only as teaching tools for staff new to the department or as a way of setting standards for care. Consider the following two examples which show how FANCAP may be used for two very different A&E patients.

5a. Patrick Dunne

Patrick was brought to the A&E department after being found unconscious in a street; he appears rather dishevelled.

AERATION
Airway. Patent.
Breathing: RR12 deep & regular, smells strongly of alcohol.
Circulation: BP110/70, P70. *Skin*: Very dirty.
Other Comments: Not expressing any emotions, uncommunicative.
ACTIVITY
Neck: No evidence of injury. *Limbs*: No voluntary movement, unresponsive, no history of trauma available, no sign of injury to limbs.
COMMUNICATION
Level of consciousness: Best response; flexes to painful stimulus, nil verbally, pupils = react briskly (see head injury chart).
Wounds: Small laceration over R eye.
Understanding of situation: Nil, unresponsive.
Eyesight: Not wearing glasses.
Hearing: Unresponsive to verbal stimulus.
PAIN
Location: Nil.
Severity 0–5: 0, unresponsive.
Type: —
Other comments: —
Anxiety: —
FLUIDS
In: Has almost empty bottle of wine in pocket.
Out: Has been incontinent of urine.
Family/friends: Nobody with him, looks to be sleeping rough.
NUTRITION
In: Appears underfed, CBG 3 mmol/l.
Out: Trousers show evidence of previous faecal incontinence, shirt soaked in fresh vomit.

This assessment should allow the nurse to deduce that Patrick's major problem is a potential threat to his airway from vomiting while unconscious and lead to him being positioned on his side, under observation, while he sleeps off his excess alcohol intake.

5b. Darren Mardon

This 18-year-old motorcyclist was brought to A&E after an RTA.

AERATION
  Airway: Tolerates Guerdal oral airway.
  Breathing: RR30 shallow, paradoxical resps. R side of chest.
  Circulation: BP80/40, P128. *Skin*: Pale, cold, sweaty.
  Other comments: Expressing nothing verbally.
ACTIVITY
  Neck: No evidence of injury but marks on crash helmet indicate substantial blow to head.
  Limbs: No voluntary movement, clinically #R shaft femur, closed.
COMMUNICATION
  Level of consciousness: Unresponsive to painful stimulus (see head injury chart). R pupil sluggish to react and dilated.
  Wounds: Nil.
  Understanding: Nil.
  Eyesight: No glasses.
  Hearing: Unresponsive.
PAIN
  Location: Unresponsive.
  Severity 0–5: 0
  Type: —
  Other comments: —
  Anxiety: —
FLUIDS
  In: Not known when last had drink.
  Out: Bladder non-palpable.
  Family/friends: Police are notifying his parents.
NUTRITION
  In: Looks within normal range ht/wt ratio. Last ate ? when.
  Out: —

This rapid assessment allowed A&E staff to identify a serious head injury, flail segment and fracture of the right femur as his main injuries. His main problems in A&E could be listed as follows:

- airway obstruction (P)
- hypovolaemic shock (A)
- respiratory failure (A)
- unconsciousness (A)
- cervical spine injury (P)
- fractured right femur (A)
- neurovascular complications of that fracture (P).

Such an assessment revealed the urgent problems needing nursing care while resuscitation was carried out and medical diagnosis of his injuries was finalized.

It is worthwhile looking at how this scheme may now be applied to Darren's care on ITU where ventilatory support was needed due to his head and chest injuries. A Steinmann pin had been inserted in his R. tibia and sliding traction applied to stabilize his fractured R. femur. The flexibility of FANCAP is shown by this different approach to its usage on ITU.

| Example 6 | Assessment of Darren Mardon on ITU |

AERATION
In
Intubated with size 9 Portex ET tube.
Ventilated on preset inspired minute vol of 8 l/min, RR12 Airway pressures 22–24 mmHg. 50% humidified oxygen.
Both sides of chest rising equally.

Out
BP120/80 P86 CVP + 4 (18:00 h).
ECG sinus rhythm.
Two chest drains *in situ*.
Arterial line *in situ* for BP

COMMUNICATION
In
Does not respond to verbal or painful stimulus, R pupil remains sluggish and dilated. According to parents has no hearing or eyesight problems.

Out
No attempt at communication with staff, unresponsive.
No wounds noted.

FLUIDS
In
NBM, peripheral and central lines *in situ*. See fluid balance chart.
Social: Family and girlfriend keen to visit.

Out
Catheter draining well 60–90 ml/h clear urine.

PAIN
In
Pt has suffered #R femur.
Psychological: No facial evidence of anxiety/fear.

Out
Showing no visible evidence of pain, unresponsive.

ACTIVITY
In
CBG 7.5.
Recreational: Keen footballer.
Work: Apprentice electrician. Works know of situation.

Out
No voluntary movement of limbs.

NUTRITION
In
NBM. Bowel sounds present.

Out
Bowels not yet opened.

Problem	Goal	Intervention
(1) Airway obstruction (P).	Pt will have a patent airway.	1. Check ET tube + connections secure. 2. ET suction hrly/prn.
(2) Pt unable to maintain adequate respiration (A).	Arterial blood gases (ABGs) within normal limits.	1. Hrly physio. 2. Monitor chest movements. 3. Monitor and adjust O_2 conc. & ventilator settings according to Dr's instructions and ABGs. 4. Give sedation as per drug chart. 5. See probs. (1)+(3).
(3) Pt may go into resp. failure due to pneumothorax (P).	No haemo/pneumothorax will recur.	1. Record chest drainage hrly. 2. Ensure drains are patent. 3. Minimal clamping of drains. 4. See prob. (2).
(4) Shock (P).	BPsyst 100–140.	1. Continuous BP monitoring. 2. Give IVI as per chart.
(5) Raised intracranial pressure (ICP) (P).	No signs of raised ICP.	1. Continuous BP monitoring. 2. Pupil obs $\frac{1}{2}$-hrly.
(6) Dehydration (P).	Fluid intake 2.5 l/day.	1. Give IVI as per chart. 2. Record urine output hrly. 3. CVP readings hrly. 4. Fluid balance chart.
(7) #R femur (A).	# will remain immobilized in correct position.	1. Check weights clear of floor. 2. Correct external rotation with padding. 3. Ensure pulley system runs free. 4. Dress pin sites as required.
(8) Neurovascular damage R leg (P).	Good pedal pulse R foot.	1. Care of traction as per (7). 2. Check pulse, skin colour warmth $\frac{1}{2}$–4-hrly.
(9) Pain (P).	No painful expression on face.	1. Give sufficient analgesia/ sedation to ensure easily ventilated & shows no pain.
(10) Pressure sores (P).	No breaks in skin will occur.	1. Pressure area care 2-hrly. 2. Ripple mattress.
(11) Stress of ITU environment (A).	Pt will suffer minimum stress and not develop stress ulceration.	1. Talk to Pt at all times as though he can hear, explaining where he is and what is happening. 2. Give ranitidine as per chart. 3. Ensure adequate periods of rest. 4. Ensure adequate sedation given. 5. Encourage visits from family & girlfriend.
(12) Unable to see to personal hygiene (A).	Will appear clean and well-groomed.	1. Bed bath daily. 2. Mouth & eye care 2-hrly.

This care plan is the broad outline of care required for Darren. The fine detail will be provided by experienced ITU staff without the need to write it down, for example the 'bag and suck' regime required to prevent the build up of secretions in the bronchial tree and ET tube. A care plan for an ITU patient needs to be flexible as the patient's condition may change from hour to hour and medical staff may order changes in various regimes, for example ventilator settings, IVIs, at the same rate or even more frequently if required. The nurse may feel there is a sufficient common core of care to make the development of standard care plans worthwhile on ITU. If so, a strong individualized component must remain.

A great deal of information is recorded at $\frac{1}{2}$-hourly or hourly intervals, so accurate charting is an essential part of the assessment–care–evaluation feedback system. This also helps to explain the brief nature of the assessment given here: many of the data are already recorded on charts, there is no point in duplication. The 'In/Out' approach to assessment was more rigorously adhered to here than in the A&E examples as this concept of homeostasis is of fundamental importance in life support.

Example 7 — The Roper model on a care of the elderly unit; Jenny Haynes

Jenny Haynes is a 78-year-old woman who was admitted after collapsing at home with a cerebrovascular accident. She has had a history of transient ischaemic attacks and has been treated for hypertension before today's episode. She also suffers from osteo-arthritis. Her daughter accompanied her to hospital and helped with the assessment.

Activity of living (AL)	Usual independent routines	Problem
Maintaining a safe environment	Cares for herself at home.	May fall out of bed (P).
Communicating	Slightly deaf, has 2 pairs of glasses for short & long sight. Speech slurred at present, though understandable, due to CVA. Conscious though drowsy, appears aware of surroundings.	
Breathing	RR14 BP180/100. Non-smoker. Has history of bad colds in winter.	
Eating and drinking	Ht 1.52 m approx, appears very overweight. 'Likes her food, always been a big eater'. Diet is low in fibre. Has not been drinking much in the evening (see elimination). Wears dentures.	Overweight (A). Dehydration (P). Poor nutrition (A).

Activity of living (AL)	Usual independent routines	Problem
Elimination	Sometimes has accidents with passing urine if she cannot get to toilet in time, so tends not to drink a lot in the evening. Prone to constipation.	Incontinence of urine (P). Constipation (A).
Personal cleansing/dressing	Able to attend to own hygiene though arthritis makes it hard to bend over and reach feet.	Is unable to attend to own hygiene at present (A).
Body temperature	T35.9°C. 'I do feel the cold in winter, it's cold now'.	Pt is cold (A).
Mobilizing	Walks slowly with aid of stick. Can manage to reach local shops which are only 50 m away but arthritis is painful.	Has L hemiplegia since CVA (A). Pressure sores (P). (Norton Scale 11)
Working and playing	Watches TV and reads, used to do needlework, but hands too clumsy and painful now. OAP. Retired.	
Expressing sexuality	Still takes pride in her appearance, widowed 8 years ago. Lives with younger sister age 74.	
Sleeping	Poor sleeper.	May now sleep well (P).
Dying	Takes each day as it comes: 'At my age you know you can't go on for ever'.	

The following plan of care was devised for Mrs Haynes.

Problem	Goal	Nursing care
(1) May fall out of bed (P).	Will not fall out of bed.	1. Orientate Pt in space. 2. Cot sides at night.
(2) Slurred speech (A).	Pt will be able to make self understood.	1. Listen carefully to Pt. 2. Ask to speak slowly. 3. Explain side-effects of CVA.
(3) Confusion (P).	Pt will be oriented in time and space.	1. Reality orientation programme.
(4) Dehydration (A).	Fluid intake 3 l/day.	1. Care of IVI. 2. Encourage oral fluids. 3. Fluid balance chart. 4. Explain need for oral fluids.

Problem	Goal	Nursing care
(5) Overweight (A).	Pt to lose 10 kg in 3 months.	1. Contact dietician. 2. Assist with feeding. 3. Discuss healthy eating when her condition has improved.
(6) Incontinent of urine (P).	Pt will not be incontinent.	1. Give Pt call bell and explain its use; check she understands. 2. Offer bedpans 2-hrly. 3. Fluid balance chart.
(7) Constipation (a).	Pt will have bowels open within 48 h.	1. Ensure hydration, see (4). 2. See (5). 3. Give suppositories if no action in 48 h.
(8) Unable to see to own hygiene (A).	Pt will state is satisfied with personal hygiene.	1. Bed bath including mouth and eye care. 2. Encourage maximum participation by Pt.
(9) Pt feels cold (A).	Pt will state she is not cold.	1. Supply extra bedding. 2. Check T 4-hrly.
(10) L hemiplegia (A).	Pt will not have contractures or injury to L limbs.	1. Discuss exercise regime with physios and carry out according to plan. 2. Approach from R side. 3. Place cups, etc. R side.
(11) Pressure sores (P).	Pt will not develop broken skin.	1. 2-hrly pressure care. 2. Check condition of skin 2-hrly. 3. Encourage Pt mobility and explain why.
(12) Lack of sleep (A).	Pt will state she had good night's sleep.	1. Ensure quiet environment. 2. Explain what is happening at night. 3. Give medication as per chart.

One final care plan using the Roper model is looked at before discussing the merits of these four approaches, particularly with reference to the criteria outlined on p. 138 for a good hospital model of nursing.

Example 8   **The Roper model in medical nursing;** William Slater

Bill Slater is a 68-year-old retired publican who has been admitted with acute shortness of breath and heart failure. He has had several admissions to hospital in the last few years and has a medical diagnosis of chronic obstructive airways disease (COAD) and congestive heart failure. He responded well to nebulized salbutamol therapy on admission and his breathing is now easier. This assessment was carried out a few hours after admission.

Activity of living (AL)	Usual routines	Problems
Maintaining a safe environment	Lives in bungalow with wife, uncertain about his medication. Admits enjoying a few drinks, evasive as to how many. Old bruises noted on arm and face 'Fell over in the dark'.	May not understand medication correctly (P). ? Alcohol abuse (P).
Communicating	Speech laboured, SOB. Hearing good, wears reading glasses, trying to make jokes.	
Breathing	RR24, BP150/90. Nicotine stains on fingers, admits smokes 10–15/day. Was using accessory muscles on admission tho' breathing now easier, sounds rattly, has coughed up some green sputum.	Chest infection (A). Episodes of respiratory distress (P). Smokes (A).
Eating and drinking	Overweight, Ht 1.7 m, weight 88 kg. Diet is high in saturated fats and refined carbohydrates, low in fruit. Drinking, see safe environment.	Overweight (A). Low-fibre diet (A).
Eliminating	No problems passing urine or faeces.	
Personal cleansing	Has bath every day, no problems.	
Body temperature	Feels hot, skin is sweaty. T37.7°C axilla.	Pyrexial (A).
Mobilizing	Gets SOB after walking 100–200 m on the flat, manages stairs slowly.	Cannot walk more than few feet at present (A).
Working and playing	Had been publican for 30 years before retired 18 months ago. Never had time for hobbies, so does little now except watch TV and read papers. Admits to being bored.	Boredom (A).
Sexuality	Sex life 'None of your business'.	
Sleeping	Used to late nights, now finds it hard to sleep. Takes tablets.	Insomnia (A).
Dying	'Never thought about it'.	

The following care plan was drawn up based on this assessment.

Problems	Goals	Nursing care
(1) Lack of understanding of medication (A).	Pt will explain medication, dose & side-effects.	1. Discuss with Pt when he is better. 2. Give written information.
(2) Possible alcohol abuse (A).	Pt will recognize he may have a problem.	1. Observe for signs of abstinence syndrome. 2. No alcohol allowed. 3. Discuss alcohol intake at later stage when better.
(3) Chest infection (A).	Chest infection will resolve in 5 days, clear sputum.	1. Antibiotics as per chart. 2. Sit upright. 3. Encourage deep breathing & coughing. 4. Monitor RR, T 4-hrly.

Problems	Goals	Nursing care
(4) Respiratory distress (P).	RR < 20.	1. See (3). 2. Medication as per chart. 3. See (8). 4. Discourage smoking. 5. Monitor BP, P, RR 4-hrly.
(5) Smokes (A).	Pt will give up.	1. Discuss effects of smoking, give leaflets.
(6) Overweight (A).	Pt will lose 3 kg in 10 weeks.	1. Consult dietitian. 2. Discuss healthy eating.
(7) Pyrexial (A).	T < 37.0°C in 5 days.	1. See (3).
(8) Limited mobility (A).	Pt will not get SOB on exertion.	1. Use commode for first 24 h. 2. Bed rest 24 h. 3. Assisted wash at bedside. 4. Allow to bathroom in 48 h. 5. Walk to day room in 48 h.
(9) Boredom.	Pt will appear to take an interest in ward activity.	1. Ensure has newspapers/books. 2. Encourage other Pts to talk to him if he is able. 3. Find time to talk to him.
(10) Insomnia.	Pt will say has slept > 6 h.	1. Ask if anything helps him sleep. 2. Minimize night noise. 3. Medication as per chart.

Discussion

It remains to conclude this chapter by seeing how the four models used compare with each other and with the criteria set on p. 138 for an ideal model of nursing in a general hospital setting.

The Orem and Roy models allowed the nurses to readily assess the key physiological aspects of the patient as did the FANCAP scheme. Flexibility in the order of assessment is essential together with a sense of priority; that is, the most urgent things are assessed first and nurses should not be afraid to vary the order in which an assessment is carried out according to the patient's needs rather than follow a fixed scheme of things set out in any textbook. The Roper model has little sense of priority and the examples in the literature seem to assess the patient always in the same arbitrary order and set out care accordingly. Nurses who intend using Roper should therefore avoid using the standard sequence of headings set out in the model as their order is arbitrary and fails to bring a sense of priority to both assessment and care planning.

The FANCAP scheme is the only assessment to highlight pain as a heading in its own right, although Roy's notion of assessing regulation brings the nurse to an assessment of pain via the nervous system. The other two models require the nurse to assess pain under a specific physiological system; thus, John Harper's pain (Orem) is assessed under aeration and pain for Jenny Haynes (Roper) is mentioned under mobilizing. The two-level assessment of Roy requires the nurse to probe for various reasons other than the obvious that may lie behind the pain. This led to the discovery that Mrs Wilkins was suffering pain post-operatively not only because of surgery but also because she was very anxious and because she was reluctant to ask for analgesia as she felt this to be a sign of weakness; she was also worried about becoming addicted.

Roper's assessment focuses the nurse's attention on what the patient could do before coming into hospital. However, in acute settings the nurse needs to assess the situation here and now. Home activity and pre-hospital problems are important, but in caring for an acutely ill patient the nurse needs to know the current problems. Time spent on investigating pre-hospital activity needs to be carefully allocated to make sure only relevant information is gathered. This aspect assumes more importance during the discharge planning phase. Roper's emphasis on 'normal routines' to use her own words may sidetrack the nurse away from important information. There are other issues here, what does normal mean? Normal for whom? What is a routine? How often does something have to be done to be routine? How important is routine? What of the danger of stereotyping the individual and losing their individuality in a grey cloak of conformist, normal routines?

The emphasis of the other models on the here and now is a strength, although the nurse must not lose track of what goes on at home as it will be equally important when planning discharge. However, we should avoid the trap of trying to reduce patients to collections of routines: patients are people not automatons.

There are some areas that do not fit easily into the various assessment schemes of these models. Consider the wound of a patient who has had surgery: it is an obvious feature and a key aspect of post-operative care, yet where do these models ask the nurse to assess the wound? The most likely candidate in Orem is the heading 'health deviancy' for that is what a wound is, while the FANCAP heading 'communication' can be interpreted in that way for a wound provides communication between the inside and outside of the body in the same way that the M4 provides communication between London and Bristol. In the Roy and Roper schemes the best that can be suggested is to consider the physiological system relevant to the wound. Thus, a patient who has had gastric surgery might have the wound assessed under nutrition or under eating and drinking, while the bowel surgery undergone by Valerie Wilkins leads to an assessment under elimination. Roy, though, does have the great advantage of ensuring that the nurse assesses how the patient feels about a wound under the notion of self-concept.

A similar problem is encountered with the notion of cleanliness and the condition of a patient's skin. Roper does require an assessment of personal cleansing and dressing – but note the limitations imposed by such terminology as 'normal routines'. This explicit statement about personal hygiene is, however, welcome. The most reasonable approach with another model might be to consider rest and activity (Roy, Orem) or just activity (FANCAP) and assess the patient's activity with regard to personal hygiene. Some nurses, though, might advocate assessing hygiene under elimination. As in the case of wounds, this flexibility is perhaps not a bad thing, but staff should reach a consensus on how they use a model's assessment scheme to ensure there is a degree of consistency in the way it is applied in order to avoid confusion, particularly among students and staff new to the model.

The use of Roy's model would require an assessment of the person's ability to adapt to their condition in pursuit of personal hygiene, while Orem directs the nurse to look at self-care ability. There seem slightly safer concepts than normal routines. Pressure-area risks can be calculated using a standard scale such as Norton or Waterlow and seem relevant when investigating the patient's ability to move about (rest and activity, mobilizing, etc.).

In writing care plans, nurses sometimes have difficulty dealing with the effects of medical interventions such as wound drains and IVIs. Such equipment presents real problems to the patient which must figure in the nursing care, but the question arises of how to incorporate essentially medical interventions into a nursing care plan. The solution requires the nurse to look beyond the IVI or wound drain and ask why is it there? The answer to that question is the real patient problem; that is, the patient is unable to maintain hydration via the oral route (IVI) or an accumulation of serosanguinous fluid may delay wound healing and become infected (wound drain). The patient's problem is then an ability to maintain hydration or the risk of delayed wound healing with typical goals being a fluid intake of 3 l/day or that the wound will heal without any complications within 14 days. The care of the IVI or wound drain then logically becomes a nursing intervention.

Invasive medical interventions such as these can be seen within the Roy model as maladaptive in so far as they breach our normal defences against infection (the integrity of the skin), while from Orem's point of view they represent self-care deficits in that the patient cannot prevent the possibility of infection occurring at the site of insertion. The risk of infection then becomes a potential patient problem.

Human physiology is a very closely integrated collection of systems which has to achieve balance or homeostasis for healthy functioning. For this reason it seems better to bring together notions of input and output and assess them together as they affect a bodily system, since one very much depends on the other. For this reason the four Orem headings of intake or air, water and food plus elimination have been reduced to three – aeration, fluid balance and nutrition, each of which is assessed from the point of view of intake and output. This reflects the FANCAP approach and avoids the duplication shown in the Roper assessment of Jenny Haynes. Perhaps the Roper model would benefit form separating the eating and drinking heading into two separate parts, and considering elimination under eating and then again separately under drinking, removing the separate elimination heading from the model.

The notion of assessing pulse separately from blood pressure and respiratory rate in Roper's model seems strange given the above observation. The cardiovascular and respiratory systems are inextricably entwined, survival would not be possible otherwise. Thus, whether it is a heading such as aeration (Orem, FANCAP) or oxygenation and circulation (Roy), both systems must be assessed together and care must be planned in an integrated way. In this way John Harper receives care that ensures there is enough oxygen getting into his arterial blood and that blood plus oxygen is being efficiently pumped around his body. Such an integrated approach is lacking in the arbitrary and disjointed headings used by Roper.

The problems discussed above indicate the need for a flexible and pragmatic approach to the use of nursing models if they are to be translated into the real world of clinical nursing and be recognized as valid tools to enable and facilitate nursing care.

The health deviancy aspect of Orem's model is an interesting concept in that it requires the nurse to look at how the patient is being affected by specific pathology and how well he or she is coping not only with that pathology but also with the effects of the medical treatment that is being given, for example knowledge of drugs being taken as in the case of John Harper. While the emphasis on health promotion and independent nursing care are welcome developments, nursing cannot ignore medical practice and illness as they affect the patient, and consequently this aspect of Orem's model is very helpful.

In using Roy, the nurse must be prepared to apply the concept of pathology and treatment to the specific systems of the body in turn, as there is no specific 'health deviancy' heading. If John Harper's care were planned using the Roy model, then his lack of knowledge about drug therapy would have to be assessed under the heading oxygenation and circulation. In using the Roper model the nurse might choose to make such assessments under the heading of maintaining a safe environment, a heading which, however, overlaps considerably with 'mobility'.

The important psychosocial aspects of care figure prominently in the Roy model with the notions of self-concept, role function and interdependence. Consideration of the two care plans, however, reveals that role function and interdependence are very closely related. Valerie Wilkins' role as a mother is bound up with her feelings about the independence of her children. At present she has no sexual partner, being recently widowed; however, if she did, consider how personal and physical self-concept after colostomy might interact with her role as a sexual partner, lover and wife, which in turn would affect her interdependence with her partner. It seems as though these three psychosocial areas of behaviour and adaptation are different but overlapping ways of looking at the same field. By analogy, to appreciate what any object looks like, a person must look at it from different points of view to see it in three dimensions. Inevitably, view A will partly look the same as view B, but view B will contain new information not seen in view A and so on for view C. In the same way, self-concept, role function and interdependence describe a whole range of aspects of a person's psychosocial functioning, inevitably with some degree of overlap because of the complexity of the ways humans think and behave.

Orem's model places emphasis on how the patient relates to others in assessing 'solitude-socialization' and the admittedly vague concept of 'normalcy' can be interpreted in terms of how anxious the patient is feeling about the situation he or she is in or likely to be in. It is important that such a vague term has an agreed common meaning for all the staff using the model if consistency of assessment and hence care is to be achieved.

The developmental component of Orem's model is a strong tool for assessing how patients are managing to cope with their stage in the life cycle. Roy's interdependence, role function and personal self-concept modes can be used to arrive at similar information, providing the nurse is sensitive to the notion of the patient moving along a life continuum of constant change associated with ageing. The views expressed by Mabel Bush in the Orem developmental assessment could be interpreted as an elderly lady with no relatives (interdependence) who feels she has outlived her usefulness and has no purpose left in life (role function), having such a low self-esteem that she just wants to die (personal self-concept). Her isolation is confirmed from the 'socialization' heading, while we note from 'normalcy' that she misses her husband badly.

The Orem model can therefore be used to assess and plan for similar dimensions of psychosocial care as Roy, although there is a different emphasis, self-care as opposed to adaptation. The question remains whether it is better to talk of self-care or adaptation in, for example, coming to terms with widowhood. Perhaps such ideas are so closely linked that they cannot be separated in practice, for to adapt the woman has to be self-reliant (self-caring), yet to be self-caring she needs to have reconciled herself to her bereavement and carried out the necessary grief work; that is, to be self-caring she has to adapt.

The FANCAP scheme is more concerned with urgent physiological problems, although a heading such as communication does open up a wide field of investigation, as through communication the nurse can learn a great deal about the patient's fears and anxieties. The assessments of Darren Mardon and Patrick Dunne both contain reference under fluids to family and friends. This may seem a little puzzling; however, it is suggested that as fluids possess a property called fluidity, this property might legitimately be included in the assessment. Fluidity corresponds to an absence of friction and may therefore be interpreted as how well does the patient get along with people, what are his or her social networks? If the nurse wishes to extend the FANCAP scheme in this way, the notion of activity might be taken to include work and recreational activity, allowing for the inclusion of further important social information about the patient and directing the care planner to think in terms of how for example, Darren, will manage in his job after this accident and whether he will be able to continue playing competitive football.

The Roper model gives the appearance of failing to get to grips with the richness and complexity of the way humans think and behave; the intricately woven tapestry of psychological and social activity is reduced to a polaroid snapshot in this model. The model as implemented usually lacks any serious attempt to understand how the patient is feeling, what their background is, why they do the things they do. Instead there is an arbitrary and disjointed check-list of physical aspects of behaviour which Bellman (1996) argues has more to do with the way nurses implement the model than flaws coherent within the model. How does Mrs Haynes feel about being elderly, possibly having to be cared for by her younger sister who she cannot get on with and has never liked? Her loss of independence has been greatly worrying her, and now comes this stroke on top of everything else. She hates herself for not being able to get to the toilet in time; it is so childish to be incontinent so she will not drink much, leading to dehydration. She used to be a very active woman, but now age has made her feel sad and useless, forced to live with a younger sister she has never liked. None of this information is likely to come out of a Roper-style assessment consisting of noting how well she could walk or cook at home before her illness. Independence is a very complex issue and the need is to look to the future not the past for Mrs Haynes.

Consider Bill Slater, an ex-publican who has a significant alcohol problem. So much might be suspected from the Roper assessment, but that is all. A different approach might have revealed that he hates being at home, has major problems in getting on with his wife, and spends most of his time in the pub. He continues to smoke despite his COAD because he believes that having a good cough helps clear his chest and smoking also calms his nerves; he is unaware just how smoky an environment a pub is because he has worked in one for so long. Information such as that might have been derived from the Roy two-level assessment approach, which is lacking in Roper. Bill spends a lot of time in the pub because that is where his friends are, the old regulars; they give him a social life he does not have elsewhere. He also has a degree of prestige as the ex-landlord that is good for his self-esteem. He cannot adjust to being retired as he feels useless, and this makes him unhappy. He gets under his wife's feet at home so they have rows and he goes to the pub to get out of the way, while their sex life fizzled out many years ago.

Bill Slater, therefore has a fundamentally unhealthy life style related to social and psychological problems. As long as he is drinking and smoking heavily, eating a poor diet and spending a lot of time in the pub, he will be prone to increasingly worse attacks of COAD, becoming severely restricted in his mobility, and at increasing risk of alcohol-related accidents and pathology, not to mention heart disease. The Orem/Roy approach is more likely to get to the root of these problems than the Roper checklist, which might only ensure that the basics of physical care are attempted by nursing staff while he is in hospital. The word 'attempted' has been chosen deliberately as Bill may well respond with hostility to having his life organized by nurses, leading to non-compliance and the 'difficult patient' label. Bill's problems are of the chronic type, and ideas of self-care and self-concept are crucial in successful management of the problem of non-compliance. An interactionist perspective may show his apparent non-compliance in a new light when he is considered as a man who has been independent all his life and who is now losing that independence owing to retirement. However, it needs an approach to nursing that will explore these psychosocial areas in a way that Roper does not, to shed that light upon the patient.

In order to have effective care, the patient must be working with the nurse. An approach to nursing that explores the psychosocial aspects of a patient is more likely to succeed in this goal as it allows the nurse to begin to see the reasons why the patient is behaving the way he or she is. Roper's physical task checklist does not provide a framework for that degree of understanding.

If we consider again the four basic components of any model – the person, environment, health and nursing – Roper's model fragments the person into arbitrary physiological systems, fails to stress the social, psychological and environmental components of life, and presents health in a negative way that leads to a focus on ill-health and patient labelling. In the light of such an unhappy performance on the first three components, it is not surprising to find the model leading to a simplistic approach to nursing that fails to recognize the patient as an integrated person.

In conclusion, the above discussion suggests that the Roper model of nursing has major weaknesses as a model upon which to base general hospital care when compared to other alternatives. Reference to the criteria on p. 138 for the ideal hospital model show that it also fails to pass most of these tests, succeeding only in being simple and in recognizing the need for the patient to function at home. Roy is perhaps stronger than Orem in showing the patient to be an integrated human being, but Orem has the advantage of stressing developmental effects and also health education. The FANCAP scheme meets some of these criteria, particularly in very acute, high-dependency situations. All models need using with the patient's point of view in mind.

There is sufficient merit in the work of Orem, Roy and also the FANCAP assessment scheme to suggest that they should be developed further in hospital care, being either refined, adapted or even partly merged. The Roper model, however, has such serious flaws that, while the underlying concept of independence is of value, the current approach should be radically reworked or abandoned in favour of more patient-sensitive models of care.

References

Bellman LM (1996) Changing nursing practice through reflection on the Roper, Logan Tierny Model; the enhancement approach to action research. *Journal of Advanced Nursing* **24**, 129–138.

Black D, Townshend P and Davidson N (1981) *Inequalities in Health*. London: Penguin.

Fawcett J (1995) *Analysis and Evaluation of Conceptual Models of Nursing*, 3rd edn. Philadelphia: FA Davis.

Ignatavicius D & Hausman K (1995) *Clinical Pathways for Collaborative Care*. Philadelphia: WB Saunders.

Orem D (1990) *Nursing: Concepts of Practice*, 3rd edn. New York: McGraw Hill.

Roy C (1984) *Introduction to Nursing: An Adaptation Model*, Englewood Cliffs: Prentice Hall.

Smith R & Draper P (1994) Who is in control? An investigation of nurse and patient beliefs relating to control of their health care. *Journal of Advanced Nursing*, **19**, 884–892.

Whitehead M (1987) *The Health Divide*. London: Penguin.

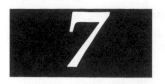

Models in Community Care

Introduction

Primary health care has increasingly come to lead the health care agenda in the late 1990s. As with other areas of the NHS there has been rapid change with practice nurses and latterly nurse practitioners growing in importance. Whatever the changes, nursing remains one of the main methods by which care in the community will be delivered and therefore community staff have to be aware of the philosophy that underpins their work if they are to meet the challenges that lie ahead. Primary health care has two important considerations; patients need to develop self-care skills and maintain as much independence as possible but in order to do so, perhaps nurses need to approach patients as partners in care rather than as recipients of care. Conceptual frameworks to help nurses in primary health care settings therefore need to embrace notions of self-care and partnership.

Characteristics needed for models in community care

Community nurses are very busy people and could be forgiven for thinking that models are all about theorizing, which is all very well for those who have the time, but the average community nurse has to get on with caring for patients. Consequently, models may seem of little value to community nurses. As nurses build up their experience in caring for patients living at home, they might also feel that they learn from experience the care that is required. Nursing models may therefore be seen as a rigid bureaucratic approach to care that could be imposed upon the nurse's own experience-based view of how an individual should be nursed. If a model is to avoid rejection on these grounds it needs relevance, flexibility and it has to be seen as something that helps rather than hinders.

This view corresponds with the description of the 'expert nurse' given by Benner (1984), who suggests that this is the final stage of development reached by nurses as they evolve from being novices to advanced beginners, competent and then proficient practitioners. Benner discusses the need for frameworks and guidance to help the nurse reach the expert stage and it could therefore be argued that the use of nursing models, at least in the early stages of a community nurse's career, helps to achieve the later stages of proficiency and expertise. The hospital nurse works in an environment where there are usually other nurses to turn to for help and advice; the community nurse, although part of a team, spends much of his or her time with patients alone. Hence the need for a framework to assist the nurse along Benner's road to expertise. That framework is a nursing model.

In discussing nurses' own informal models of care, Luker (1988) commented on how important they are in pointing the direction that individual nurses are likely to follow in carrying out care but also noted that they tend to lead to an informal and unsystematic way of working which she considered characteristic of many community nurses. Luker went on to point out that it is very difficult to share such informal models of care with others.

When this is considered in conjunction with the often single-handed nature of the community nurse's work, and Benner's analysis of how nursing expertise develops, an argument in favour of nursing models starts to emerge. It is essential, given the different members of the community team that everybody is using the same approach to care. Care must be consistent and not contradictory as different members of the primary health care team (PHCT) come into contact with the patient and their family. The dangers of interprofessional rivalry and territorialism are well recognized by James (1995) who urged that the PHCT environment must be one in which these problems simply are not an option. She urges good communication and the investment of time in building up working relationships while stressing the importance of education in avoiding these pitfalls. Littlewood (1995) considers that the situation is likely to be brought to head soon as a result of reprofiling and major skillmix exercises which will fundamentally alter the make-up of the PHCT and how it works.

The PHCT has several nurse members who historically come from different backgrounds as well as members of other professions such as medicine and social work. If the nurse members of this team have different philiosophies underpinning their care and are jealously guarding their own turf, the result is likely to be confusion for the patient and a lack of effective teamwork. Unfortunately, there is research evidence of precisely this lack of agreement. It has been provided by Wiles and Robison (1994) who studied teamwork in a sample of 20 practices in one Family Health Service Authority (FHSA) by interviewing members of each staff group in each practice.

The researchers found that while the philosophy of care described by practice nurses and district nurses had a lot in common with each other and also with the GPs, there was a significant divergence when it came to health visitors and midwives. If two such important members of the PHCT do not share the philosophy of other members, this is potentially fertile ground for disagreement and confusion. The health visitors and midwives also reported much higher levels of disagreement with regard to the roles and responsibilities of other colleagues when compared to district and practice nurses. It should also be noted that there was a general assumption among all staff that the GP was the leader of the PHCT, though the researchers felt that as a result of the extensive programme of interviews they undertook, if anybody had the potential to challenge GPs in the future it was the practice nurses, especially as they develop nurse practitioner roles.

Models of nursing offer a potential way of helping to bring together this fragmented picture as they can give staff working in the primary health care team a shared philosophy of care. The UKCC have chosen to perpetuate this divided approach to community care by opting for eight different types of specialist community nursing qualification (and yet they opted for no differentiation among the much more specialized field of hospital nursing – very strange?). Educationalists in this field could help minimize the divisiveness of the UKCC approach by ensuring that common philosophies of care underpin the educational programmes preparing staff for these different qualifications. The study of several models of nursing offers the opportunity for students to work towards such a common philosophy.

Such a model for the community needs to reflect the experiences of many different practitioners and their patients, allowing nurses to structure care in a logical way that is easily shared with others. The model therefore needs to be based in reality and be derived from that reality. It needs to be as unambiguous as possible – jargon is positively harmful in this respect.

Community care involves the patient (and family) dealing with his or her own health care needs. This leads towards a philosophy of self-care or independence. It is essential for continuity of care that the approach of the family and patient should reflect the philosophy of the nurse. In order to achieve such harmonization, a simple model that is readily grasped by lay carers is essential. Simplicity and a focus on independence therefore emerge as key ingredients of any community model.

A nursing approach that is aiming at self-care or independence can, however, be misinterpreted by the patient or family as neglect or a lack of care, There is a thin dividing line between the nurse saying 'You must learn to do this for yourself Mrs Smith' and the perception that this is because the nurse cannot be bothered to do whatever it is for Mrs Smith herself. This points to the need for an open discussion about the main aims of care with the patient and family so that the model or philosophy of care is fully understood.

The model may, however, be rejected by the patient, which leaves the nurse in a difficult position, being very much a guest in the patient's home, seeing the patient perhaps for half an hour every other day. Tactful negotiation and compromise, coupled with recognition of the patient's own rights of self-determination are essential in this situation.

The involvement of the family in care, and the recognition that such care is carried out in the home, requires that any model should address the importance of family relationships and other social factors relevant to the patient's domestic situation. Unless the model directs the nurse to assess such areas and formulate goals that are appropriate, it is of little value in community nursing. This argument has been pursued by Haggart (1994) who considers that Neuman's systems model offers a sound basis for public health nursing (see p. 211 for a brief account of this model). In her view, the wellness-oriented approach of Neuman which seeks to involve clients in their health care and which focuses on prevention as a key means of intervention all make for a model which is congruent with the needs of community nursing. Involving patients in their care is a key characteristic of several other models which have developed in the field of mental health such as King's model (see p. 215) and this partnership in care is a highly desirable aspect of community nursing (Kenrick and Luker, 1995).

However, what is desirable may not translate into performance. The Porter in Shakespeare's *Macbeth* famously tells Macduff that drink 'provokes the desire but it takes away the performance'. Do exhortations by academics urging community staff to involve patients as partners in care lead to staff agreeing it is a good idea but not translating this into practice as they distrust academics? In short, it 'takes away the performance'! There is interesting evidence in this area from a study by Kendall (1993). She investigated the interaction between health visitors and mothers in a sample consisting of 62 taped interviews. Kendall found that client participation was rarely initiated by the mother or sought by the health visitor who dominated the conversations. Health visitors appeared to consider their advice giving constituted legitimate health promotion activity in a one-to-one relationship with the mother, despite the fact that they did not allow the mothers to play active parts in the consultations. The much-espoused notion of involving patients as partners in their care was not happening in this study. It has to be acknowledged that this is only a single study and would need replication to be more confident about the significance of the findings; however, it does provide some evidence showing health visitors do not engage clients as equal partners in care, however desirable that may be.

Perhaps an educational preparation founded upon an explicit philosophy of client involvement as found in participative models such as those of King of Neuman might make for more evidence on the ground that community staff really do regard clients as partners in care? Normandale (1995) has written of just such an approach in her health visiting practice in which she based her work upon the model of Peplau (see p. 212). She stresses the ideas of developing relationships and partnerships with clients were ideally suited to her practice and found using Peplau's ideas allowed her to develop therapeutic interpersonal relationships with mothers. Although her work has not been formally externally evaluated, Normandale reports in a critically reflective vein that her clients and herself feel that this approach has greatly enhanced her practice. This contrasts with the health visiting practice described above by Kendall (1993).

Hall (1994) offers a single case study describing an attempt to use Peplau's model in the community care of a middle-aged man with haemophilia who acquired AIDS as a result of infected blood products. Her case study is instructive in that she was forced by local policy to use the Roper Logan Tierney assessment schedule to try and derive a plan of care based upon Peplau's conceptual framework. This is clearly absurd as it fails to recognize the internal validity and consistency of a model such as Peplau's. It also demonstrates the folly of blanket and rigid implementation of nursing models, particularly the Roper model. It is equivalent to planning a shopping trip to the DIY store based upon an assessment of what you need in the bakers! Single case studies of this type are unfortunately of little value anyway unless there is an accumulation of similar studies which can be analysed together.

The patient discharged from hospital may have received very variable amounts of discharge information and health education. Ever-earlier discharges reduce the amount of time available for ward-based patient teaching. The community nurse, therefore, can usually expect that patients will need a substantial amount of teaching and education in the immediate short term after discharge, followed by encouragement and reinforcement to sustain health-oriented interventions such as dieting, giving up smoking or reducing alcohol intake over a prolonged period of time. A strong health education component is therefore seen as an essential ingredient of a successful community model of nursing care.

A philosophy of self-care underlies much community nursing activity with the aim being the promotion of independence. This leads Kenrick and Luker (1995) to raise the interesting point that control over health education should not rest with the nurse, but with the client, who will use the nurse as a resource to learn what-ever the client feels he or she needs to know and who may look to the nurse more in a counselling and supportive role. Nurses may find this difficult to come to terms with, especially as their own experience of education has tended to be didactic (i.e. the teacher tells the student what he or she needs to know, usually via a lecture, rendering the student a passive receiver of knowledge). Exposure to the ideas of writers such as King, Neuman and Peplau may make it easier for the nurse to fully implement the self-care concept of Orem which underpins much community practice. Then, as Haggart (1994) argues, community nursing really could start to empower communities and individuals in the pursuit of better health.

Continuity of care requires that just as the family and community nurse should try to harmonize their care philosophy, so too should the hospital and community team. A nursing model that is to be applied in the community should ideally be consistent with that used in hospital in order to avoid the confusion that may follow in the patient's own mind on seeing the nursing care given after dis-charge contradicting the care given in hospital. It may be argued that the environment and health status of the patient after discharge are very different from in hospital and that, therefore, it is inappropriate to try to use the same model of care. This is true, but in many cases a change in emphasis or in the way the model is interpreted can accommodate this change rather than switching model. The reverse is also true if a patient is hospitalized after a period of community care. Orem's model is particularly striking in this respect as the model has the built-in notion of different systems of nursing care which reflect the whole continuum of dependency.

This requires of models that they be flexible enough to apply equally well in hospital and community settings, but it also requires nurses to be flexible and creative in the way that they use models if this goal is to be achieved. A piece of rubber is very flexible, but only if a person bothers to try to bend it; so too with a nursing model, even if it is flexible, it will only meet the patient's needs if the nurse has the wit to utilize it individually and creatively.

However, if the nurse feels that a change of model is justified upon discharge, it is important to discuss this change in philosophy with the patient in order that the patient fully understands the changes which may occur in care and the reasons behind such changes.

Community nurses therefore need a common repertoire of nursing models shared with their hospital colleagues in order that the care required for differing patients after discharge may be continued without any major hiatus or contradiction. Hospital and community nurses need to discuss conceptual frameworks for care in order that disruption may be minimized when patients are transferred from one environment to another.

Among the many changes that have occurred in community nursing in the last few years perhaps none is potentially as revolutionary as the development of the nurse practitioner (NP). This is not the place to launch into a full discussion of their role but it is important to recognize that despite the difficulties the UKCC appear to have had in including NPs into the family of nursing, the Royal College of Nursing's description of the role has no such problem (RCN, 1996). The NP therefore works within a nursing conceptual framework even though their role includes being the first point of contact for patients with undifferentiated medical problems, utilizing expanded assessment and physical examination techniques to arrive at a likely cause of the patient's health problem and the authority to act autonomously, if appropriate, in resolving that problem using a holistic patient-centred approach. NPs therefore are not doctor substitutes and do not have a disease focus. They operate in such a way as to have a clear focus on health, to see the whole person and the family environmental context and to always remember that they are nurses providing a service called nursing. This approach complies with the four key dimensions of any nursing model; that is, statements about health, the person, the environment and nursing. The RCN Institute nurse practitioner degree programme includes coursework on nursing models in its curriculum to further emphasize the point. The NP therefore firmly sits within a nursing conceptual framework.

The basic requirements of nursing models that are applicable to community care can therefore be summarized as follows:

- They must be simple, flexible and jargon-free if implementation is to be realistically expected in the busy community environment.
- Any model must be rooted in the shared experience of other community nurses if it is to help beginners achieve expertise.
- The importance of family and social networks must be emphasized.
- The philosophy of the model should reflect the real world of the patient having to care for him or herself therefore notions of independence and self-care should figure prominently.
- Patient participation as a partner in care and in mutual goal setting are strong characteristics of mental health nursing models (see Chapter 8). These characteristics also commend themselves in the field of community care and offer a valuable philosophical underpinning to education for all members of the PHCT.
- Health education and long-term support must figure prominently.

One other recent development referred to in Chapter 4 concerns the replacement of time-consuming care plans with critical pathways (CPs). These new tools for planning care are not confined to hospitals and work is underway in developing them for community use in the USA, including nursing home settings (Ignatavicius, 1995). In recognition of the long-term nature of some community care, the time line in community CPs may be best drawn in terms of weeks or even phases of care such as numbers of home visits. CPs may also be extended from hospitals into the community although this would require a high level of interdisciplinary co-operation by both hospital and community staff. Perhaps in the era of a 'primary care led NHS' this might be no bad thing! CPs may also provide an interesting stimulus to the debate about who should be the leader of the PHCT.

In the following care plans, some of the patients encountered in Chapter 6 will be studied in their home environments to see how the models used to plan care in hospital may be extended into the community setting. How well they measure up against the above criteria will be considered at the end of the chapter.

The Roper model and Jenny Haynes

In Chapter 6 we saw how the Roper model could be used to construct a plan of care for this 78-year-old lady who had been admitted to hospital after suffering a CVA. The next step is to look at how a community nurse might use Roper to plan care for this lady after discharge.

Continuity of care was discussed in the preceding section and in the interests of achieving this goal we hypothesize that a copy of the patient's hospital nursing care plan (pp. 170–171) has accompanied her home. This would allow the community nurse to immediately note the patient's level of independence in the various activities of daily living (ADLs) prior to her CVA without lengthy questioning. The hospital admission assessment also gives the community nurse a baseline to work from, as it should show how much progress has been made by the patient in recovering independence.

The following care plan has therefore been derived, from comparing the level of independence demonstrated by the patient upon returning home with the usual independent routines outlined in the hospital assessment in order to discover problems. The plan is by no means exhaustive; rather, it is a sample of the sort of problems that may be taken as representative of such a patient when the Roper model is applied in this context. Clearly, this plan will change with time as frequent reassessment of the progress being made by the patient occurs.

Care plan: Jenny Haynes

Problem	Goal	Intervention
(1) Access to bath/bedroom limited by risk of falling on stairs due to L-sided weakness (A).	Pt will toilet and sleep downstairs.	1. Rearrange furniture downstairs. 2. Order commode.
	Pt will return to use of bed/bathroom (L).	1. OT Assessment for stair handrail. 2. Encourage physio at day hospital.
(2) Anxious about stairs due to L-side weakness (A).	Pt will state less anxious about falling.	1. Let Pt talk about fears. 2. See above.

Problem	Goal	Intervention
(3) Slurring of speech persists (A).	Pt will improve verbal communication.	1. Listen carefully. 2. Encourage speech. 3. Discuss with Pt's sister. 4. Arrange speech therapist appt.
(4) Discharge Wt 73 kg Ht 1.52 m. Obesity therefore restricting movement (A).	Pt to lose 8 kg in 3 months.	1. Discuss diet with Pt and sister. 2. Give reducing diet sheets.
(5) Reluctance to drink due to fear of incontinence may lead to dehydration.	Fluid intake of at least 2 l/day.	1. Explain importance of drinking; see (7). 2. Maintain fluid chart as reminder.
(6) Constipation (A).	Pt will have bowels open every 2 days.	1. (4) 1, (4) 2 above to include fibre. 2. See (5) above. 3. Mild aperient prn.
(7) Incontinence of urine (A).	Pt will not be incontinent	1. Order commode for downstairs. 2. Pelvic floor exercises. 3. Reduce fluid intake in evening; see (5).
(8) Unable to maintain personal hygiene (A).	Pt will state she is happy with personal hygiene	1. Arrange 3 baths/wk with DN. 2. Strip wash with help of sister x4/wk. 3. Deliver bath board and seat. 4. Encourage maximum Pt participation.
(9) Unable to dress self (A).	Pt will be able to dress unaided in 1 month.	1. Reinforce and encourage skills learnt in hospital. 2. Discuss clothing adaptation, e.g. Velcro.
(10) Hypothermia (P).	Pt will not develop hypothermia.	1. Teach Pt & sister. 2. Give leaflets, etc. 3. Wall thermometer. 4. Refer social worker re benefits.
(11) Restricted mobility. Cannot walk without another person to help (A).	Will be able to walk 20 m with walking aid only.	1. Day hosp. physio. 2. Teach passive exercises to Pt & sister. 3. Encouragement and practice each visit.
(12) Pressure sores (P).	Pt will not develop any pressure sores.	1. Teach Pt & sister about pressure care; devise care plan.
(13) Restricted activity may lead to boredom and frustration (P).	Pt will develop new interests.	1. Provide wheelchair. 2. Son-in-law to build ramp to front door. 3. Refer to voluntary community visitors. 4. Contact local day centre, arrange transport. 5. Explore potential skills with OT.

Problem	Goal	Intervention
(14) Difficulty in sleeping downstairs (A).	Pt will have min. of 7 h sleep/night	1. Hospital medication to continue in reduced dose. 2. Review in 1 week.
(15) Pt stated 'I would have been better off dead'. Depressed (A).	Pt will talk positively about the present and tomorrow.	1. Allow Pt chance to verbalize fears and anxieties.

The Roy model and Valerie Wilkins

In Chapter 6 the Roy model was used to plan care for Mrs Wilkins after she had undergone bowel resection due to cancer and the formation of a colostomy. If a copy of her hospital care plan was sent to the community nurse this would facilitate care by allowing the community nurse to see how Mrs Wilkins felt about her surgery and how well she adapted in hospital. The assessment follows the convention of identifying what Roy calls 'maladaptive behaviour' by underlining it, in order that problem statements may be formulated reflecting these areas. The problems identified and their causes give the DN a framework for psychosocial support in addition to physical care.

First-level assessment	Second-level assessment		
	Focal	Contextual	Residual
PHYSIOLOGICAL MODE *Oxygenation*: RR16, P74. Non-smoker, no cough. *Fluid balance*: Drinking freely, looks well hydrated. *Nutrition*: Ht 1.6 m Wt 45 kg.			
Lost 5 kg since surgery.	Surgery.		
Anxious and uncertain about diet, eating little.	Lacks knowledge of what to eat.	Dislikes stoma functioning.	Worried bag will leak.
Elimination: Stoma is pink, looks healthy, functioning 2–3 times/day. Pt unhappy about changing bag.	Disgust at contents.	Dislikes smell in house.	Afraid 'may catch something'.
Abdominal wound healed but has discharging sinus.	Wound infection.		
Frequency and pain on p.u.	UTI.		
Rest/exercise: Sleeping very poorly.	Anxiety.	Afraid bag will leak in her bed.	
Feels fatigued.	Major surgery.	Anaemic.	
Regulation: Still has some pain and discomfort.	Surgery.		
SELF-CONCEPT MODE *Physical*: Disgusted at the stoma. 'Thought I could cope as it was only temporary, but it's so horrible'.	Apperance of stoma.		Beliefs about normal bowel function
Worried about weight loss.	Loss of 10 kg in 4 months.	Clothes lost fit and shape.	Belief it's a bad sign.
Personal: Feels worthless and powerless.	Stoma.	Loss of control over body function.	Afraid to meet people. Ashamed of stoma.

First-level assessment	Second-level assessment		
	Focal	*Contextual*	*Residual*
Fears the cancer may return.	Knows surgery was for cancer.		'You can't cure cancer, it kills you in the end'.
ROLE FUNCTION MODE Anxious about returning to work, loss of income.	Surgery will mean off work for 4–6 weeks.	How will others at work accept her stoma?	
Worried stoma will stop her enjoying grandchildren. Isolation from family.	Fears she cannot play with them.		Fears family may reject her now.
INTERDEPENDENCY MODE Depressed about future relationships.	Fears nobody will want to know her with stoma.		
Fears will lose independence if cancer returns.	Knows diagnosis.		Belief cancer will return.

The Orem self-care model and Mabel Bush

Mable was discharged home 2 weeks after surgery, still in need of a significant amount of nursing care. Her self-care ability needs to be examined in the light of her pre-hospital, as well as her present, abilities. Discharge home with a copy of her hospital care plan for the community nurse will greatly facilitate this process and in constructing this assessment and care plan it will be assumed that this was the case. The community nurse therefore already has a baseline of her pre-illness self-care ability to work from.

Post-discharge self-care ability

AERATION

Very SOB on exertion, cannot manage steps. P88 irreg., RR22.

FLUID BALANCE

Remains anxious about incontinence and is reluctant to drink. Admits she had several 'accidents' in hospital.

NUTRITION

Cannot now get to the shops and admits to still being worried about her constipation. Can cook for herself although preparing some food will be difficult (e.g. vegetables).

ACTIVITY AND REST

Lacks confidence in walking, can only manage a few metres with the aid of a stick. Admits she is frightened of what will happen to her if she falls over again. Cannot manage steps (see aeration). Sleeping is only possible if she is sat upright as she gets breathless; tends to prefer dozing in a chair. Hopes she can resume her embroidery. Is aware that she cannot now manage to bath herself or use the bathroom. There is a pressure sore on the back of her R heel, dressed with Opsite.

SOCIALIZATION/SOLITUDE   Is very concerned about being a burden on her neighbour. Does not think family will be bothered with her; fearful of living alone and how she will manage the house.

HAZARDS   Feels she may fall again; worried about security of house with her on her own inside.

NORMALCY   Relieved to be out of hospital, acknowledges everybody was very kind and helpful, but did not like it there. Glad to be home, but unsure of the future now, feeling sad and wondering what will happen to her. Is thinking about selling up and moving to a nursing home, but she and her husband had lived in this house for nearly 50 years so she is very reluctant to do so.

DEVELOPMENT   'My body is letting me down, you get so useless when you are old'. Mabel seems depressed and unable to carry on with life alone, feels this is the beginning of the end. (See admission assessment.)

HEALTH DEVIANCY   Remains uncertain about her medication. Her hip is still painful and there is some ankle oedema, she is sitting with her feet on a foot stool with the pressure over the back of her heels, including the area that has a pressure sore dressing. Is unaware of the cause of her pressure sore. Does not know how she will adapt to her reduced mobility as she does not think she will be able to get out of the house again or walk more than a few metres.

By putting together information contained in the hospital care plan and knowledge gained from the above assessment, the community nurse may devise a plan of care similar to that given below. The whole strategy is centred around improving Mabel's self-care abilities and developing the nursing role away from a partially compensatory mode towards a more educative consultative mode.

Self-care deficit (problem)	Goal	Intervention
(1) Unable to prevent pressure sore formation (P).	Pt will avoid pressure sore formation.	1. Teach about pressure sores. 2. Encourage mobility. 3. Spenco cushion L heel. 4. Sit on settee, or teach correct use of foot stool.

Self-care deficit (problem)	Goal	Intervention
(2) Uninfected pressure sore R heel 3 cm diameter.	Sore will heal within 3/12.	1. Granuflex dressing. 2. See (1).
(3) Unable to maintain own hygiene.	Will be able to carry out own hygiene to a standard acceptable to Pt.	1. Order commode, discuss emptying with neighbour. 2. Work out strip-wash routine with Pt. 3. Daily visits to help with (3)2 but encouraging more self-care per visit.
(4) Occasionally unable to maintain continence of urine.	Pt will be continent at all times.	1. Teach pelvic floor exercises. 2. Review diuretic regime teach Pt re diuretics. 3. Pt to keep own fluid chart. See (3) & (9).
(5) Inadequate diet due to lack of knowledge and Pt's inability to shop for self.	Pt to eat healthy well-balanced diet.	1. Discuss difficulties in food preparation. 2. Teach about healthy diet and food prep. 3. Give leaflets on diet. 4. Refer for meals on wheels assessment. 5. Discuss shopping with neighbour.
(6) Pt unable to have normal bowel motions due to constipation (P).	Pt will have bowels open every 2 days.	1. See (5). 2. Fluid intake 2.5 l/day; see (4)3. 3. Mild aperients prn.
(7) Pt is unable to maintain social contact (A) which may lead to loneliness and possible disorientation (P).	Pt will engage in social contact and comment favourably on this.	1. Suggest friends visit. 2. Discuss referral to Help the Aged voluntary visitors and luncheon club. 3. Discuss news/current affairs on visits. 4. See (11)3.
(8) Pt does not understand her medication	Pt will achieve self-medication and show safe level of knowledge of her drugs.	1. Discuss and teach. 2. Measure out daily needs in labelled egg cups. 3. Reinforce importance of medication at each visit. 4. Suggest purchase of tablet dispensing aid.
(9) Pt unable to walk > 7 m due to fear of falling, pain and SOB (A).	Pt will be able to walk 20 m, with stick, in 4/52. Short term: 10 m 1/52, 15 m 2/52, 15 m outdoors at 3/52.	1. Discuss how Pt feels about her walking. 2. Encourage walking at each visit, give +ve reinforcement. 3. Check correct use of walking stick. 4. Check safety of floor coverings, furniture, etc. 5. Refer domestic physio? 6. See probs. (7) & (10).

Self-care deficit (problem)	Goal	Intervention
(10) Pt has pain in hips which she cannot relieve (A).	Pt will be able to relieve any pain herself. Pain free in 5/7.	1. Review analgesia with GP. 2. Teach about analgesia 3. See (8)2. 4. Check positioning for comfort. 5. See (11).
(11) Pt very anxious about how she will cope on her own (A).	Pt will talk of future plans in a positive way, state less anxious in 2/52.	1. Encourage Pt to talk of worries and how she sees the future. 2. Help Pt explore possible strategies for future. 3. Encourage contact with son living in UK. 4. Check security of house, arrange visit from crime prevention officer. 5. Refer social worker. 6. See (7).
(12) Pt may be demoralized and neglect herself (P).	Pt will achieve maximum self-care and express a +ve view of the future.	1. See (7) & (11). 2. Give +ve reinforcement and encouragement for all self-care. 3. Monitor appearance of Pt and house.

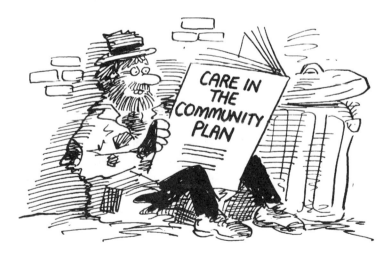

Discussion

The experienced community nurse will be aware that there are many social networks supporting the patient at home, some obvious and some not so obvious. These range from immediate family through to neighbours and on to people such as sympathetic local traders, for example the milkman or owner of the corner shop. The patient's survival and level of functioning may depend heavily on such networks; it is therefore appropriate to consider how the three models reviewed here treated such networks.

The Roper model, focusing as it does on physiological aspects of independence, clearly failed to point the nurse in the direction of the patient's social networks, which remained largely unexplored in the case of Jenny Haynes. On the other hand, Roy's assessment looked into interdependence and role function and in the case of Valerie Wilkins allowed the nurse to explore these areas, outlining a variety of problems and possible interventions. By the same token, Orem required the nurse to assess solitude/socialization, which brought out Mabel Bush's fears of becoming a burden and her concern that her family would no longer be bothered with her.

The experienced community nurse using Roper's model may well enquire into such areas automatically, but this should not be taken for granted. Roper's failure to explore social networks compared to the explicit way these areas are to be assessed when using Roy or Orem is unsatisfactory if this model is to be used in the community.

Closely allied with social aspects of care is the question of how patients feel about their problems, what are their fears and anxieties? The psychological dimension of the patient must be considered, and here again we find Roper deficient as there is a lack of room in the assessment to explore feelings. Jenny Haynes stated that she felt she would be better off dead, a chance remark that arose because Roper requires the nurse to explore the patient's views about dying. Setting aside the difficulty of broaching such a subject to a patient, we have only the tip of the iceberg in this despairing comment. Does Roper's model offer the nurse any help in dealing with a patient expressing such views? Could another approach to Jenny Haynes have led the nurse in through easier ground to explore her psychological problems?

Consider the following differing avenues offered by Orem that might permit a gradual opening up of the patient's problems.

- 'How easy is it going to be to meet people from now on?' (Solitude/socialization)
- 'How do you think you will be able to manage on your own?' (Hazards)
- 'What are your feelings about going to a day centre once a week to meet others?' (Normalization)
- 'How do you feel your life is changing now?' (Developmental)

Somehow this seems a less direct and confrontational way in to the patient's problems and the philosophy of a continuum of self-care/dependent care gives the nurse some clear ideas to use in trying to develop interventions to meet the patient's needs as they unfurl within this assessment framework. Roy's model might also offer a more perceptive and gradual approach to Jennie's psychological problems, as the nurse can explore how she feels about herself and her relationships with others via the psychosocial modes of the assessment. The care plans for both Valerie Wilkins and Mabel Bush show a more sensitive and perceptive approach to the patient's psychological problems because the relevant models open the subject area up gradually in the assessment stage and give the nurse a clear and relevant philosophy to work with in planning care.

This difference of approach poses questions such as how well-qualified the nurse is to use the model and whether the nurse has the time and skills to utilize the assessment tool fully. Taking the second question first, it is apparent that Orem and Roy's assessments require the nurse to have considerable skills in questioning in order that various sensitive areas may be explored. Time is also at a premium. Valerie Wilkins' ability to cope with her stoma is going to depend upon a lot more than mastering the simple mechanical skills of changing a bag, and to help her nursing as a profession must recognize this crucial fact and begin to tackle these difficult areas with tools that are sensitive enough to do the job. Nursing, therefore, will need to develop considerable sophistication if models such as these are to be used in preference to the rather simplistic and naïve approach of Roper.

The issue of how the nurse's view of patient problems differs from the patient's is nicely illustrated by Mabel Bush. The nurse sees occasional incontinence as a problem and hopefully sets a goal of trying to minimize accidents in the short term and aiming for a completely dry patient in the long term. However, Mabel might be unconcerned by the odd bit of dampness 'After all I've been through, it's a minor thing' and not see incontinence as a problem. Alternatively, she might cope with the problem by denial, hence the importance of the community nurse using all her senses in assessing a patient. The unmistakable odour of incontinence might have to be reconciled with a patient steadily denying having any problems. Jenny Haynes may view her house as adequately heated, having become unaware of the real cold, and may consider her weight no problem at all while Valerie Wilkins may be convinced, despite all assurances to the contrary, that her stoma bag smells offensively.

In each of these three patients, it can be seen that, whichever model is used, the patient's perception of a problem may be very different from the nurse's. Unless the nurse is aware of this and is prepared to try to see things from the patient's point of view, then progress will be very limited. All three models used here lack a patient perspective as they were originally formulated and the nurse must be prepared to graft on to these models a notion of the patient's point of view.

Alternatively, the nurse may start out with a conceptual framework which places partnership with the patient at the centre of care (see p. 185 where the value of writers such as Peplau, Neuman and King in community care has been stressed). A nurse working from such an approach would concentrate upon obtaining the patient's point of view, understanding the significant forces at work in the individual's life which will probably affect diet or attitudes towards continence to a greater extent that the nurse's simple exhortations ever would. This could then lead to negotiating mutually acceptable goals in connection with weight loss or continence which might have a greater chance of success as interventions would acknowledge the social circumstances of the individual and the patient would have agreed that this was a worthwhile goal that she would like to achieve.

The practice nurse, and increasingly the nurse practitioner, often manages groups of patients in nurse-led clinics for conditions such as asthma or hypertension in addition to women's health. Nurse-led clinics often have a common theme therefore of patients with a chronic condition requiring self-management to maintain health. The nurse must work with a complex interplay of psychosocial factors, drawing upon significant biomedical knowledge and deploying a wide range of communication skills in order to assist the patient to maintain health. Lecturing the patient about the benefits of weight loss or smoking cessation will achieve little; however, a holistic nursing approach based upon the twin notions of partnership and self-care offers a much greater chance of success. The practice nurse therefore can also benefit from drawing upon interactionist conceptual frameworks rather than the physiological emphasis attributed to Roper, Logan and Tierny. The inclusion of *relevant* conceptual frameworks within community nursing education is therefore highly desirable, especially if they are taught as conceptual frameworks to guide practice rather than as something that comes out of a recipe book. Dogmatic detail is no substitute for intellectual freedom and creativity.

Practice nurses (and nurse practitioners) are also free from the bureaucratic nonsense described by Hall (1994) of NHS Trusts imposing single models such as the Roper model on all staff as at present they do not work for NHS Trusts. Cumbersome care plans are not required, although some record of care is needed; rather, it is about taking on board the philosophy that underpins the writing of nurses such as Peplau, Neuman and King that matters. By truly valuing patients as partners in care, practice nurses can give a clear lead to hospital nurses in what is increasingly becoming a 'primary health care led NHS'.

In the introduction to this chapter we emphasized the fact that the community nurse is operating as part of a team of carers, and how important it is for all members of that team to share the same philosophy of care. There is little value in the community nurse aiming to make patients as independent as possible or to maximize their self-care ability if other members of the team such as the nursing auxiliary or health care assistant carry out all care for the patient at the expense of self-care or independence.

It is easy to see how, in the case of Jenny Haynes, goals and interventions for problems (8) and (9) in the care plan could easily be undermined by a well-intentioned assistant who washed and dressed the patient totally because it was simply quicker than spending the time involved in letting the patient do as much as possible for herself. Similar observations relate to Mabel Bush (e.g. problems (3) and (9)). Unless all the care team and the informal carers of the patient are speaking the same language and sticking to the same plan of care, then chaos and confusion will result, with the patient picking up mixed messages and the district nurse's plans coming to nought, whatever model they are based upon.

It may be argued that Roy's model is the most complex and that therefore it is here that misunderstandings may occur. It is the author's experience in teaching this model that students often disagree whether a stimulus is focal, contextual or residual. Consideration of the nutrition part of Valerie Wilkins' assessment is a case in point, as it is a matter of opinion whether the prime cause of her eating little is a lack of knowledge (as stated here and therefore the focal stimulus for the problem) or whether it is a dislike of the stoma functioning (here assumed to be a contextual stimulus). If these two causes or stimuli were reversed and her dislike of the stoma functioning was considered to be focal while the lack of knowledge was considered contextual, would it make any difference to the plan of care?

The answer of course is no. What matters is that we have identified a problem – the patient is eating little and is very anxious and uncertain about what she should be eating – and have discovered that this is due to a combination of a lack of knowledge about diet and a dislike of the stoma functioning (and also a fear of the bag leaking, the residual stimulus). Roy's model urges intervention wherever possible around the causes of the problems and that is what the care plan sets out to do by teaching her about her diet and helping her adapt in a variety of ways to the stoma. The title 'focal' and 'contextual' became academic in this context; what matters is that we have identified a problem, worked out the causes of the problem, and are directing nursing care at those causes.

The community nurse should not, therefore, become too preoccupied with the academic minutiae of models, particularly the more complex ones such as Roy, but should adopt a more pragmatic approach to making the general principles work. Having said that, it is still a fact that Roy's model makes the nurse consistently look into the causes of the patient's problems in a way that none of the other models do. To some extent this might leave the nurse guessing at the causes of some problems; there has always been a place in nursing for hunches and the experienced community nurse probably relies upon such hunches from time to time, such is the art of nursing.

This chapter would not be complete without acknowledging that access to hospital-based information and care plans for community nurses is often not all that it should be. It has been assumed that the community nurse had access to hospital care plans for the three patients studied in this chapter, a factor which would save a great deal of time if this were standard practice.

The fragmentation of the NHS that has occurred with the setting up of community and hospital Trusts is not helping the delivery of integrated care. Access to care plans is therefore potentially very benefical for both hospital and community staff. CPs have a great deal to offer as it is not difficult to see how Mabel Bush could have come out of hospital with a CP written to cover the next 3 months. Jenny Haynes may also have had a stroke CP written to continue her care and rehabilitation from hospital into the community.

In conclusion, it seems that Roper's model probably would not deliver the depth and range of holistic care needed to support these three patients in the community nor would it help the practice nurse or nurse practitioner in his or her work or running nurse-led clinics to manage chronic health problems. The self-care orientation of Orem and the emphasis on adaptation which is derived from Roy coupled with the interactionists' perspective all suggest a more useful framework of ideas within which the nurse may operate in the community. The community nurse should have the freedom as an accountable practitioner to use documentation that reflects his or her philosophy of care, rather than an imposed set of documents. They should also recognize that Orem and Roy's models were hospital based and therefore not be afraid to adapt them as necessary to fit the needs of the primary health care environment. This is particularly true if an interactionist perspective, involving working with patients towards mutually agreed goals, is adopted as a major part of the nurse's philosophy.

References

Benner P (1984) *From Nurse to Expert.* Menlo Park, CA: Addison Wesley.

Haggart M (1994) A critical analysis of Neuman's systems model in relation to public health nursing. *Journal of Advanced Nursing,* **18**, 1917–1922.

Hall K (1994) Peplau's model of nursing caring for a man with AIDS. *British Journal of Nursing,* **3**(8), 418–422.

Ignatavicius D (1995) *Clinical Pathways for Collaborative Practice.* Philadelphia: WB Saunders.

Kendall S (1993) Do health visitors promote client participation? An analysis of the health visitor–client interaction. *Journal of Clinical Nursing,* **2**, 103–109.

Kenrick M & Luker K (1995) *Clinical Nursing Practice in the Community.* Oxford: Blackwell Science.

James E (1995) Primary health care in the community. In Sines D (ed.) *Community Health Care Nursing,* pp. Oxford: Blackwell Science.

Littlewood J (1995) *Community Nursing.* Edinburgh: Churchill Livingstone.

Luker K (1988) Do nursing models work? *Nursing Times,* **84**(5), 27–29.

Normandale S (1995) Using a nursing model to structure health visiting practice. *Health Visitor,* **68**(6), 246–247.

Royal College of Nursing (1996) *RCN Council Policy Statement on Nurse Practitioners.* London: RCN.

Wiles R & Robison J (1994) Teamwork in primary health care; the views and experiences of nurses, midwives and health visitors. *Journal of Advanced Nursing,* **20**, 324–330.

8 Mental Health Nursing and Models

Mental health nursing today is under tremendous scrutiny and is experiencing an ongoing period of change. As a result there has been close examination of both its future and its role (Peplau, 1994). Not only is there an apparent move away from the title 'psychiatric nurse' to the more politically correct 'mental health professional' but also an associated and long-awaited review of philosophy and approach in general (DOH, 1994). As a result, the relevance of dated and adopted models of care is being questioned for a variety of reasons, not least of which is the move away from institutional to community-based care and the major implications this has for mental health nursing.

In order to explore the value and direction of nursing models in mental health care, the following key issues warrant examination and discussion in a present-day context:

- The increasing transition to community care and related implications for clients, carers and nurses alike.
- An examination of models commonly associated with the mental health nursing role and their critique/evaluation in the light of present-day needs.
- A general discussion of recommendations for practice and the inclusion of essential issues such as advocacy, participation, communication, patients' rights and the 'user movement'.
- A summary of implications for future practice.

It is widely acknowledged that a large proportion of the community will probably have mental health problems at some stage in their lives. It is therefore interesting to note that 95% of these people will *not* see a psychiatrist, but instead have treatment from their GP and a wide range of other professional groups in which nursing figures very prominently (Wilkinson, 1988). Various studies (Paykell, 1982; Mangen *et al.*, 1983) have demonstrated clear benefits to patients who were cared for by community psychiatric nurses in particular, rather than psychiatrists on an outpatient basis. More recent work in Manchester confirms the view that patients treated in day hospitals will have a lower relapse rate than those admitted to hospital as inpatients for treatment of acute episodes of mental illness, although this latter group may show a more rapid short-term improvement (Rae, 1990).

The continuing policy of discharging patients from mental hospitals to the community has only served to further increase the already heavy workload of nurses and other professional groups in providing care for the mentally ill. We are now seeing, therefore, that a major component of care for the mentally ill is carried out by nurses, increasingly in the community. The issue of models of nursing is therefore very relevant to mental health care in the 1990s, and one that has implications for the future role of the mental health nurse.

Community care and related issues

For more than a decade now there has been a growing escalation of debate about the realities of community reforms and resulting community mental health nursing approaches. These have often been associated with a negative as opposed to positive critique (McFayden and Farrington, 1996) and their resulting questionable, influence over the positive or negative mental health of clients (Burrows, 1996). There is no doubt that such reforms, spurred on by the emergence of the NHS and Community Care Act 1990 and the much maligned but associated care programme approach, have been influenced by a mixture of social, clinical, market and public trends (Beecham *et al.*, 1996). However, society's belief in the rights of each individual, well or otherwise, has most certainly shaped the nurse's role in relation to patient advocacy, participation and overall negotiation. This has coincided with a move away from the heavily criticized, historical, medical model.

Community care, irrespective of the arguments, is now undoubtedly a reality. Institutions are closing and mental health nurses are being increasingly deployed in alternative settings such as group homes, crisis intervention centres, GP practices, day hospital services (which incidentally are extending their hours in many cases) and community psychiatric services. There is a distinct mood of unease among some nurses who feel ill-prepared for their changing and often uncertain role. This is coupled with a dramatic shift away from short-term, frequently anxiety-based mental health problems and all that entails. Such a shift has resulted in a lack of definition and direction today. As a result there is a need for mental health nurses, in general, to redefine and reprofessionalize their role with the principles, professional practices and philosophies that are in tune with the needs of those they care for and the setting in which they care (Peplau, 1994; McFayden and Farrington, 1996). Such a call has not gone unnoticed and is reflected in the fairly recent and long overdue evaluation of mental health nursing/services with a host of recommendations being made for the future (DOH, 1994). Not least of which is a change in role title from psychiatric to mental health nurse and an emphasis upon individuals with long-term problems who are usually the responsibility of the community and their long-suffering carers. The approach to caring for such people so far, has been intensely criticized for its ongoing failure and lack of professional input (Zito, 1994). Ultimately, as a result of failing services and inadequate resources, there is also increasing criticism of unproductive, inpatient services by patients, carers and advocacy groups (Rogers *et al.*, 1993). This in itself speaks volumes. However, the future for mental health workers, although in question, has a positive outlook and great opportunity for innovative revision, adaptation and responses to need, if only nurses are willing to take control of their professional arena.

Nursing models are, in part, the key and must reflect such trends and needs and warrant more than a token change in title but a combination of skills, knowledge and ability that ensure the full spectrum of mental illness is both recognized and catered for in a therapeutic relationship (Barker and Johnson, 1996). This may mean the utilization of a combination of models already well defined or the development and integration of new approaches into the sought after, holistic, nursing paradigm.

The changing face of basic philosophy

Within the field of psychiatry there are already a range of models of mental illness which Collister (1986) feels most nurses are familiar with, listing the medical–biological, behaviourist, psychoanalytical and socio-interpersonal models as four main models. There are various other ways of looking at or modelling mental illness besides these four approaches, which were described by Siegler and Osmond (1966). Differing views of mental illness will lead to differing approaches to therapy, the nurse–patient relationship and a whole range of other variables.

The literature, and also the reality of practice, frequently gives less prominence to nursing models of mental health care as the medical model remains in the ascendancy in many areas. Nursing models should not be thought of as alternative models of mental illness to those cited above, but rather as models of caring for patients with a mental illness, however that illness is conceptualized.

Smith (1986) has commented that what is lacking from nurses is a body of knowledge and opinion about psychiatric nursing care. The dominance of the medical model, with its reliance on physical treatment and chemotherapy aiming at a cure, has had profound effects on nursing. It is true that some patients present for treatment in such a disturbed condition that drug therapy is needed to stabilize the situation before any further progress in care or therapy can begin. Nurses have frequently tended to work with specific disease labels in institutional settings, with the emphasis often on custodial care. The dehumanizing effects of the large institutions is well known and focusing on a disease only leads to losing sight of the whole person. This is the history that mental health nursing has been trying to grow away from in the past 10 years.

In fairness to the medical profession, it has to be said that they have their point of view as well as nurses, and this can be very imaginative and creative in many cases. The biomedical model continues to influence both the world of psychiatry and mental health nursing and, in fact, is presently receiving renewed enthusiasm as research increasingly supports neurochemical hypotheses in relation to the development and/or precipitation of mental illness. Gourney (1990) advocates the crucial recognition of such findings and the essential integration of biophysiology into planned nursing care and management as part of the nurses on-going role. In contrast, nurse theorists continue to emphasize the importance of psychosocial complexities so readily ignored historically. The words holism and eclecticism have now become household nursing terms, so to speak. Dawson (1994) in a recent passionate paper condemns the biological approach to mental health nursing altogether, particularly, the professional, uncritical acceptance of this paradigm. It may be that while such contrasting debates continue, holism may never truly become a reality in nursing. It appears, somewhat confusingly, that although the welcomed philosophies of holism, therapeutic communication and self-transcendence have been taken on board (at least theoretically) by the mental health nursing world (Dawson, 1994), the practicalities of how to translate these into practice is still open to debate. Hence the continued acceptance of medically biased treatments and models, albeit with the increasing nursing skill and evaluation needed for such approaches. However, an independent profession of mental health nursing requires the creation of a body of professional knowledge and a view of health care that is unique to nursing, hence the growth of nursing models to try to give a theoretical framework to this effort. Inevitably this might lead to differences with other groups of staff who have different views of mental illness and therapeutic models. But an independent profession should be mature enough to handle such potential conflicts and find negotiated solutions.

Just as general nurses are wrestling with the question 'What is nursing?' so too nurses in the field of mental health must tackle this question. General nursing faces the problem of increasing numbers of paramedical and technical staff taking away bits and pieces of care and treatment, leading to the risk of fragmentation of patient care and the deskilling of nursing. The notion of a nursing body of knowledge and nursing models of practice is an attempt to define the boundaries and profession of nursing. Mental health faces similar problems as various professionals such as clinical psychologists, social workers and occupational therapists increasingly take over aspects of patient care, leading to a loss of continuity and the erosion of the nursing role until little more than a custodial function involving meeting basic physiological and safety needs remains. The development of lay advocacy groups acting to protect the patient's interests is a further challenge to the nursing role.

General nursing has learnt a great deal from mental health nursing in terms of seeing the patient as a whole person rather than a piece of pathology (the medical model). It would be ironic if mental health nursing were now to ignore the lessons that general nursing could teach; that is, the need to define an integrated profession of mental health nursing with its own body of knowledge and models of practice unique to nursing, rather than borrowed from elsewhere. Fitzpatrick *et al.* (1982) have pointed out that nursing's willingness to embrace non-nursing models in psychiatry has done psychiatric nursing a disservice, while McKenna (1989) in a discussion of this issue urges nurses in mental health to strive to develop nursing models of practice rather than rely exclusively on the views of other, different professions. In making this plea, McKenna cites the work of Reed (1987), who argues that only nursing models can lead to a clear understanding of the theoretical and conceptual basis of psychiatric nursing.

If nurses in the field of mental health wish to move once and for all away from the custodial role, then they have to be prepared to move away from the safe ground of the medical model and following doctors' orders to explore new territory, claiming this as mental health nursing. Failure to do so now will mean that in the future most of that territory will have been partitioned out among a wide range of other groups of staff, particularly in the community, leaving mental health nurses as guardians of the keys and the doers of messy jobs that nobody else wants. Ultimately, mental health nurses, whatever the clinical and social setting, must care enough to step out of the shadows of medical imperialism and control and become proactive in giving a voice to those who have none (Dawson, 1994).

Smith (1986) is only one of many authors who has highlighted the traditionally low prestige of mental health nursing, pointing out that the development of a uniquely nursing knowledge base and the use of nursing models as a conceptual framework would be an essential part of a programme aimed at professionalizing this branch of nursing. If it wishes to develop a professional identity of its own, which should benefit both clients and practitioners, then there is a need to

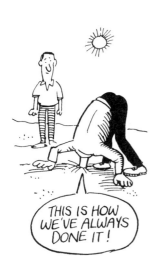

THIS IS HOW WE'VE ALWAYS DONE IT!

develop a unique body of knowledge of which nursing models would form a key part. The phrase mental *health* nursing is chosen quite deliberately in line with modern-day thinking (Peplau, 1994), as another prime factor would be an emphasis upon health rather than illness in such a nursing approach (DOH, 1994). An alternative choice is to continue as before, making the best of other people's views of mental illness, such as the medical model, but aware of the possible retrograde steps towards a deskilled, custodially oriented labour force this may involve.

Existing models – priorities and pitfalls

In the next section of this chapter, models of nursing and some of their basic characteristics are reviewed to see which have most commonly lent themselves towards use in the field of mental health nursing. Traditionally, theoretical frameworks within the mental health field have been handed down from other disciplines and those congruent with mental health nursing practice itself have been poorly articulated (Onega, 1991). Holdsworth (1995) argues that if mental health nurses are to integrate the skills and underlying philosophies necessary to accomplish the diverse task that compromises their professional role, then what is required is an eclectic model based upon the principles of what they term 'folk psychology'. By this they mean an approach that epitomizes the rich and extensive, but unsystematic (as advocated by Peplau) network of verbal descriptions of subjective states found in the language of everyday life. Such a paradigm from which to nurse can already be found in advocates of the patient-centred approach that is so clearly emerging today as a result of increasing criticism of the present service (Brearley, 1990; Rogers *et al.*, 1993). Present-day models must take on board such a view whereby any nursing accounts of mental illness are couched in the language of service users and their subjective experiences of ill health (Holdsworth, 1995).

Discussion elsewhere has identified that models of nursing contain four basic components: a view of the person, how that person reacts with their environment, an understanding of what is meant by health, and finally how nursing comes into play to help the person. These four components are all consistent with mental health nursing, which must focus on the person as a holistic individual who has both physical as well as mental health needs. General nurses have rightly been accused in the past of only seeing the physical at the expense of the psychological needs of the patient; mental health nurses should beware the reverse situation and the risk of neglecting the patient's physical health, biological needs and related physical therapies (Gourney, 1990). The way a person interacts with both the physical and social environment influences their state of mental and physical health and is therefore of great concern to the fourth component of a nursing model, nursing itself. Nursing models, therefore, are built from components which are wholly consistent with mental health care.

We have also seen (p. 29) that models may be broadly grouped into one of three categories; those that are concerned with achieving a balance between systems (homeostatis), be they physical or psychosocial (systems models); those that are concerned with patient development; or those with an interactionist perspective. These three broad approaches to building nursing models are again compatible with mental health care.

Models based on systems run the danger of becoming reductionist if they only focus on physiology, and if this approach alone is used then it would be true to say this is not a suitable way forward (see p. 130 for a critique of Roper's model in this regard). However, systems and the concept of balance operate at many other levels other than cellular biology, particularly in the field of family and community (i.e. social systems) and it is in this area that many patients have problems. Systems in terms of nursing models have been described by Pearson and Vaughan (1986) as continually interacting with each other and also being susceptible to the effects of change both within and without the system, a description that applies to groups such as the family, networks of friends or employees. Viewed in this light, systems are clearly relevant to mental health.

We have already counselled caution about neglecting the person's physical health; health is a complete state of well-being that involves physical as well as psychological and social dimensions. Mental health nurses must also be prepared to promote physical health, and this needs attention to physical systems involving, for example, nutrition, elimination and cardiovascular function. Systems models have a place in mental health nursing providing they stress the importance of social systems, and also as a useful reminder to the nurse to think also about the patient's physical health. This point is illustrated further on.

A significant number of mental health problems stem from developmental difficulties involving growth and change. These processes are characterized by identifiable stages but do not necessarily flow in a smooth, constant, linear way. Progression can involve going backwards to go forwards (cyclical) or may involve a series of branching pathways leading to different goals or a spiralling in towards an eventual goal via a circuitous route. A variety of forces drive change onwards, perhaps in differing directions as the nature of the forces in a person's life change. This analysis of development, due to Chin (1980), seems appropriate for many mental health problems, while engaging in nursing care with a client itself involves development of the nurse–client role through a series of stages.

Interactionist models are based around the way people interact with others and their environment. They seek to discover the meanings that people give to experiences and events and acknowledge the uniqueness of these meanings to individuals, stressing the importance of the nurse's understanding how the patient sees things. In the interactionist view people learn meanings and values through the way they interact with others and also take upon themselves various social roles. This approach to nursing seems to offer a potentially very useful tool in the field of mental health and reflects the increasingly noticeable trend towards psychosocial needs and related therapies.

Having established that the various key principles used in the construction of nursing models are at least consistent with the sorts of problems mental health nurses will encounter, let us now focus on some specific models. It is particularly important to establish the fluidity and adaptability of the four models outlined. There has been a distinct lack of new nursing models in the 1990s which highlights possibly one of three things:

- that existing models encompass the crucial elements of nursing, and therefore, possess an ageless quality already incorporating vital agendas of today such as advocacy, participation, communication and holism;
- that nursing models are just another passing fad that have since lost their impetus in nursing; or
- in the face of increasing criticism regarding the theory/practice gap (Scott, 1994), related difficulties (Kenny, 1993) and new nursing agendas such as community care, nursing models are on hold, so to speak, with a view to review, reflect and rethink the nurse's future role (DOH, 1994; Benton, 1995). This would not be an unwelcome notion as the nursing world has frequently been criticized for the impulsivity with which it has uncritically accepted unworkable or non-British-based frameworks on which to base care (Kenny, 1993).

Certainly, if the former and latter possibilities are to be believed, then the future may see the re-emergence of 'model' development with an increasing emphasis upon reflective practice, primary care, a needs-driven service and independent users (Benton, 1995; Johns, 1996) in the not too distant future. This is not to say that existing models do not hold the key to patient-centred care, whatever the context. After all, there are a handful of models such as those that follow, that continue to dominate, encouraging research, manipulation and application and as such most consistently hold some valuable insights into the world of mental health nursing and universal elements.

It is important for the reader to welcome and embrace the key ingredients of these universal elements: person, environment, health and the nurse's role, which are the pillars on which to base, analyse and apply both existing and newly developing philosophies of care and the models that represent such values (Pearson and Vaughan,

1986). Jooton and McGhee (1996) argue that ultimately 'care involves social, physical or psychological categories and the idea that it can be delivered without a proper infrastructure that promotes these values is a myth'. Hence, nursing models live on and are built mainly on a consistent infrastructure that is universal to most health care needs, care settings and therapeutic relationships. It is generally the emphasis that shifts from one decade to the next, as one priority receives more attention than another.

Elsewhere in this book care planning and the models of Roper, Roy and Orem together with the FANCAP assessment scheme have been discussed in detail in a variety of clinical settings. These approaches are often more suited to the general nursing field with their emphasis on physical care, a criticism particularly valid in the case of Roper. In this chapter, therefore, it is intended to introduce some other models which appear to be more applicable to the mental health setting starting with that of Orlando.

Andrews (1983) considers that the importance of Orlando's work is that she was one of the first theorists to emphasize patient participation in planning care. Orlando sees the main aim of nursing as identifying and helping the patients meet their needs. Schmeiding (1986) has pointed out that the core of this model is the relationship between patient and nurse which allows problem identification and therefore the meeting of patient needs. The importance of this step is not just confined to mental health and is of fundamental importance in all aspects of care.

A view that characterizes Orlando's work is that a patient's presenting behaviour, whatever form that may take, is a plea for help. This requires the nurse to attempt to discover the meaning to the patient of their behaviour stating that while the person's perceptions, thoughts and feelings are internal and therefore not observable, only their behaviour and speech might give clues to these internal processes. The importance of the nurse–client interaction is stressed, with the nurse seeking to fully understand the patient's perceptions and feelings through in-depth conversation and exploration. It is a fundamental understanding of the aims of professional nursing that gives this exploration its sense of direction and makes it unique to nursing, rather than merely conversation.

The failure of nurses to explore the meanings of behaviour with patients and the problems that flow from nurses assuming they know what the behaviour means have been well described by Schmeiding in a review of the research. She is also able to give a series of real anecdotes, some of which are based in mental health care, to show how problems have arisen and been resolved by using this approach.

In summarizing the model, Andrews (1983) considers it to be a valuable guide for nursing practice, though not fully developed as a model and rather narrow in scope. It is an approach to nursing that may clearly be of benefit in many situations in mental health, although it lacks a clearly defined structure for assessment and has little to say about the patient's physical needs.

Another model deserving of attention is the Neuman model, which, according to Whall (1983) may be applied to mental health settings. This is basically a systems model but can be interpreted to include social as well as physiological systems that see the goal of nursing as maintaining equilibrium within the various systems leading to the whole person being restored to health. One problem with this view is the danger of seeing equilibrium as a static rather than a dynamic state of affairs. In the same way, health can be seen as a static state of wellness or as an active state of seeking well-being and improvement, leading to self-actualization. If this latter view of health is subscribed to, then care must be exercised in using systems models not to fossilize the client but to achieve equilibrium in a dynamic sense. The institutionalized long-stay patient may be said to have achieved a state of equilibrium, but it is a static, dependent state leaving the person unable to cope with the changing world outside.

Consider the analogy of a car parked at rest. It is in a state of equilibrium, but it is going nowhere. Now consider that same car driving along at a steady 30 mph: This is a state of equilibrium but is a dynamic state as the forces of friction balance its tendency to accelerate: the key difference is that this car is going somewhere. Note also that if the forces acting on the car get out of balance it will either grind to a halt or accelerate out of control into a crash. In using systems models we are trying to establish equilibrium so that the client neither grinds to a halt nor has a crash, but we should be aiming for a dynamic not a static equilibrium that allows the client room for growth, development and self-actualization.

After this digression into the realms of physics we must return to the Neuman systems model and mental health! This view sees humans as whole persons constantly reacting with stressors in their environment, striving to achieve health, which is seen as a state of wellness determined by physiological, psychological, sociological and developmental factors. This concept of health appears to be a static state of affairs. The stressors to which the person responds are from within the person (intrapersonal), between persons (interpersonal) and on a larger scale in society as a whole (extrapersonal).

The key to understanding the patient's problems lies in identifying these stressors and in discovering the patient's perceptions of them, and Neuman offers a semistructured assessment schedule with which to explore these issues. The goals of nursing are to allow the patient to cope with these stressors and restore equilibrium by working within one of three areas. Primary prevention involves preventing a stressor coming into contact with a person or strengthening the person's defences against that stressor to enable them better to deal with it. This might involve teaching strategies to avoid stress-provoking situations or teaching coping strategies should they arise. Desensitization techniques to help patients with phobic states might also come under this category. Secondary prevention involves helping the patient once a problem has occurred to try to restore stability. This may be thought of as helping the client put the pieces back together, a familiar situation in mental health nursing. Tertiary prevention looks to the future and asks what lessons can be learnt to avoid a recurrence of this problem? There is great potential here for mental health nurses to make a major contribution towards the patient's health.

A different perspective on these three groups of goals is offered by Whall (1983), who, in reviewing the application of the model to psychiatric nursing, suggests that primary prevention consists of helping patients understand that life is full of problems and can be very frustrating and difficult while the secondary level consists of working through feelings. Since admission to hospital is often in response to crisis, many patients are only too aware that life is full of problems. Crisis intervention and stabilizing the situation often take priority after admission, with working through feelings coming later. The tertiary level is described as assisting the client in a crisis by working with available environmental supports. Whall thus sees the tertiary level in the mental health field as working with problems once they have occurred rather than a teaching and learning process to help the patient prevent future recurrence of problems as suggested by Neuman. Whall's analysis is therefore less applicable to a hospital situation than perhaps to others and may be a useful tool in the transition to community-based care and priorities.

Neuman's views on nursing are consistent with the needs of a significant number of clients with mental health problems. The danger is that it may lead to a *status quo* and not emphasize sufficiently the need for the client to achieve and grow in a dynamic way. It is difficult to see how this model may be applied to the situation in which a person has lost contact with reality and is therefore unable to give answers that are rational within the nurse's own frame of reference. This same comment also applies to Orlando's approach. The key question in Neuman's assessment is to ask the patient what they consider to be their main problems; an answer to the effect that the client considers there are no problems, or answers framed within a logic that has lost touch with reality, may leave the nurse wondering which way to turn next. Undoubtedly, client participation is crucial at whatever level. To assume that clients are unable to contribute to their care is prejudicial and untherapeutic. A view not held by clients themselves (Rogers *et al.*, 1993) nor advocated by changing, modern-day philosophies of care (Brearley, 1990).

The third model to be reviewed here is that of Peplau, which with its emphasis on development and growth immediately answers the criticism made of Neuman's model above; that is, the danger of stagnation. Peplau, according to Collister (1986), focuses on the personal interaction between client and nurse and is concerned with the development of this relationship. Anxiety and communication are key ingredients in Peplau's understanding of health for the perception of any threat, which is a process that involves communication, provokes anxiety in the person. Anxiety can be a useful coping tool that allows us to mobilize resources to deal successfully with a threat; however, it can also overwhelm the person leading to anxiety states, preoccupation and a withdrawal from the real world.

The nursing interaction with the patient first involves orientation; that is, making the client aware that help is available and beginning to discover the reasons why the person feels in need of that help. There is a danger of relapsing into the medical model at this stage, with the interaction focusing on disease labels and means of overcoming or attempting to cure a disease entity. Peplau argues that instead the focus should be on the person's situation and problems and seeing these as part of life and an opportunity for learning. In this way the person can grow and develop through their problems in a richer and fuller sense; the experience becomes a positive life event in which the person played a major role and one which is meaningful to their life style in a community setting.

This phase is followed by the process of identification, in which the client begins to identify the nurse as someone who cares and who is able to help. This in turn allows the client to express their feelings although this will be influenced by the degree of dependence the client may feel upon the nurse. The stage is now set for exploiting the strength of the nurse–client relationship and the feelings and patient perceptions that have been uncovered in an attempt to resolve problems. The meanings behind events and behaviours may be explored and goals set at this phase. This problem-solving phase is therefore known as the exploitation phase and leads on to the client leaving the relationship with maximum independence, the resolution phase.

Peplau's model does not offer a structured assessment tool and has been criticized by some for lack of definition and direction (Scott, 1994). However, this is not a criticism directed at Peplau alone. Pearson and Vaughan (1986) have observed that it would be inappropriate if structure did dominate as the core of her model is the forming of a relationship with the client, particularly during the orientation phase. The mental health nurse uses a whole range of skills, and his or her own experience base, in exploring the patient's mental state. This approach does not lend itself to a rigidly structured assessment tool since the assessment is as much patient-led as nurse-led. It is essential, however, that written records be kept and consequently Pearson and Vaughan suggest using Maslow's hierarchy of needs and the SOAP process (see below) alongside Peplau's model as a means of planning and documenting care.

The letters in SOAP stand for Subjective experiences and feelings of the client (S); Objective observations made by the nurse such as height and weight (O); Assessing the client using subjective and objective information that has been gathered to formulate problem statements (A); and finally deciding on a Plan of action (P). We have already seen that an excellent assessment form consists of a blank piece of paper and such a form is ideally suited to a wide range of nursing situations including the SOAP format.

According to Reed and Johnston (1983), Peplau's model has served as a basis for psychodynamic nursing since 1952, when her early work was first published, and has remained a valid model for nursing psychotherapy ever since. It may be said that the model is limited in the number of situations in which it can be applied as it requires a great deal of one-to-one interaction and is therefore time-consuming and its use depends upon the client's ability to recognize that he or she has problems. However, we have argued elsewhere that models should be chosen to suit individual client's needs, there can be no universal model, and it has to be said that whatever approach is followed, it is difficult to help a client who does not recognize that he or she has a problem in the first place.

Peplau's emphasis on good communication is a lesson that all nurses should take on board whatever their speciality and she should also be given credit for being one of the first nurse theorists to try and expound a model of something that is uniquely nursing-based on inductive reasoning from a great deal of observational work.

Peplau's main emphasis is on the way people relate to each other and, as Collister points out, this requires the nurse to 'know thyself' as a person and also maintain a neutral non-judgemental attitude to the client throughout the interaction. The need for a high degree of self-awareness on behalf of the nurse in this model has implications for nursing education as self-awareness training needs to be included in curriculum design if Peplau's model is to be used. Nurses in the general field might also benefit from such an approach since criticisms abound of the inadequate communication skills of nurses (Faulkner, 1993; Arnold and Boggs, 1995). Peplau's work and her emphasis upon the nurse–patient relationship is, therefore, of great relevance to all nurses whatever their speciality and years of experience.

The final model that is reviewed briefly is that of Imogene King. She places the emphasis again on social interaction, although there are strands of systems theory present in her work. King is concerned principally with the way social systems, interpersonal relationships, perception and health are linked together through interactions between people. Problems in the field of mental health commonly arise out of interpersonal relationships and also the social setting of the individual, while the client's perceptions of reality may also lead the person into severe difficulties. Health is seen as coping with stress and being able to function within social roles. The model therefore seems relevant to mental health problems and has a view of health that should be acceptable to nurses in this field.

Interaction with other people in pursuit of common goals leads to three sets of systems, personal, interpersonal and social, and according to Aggleton and Chalmers (1990), the nurse must understand each of these systems and how they affect each other in order that high-quality care may be delivered with the King model.

The personal system is about the client's self-concept, while the interpersonal system relates to communication and interaction with others. The final system, the social system, is concerned with groupings within society which in their turn influence the individual, such as family or the health-care service itself. Notions of power and authority are inherent in this system and may be very relevant to the problems experienced by some clients.

The nurse needs to explore King's three systems with the patient in the assessment stage, seeking both objective and subjective information. This process of interaction should be geared towards arriving at a mutual, shared understanding of problems and goals as the three systems are explored. This process allows the agreement of common goals, and it is this process of mutual goal setting between nurse and patient that is fundamental to King's model. The interaction of human beings with each other and their environment which leads to goal attainment is defined by King (1986) as transaction, the fundamental goal of nursing intervention. King emphasizes the need to prevent health problems occurring as well as the need to help the client once problems have arisen, a fact that should be borne in mind during client–nurse interaction.

Various writers have made the point (e.g. Pearson and Vaughan, 1986) that communication and perception are crucial to the successful outcome of nursing care using King's model. King (1986) herself proposes that the interaction process will be influenced by the perceptions of nurse and client. Major difficulties in working towards mutually agreed goals may unfortunately arise if the client's perceptions of reality are seriously distorted. However, an appreciation of the client's perception of reality is clearly a prerequisite for nursing care and in this sense King's emphasis on this facet of nurse–client interaction is a strength. Mutual goal setting or transactions may have to be postponed until the client has a clearer perception of reality, as King herself states that perceptual accuracy is necessary in nurse–client interactions, along with an accurate perception of time and space, for transactions to occur. This of course raises the issue of what reality is, a debate that has exercised the minds of great philosophers since human beings first evolved the ability to think!

King therefore requires nurses to explore the client's world in terms of the client's self-concept, relationships with individuals and with the larger social groups and forces within society. Nursing interventions involve transactions with the client; that is, setting goals that both parties agree will be helpful in allowing the patient to reduce stress and function within his or her various social roles. A wide range of nursing skills is necessary in this context, particularly drawn from the field of counselling. Change and development of the relationship is to be encouraged, with the client increasingly taking the lead in interactions; however, the nurse needs to ensure that transactions remain realistic.

As we saw with Peplau's model, the assessment lacks structure and it would be very easy, while concentrating on the client's personal, interpersonal and social systems, to miss important physical aspects of his or her well-being. Physical health problems may exist concurrently with mental problems and be closely linked. Examples of a few such common problems are listed below:

- A depressed client may, for example, have neglected eating and drinking, leading to weight loss, dehydration and a poor nutritional status, which can lead on to many other health problems.
- Chronic pain can lead to clients feeling low and depressed.
- Problems such as constipation, stress incontinence or a urinary tract infection may exert a negative effect on the way a client feels.
- Inactivity may be reflected in poor standards of personal hygiene and neglect.
- Smoking leads to many health problems of which those affecting the respiratory and cardiovascular systems are the most obvious.
- Frustration, anxiety, depression and feelings of worthlessness are commonly observed among patients in general hospital and community settings suffering from severely limiting physical disorders.

In view of the key role played by communication in King's work, it is suggested that the assessment be structured around the FAN-CAP scheme (p. 127). The 'C' stands for communication and it would be appropriate therefore to commence the assessment by exploring the patient's mental status in a general way with the aid of King's systems under that heading, before moving on to a more structured assessment of the physically oriented headings of fluids (F), aeration (A), nutrition (N), activity (A) and pain (P).

Communication should start with the patient's personal system, looking at his or her perceptions, self-concept and body image, growth and development along with the client's views of space and time. The interpersonal system requires the nurse to discover the client's views on roles, significant others in the person's life and interactions with others. Both verbal and non-verbal communication should be assessed along with stress reactions and coping mechanisms before moving on to see how the client feels about larger-scale social systems such as relationships within the family. The route the nurse follows to explore these areas will be unique to each individual patient and should be as flexible as possible before moving into the more structured, physically orientated, assessment.

The extent to which the model depends upon interpersonal relationships and such culturally sensitive areas as communication suggests that it may not be very applicable in other cultures. However Frey *et al.* (1995) are able to claim that through their work they can show King's principles have a high degree of validity in such diverse cultures as Japan and Sweden. These authors cite the strong goal attainment aspect of Japanese culture and the philosophical orientation of Swedish culture towards the interaction between person and environment as supporting the relevance of King's model to these countries where Frey *et al.* are currently developing and expanding upon King's work.

King's model has various implications for nursing, the most obvious of which is a willingness to treat the client as an equal partner in care, which marks a major divergence from some of the more traditional schools of thought. Without this concept of equality, mutual goal setting and meaningful transactions will be hampered. King emphasizes individuals' rights to have knowledge about themselves and their right to participate fully in decisions affecting their health and lives, including the right to refuse health care.

The principles that underlie King's model can also be applied outside mental health settings. Woods (1994) provides a detailed case study showing how the model was used to meet the needs of a group of elderly residents (all aged over 80) in a nursing home environment. Group discussions, video presentations and other teaching techniques were used to deal with the identified need among the residents to understand stress and hypertension while the important developmental task in the elderly of achieving integrity (rather than despair) was approached using a range of reminiscence and music therapies. Woods concluded that King's approach had indeed worked for this group of elderly residents suffering from chronic health problems and that meaningful interaction and transaction had occurred leading to improved health status.

A logical step from this position is the right of the client to share access to information held about the client. It is interesting, therefore, to note the results of research by Essex *et al.* (1990) into shared care records for mentally ill patients. They studied a situation in which clients' information was recorded in non-technical language and the clients themselves were invited to make entries into the records. Of the 51 persons involved almost all said they liked to see what was written about them and being asked for their comments. GPs were also enthusiastic about the scheme, but psychiatrists involved were unhappy about the project. Community nurse managers were sadly recorded as lacking in any interest in the idea. Does this mean that the nurses in question were not prepared to accept clients as partners in care?

The use of King's model also requires nurse education to embrace communication skills as a major aspect of care while challenging traditional ideas of the nurse as in some way superior to the client. For a nurse to feel comfortable in a joint goal-setting exercise, that nurse must also feel comfortable in himself or herself. Self-awareness is a key element here, as in the work of Peplau. The education of nurses in the field of mental health already embraces communication skills and self-awareness, so their requirement as part of a curriculum based on King's model should be no barrier to such developments as advocated by Faulkner (1993).

King's model, in conjunction with the FANCAP scheme, has been successfully used for teaching mental health nursing as part of undergraduate nursing studies at the University of the West of England (Bristol) for many years. It clearly has great potential in a wide range of fields of mental health nursing, and Gonot (1983), after a rigorous analysis, has concluded that it has great practical value in terms of contributing to nursing research, education and clinical practice.

In briefly reviewing these four models it has become apparent that the concepts and ideas they embrace have a lot to contribute to mental health nursing, and also should give general colleagues food for thought. Key ingredients such as notions of growth and development along with respect for the individual and the effects of social and environmental factors in producing behaviour prevail. The client's view of the world and the meanings attached to those views are emphasized while the nature of interpersonal relationships is explored on many levels. There is therefore a rich framework of ideas contained within these four models alone that could form a basis for the development of mental health nursing as a profession in its own right, growing away from the traditional domination of the medical profession. Given the huge problems facing mental health care today and a shift in location and emphasis of care priorities, a combination of existing models and adaptation to incorporate new key issues is essential.

The discussion so far has suggested that there are some potentially very useful conceptual frameworks available for development in mental health. The reader is reminded of the discussion earlier in this book about the need to be flexible, adapting, maybe mixing parts of models as part of the process of development to suit particular requirements. That is equally as valid in mental health care as in any other field of nursing endeavour.

Models of care today and in the future

Undoubtedly, the stark reality that now faces mental health nurses and their community role means that the time for preparation and deliberation is over. The DOH in 1994 recognized the urgent need to act and promote the nurse's role as a positive move forward, no longer relying upon his or her medical colleagues.

If nursing models are to be effective in the new and developing mental health centres of today and tomorrow, then the nurse–patient relationship and the psychological needs of the individual and his or her family must feature predominately and clearly in underlying philosophies and plans of care. The medical model cannot be ignored given the increasing debate concerning biochemical imbalance and neurological abnormalities (Gournay, 1990). Holism would not be holism, indeed, without recognition of physical elements. However, as with many of the models discussed, the maintenance of the equilibrium at an optimum level must continue to incorporate the fullest possible picture in relation to the health of the individual as perceived by everybody, the environmental context and the dynamic nature of the nursing role be it specialist, institutional or community based. Whatever the focus, the most important element must be a nurse–patient-led partnership irrespective of boundaries, physical or otherwise, imaginary or real as implied by the folk psychology approach mentioned earlier.

One approach that has more recently been advocated to meet present-day trends and needs is the quadratic model proposed by Holdsworth (1995). This four-part model of the mind focuses on a four-part classification of subjective patient experience – thought; belief; desire and sensation – and relies upon and incorporates the everyday language of 'folk psychology'. The origin of this classification lies originally with the work of Swinburne (1986). As with Peplau's model this quadratic model relies heavily upon the nurse–patient encounter/relationship and emphasizes the use of structured interviews to gain access to the individual's subjective life by exploring the following:

- What is this person thinking?
- What are this person's beliefs and desires?
- What sensations is this person experiencing?

Once examined, appropriate interventions can be geared towards particular needs in an eclectic approach as shown below. This then means that nurses must not only have a full and true understanding of their patients' perceptions of their needs, but an understanding of their own skills and knowledge in relation to various interventions and the ability to know when and where to refer.

Draper (1990) has proposed four goals for any adequate theory of nursing:

- to provide a language with which nurses can discuss nursing;
- to describe nursing by describing nursing phenomenon;
- to provide tools for the professional practice of nursing;
- to form a realistic basis for curriculum design.

The flexibility of the quadratic model means that nurses can have the structure of the holistic framework as seen when exploring the elements of thought, belief, desire and sensation, use language that is both meaningful and accurate to both patient and nurse alike and utilize and develop existing and valuable therapies in line with the present atmosphere of expanding roles.

If the physically oriented, 'doing things for the patient' models are thought valid in an institutional setting, then let us be honest about this and ask how appropriate community care would be for such patients? The indications would appear to be that a very high degree of support would be necessary to sustain patients coming directly into the community from care under such a nursing philosophy. Those resources have clearly not been available in the rest of the UK, as the sorry state of many long-term patients eloquently testifies.

The purpose of this chapter has been to review the position of mental health nursing as a professional discipline in its own right, to briefly discuss and review four of the various nursing models that offer significant potential as tools to help build a body of knowledge unique to mental health nursing and to examine key issues that need to be incorporated into new or adapted models in light of recent and ongoing developments. Community care, enduring mental health problems and their management (Kwakwa, 1995), advocacy and its promotion (Gates, 1994), psychosocial and alternative interventions, therapeutic communication (Faulkner, 1993) and the re-emergence of the medical model as a valid concern being just some of the topical aspects open for present-day debate and integration into care.

It is hoped that this chapter will stimulate thought and debate of the issues involved and also show that while mental health nursing is different in some ways from general nursing, nurses in these fields can and must learn from each other as we each face a significant number of similar problems. Nursing in any situation exists for the benefit of patients and clients whose needs derive from a mixture of physical, mental and social problems. Nursing must be flexible and integrated enough to meet that challenge of the millennium and the community-based focus of both the acutely distressed and long-term suffering.

McFayden and Farrington (1996) conclude that it is time for community mental health nurses, in particular, to set the scene and redefine and reprofessionalize their role with the principles, practices and philosophies that reflect public need (Gourney, 1994; DOH,

1995; Beese and Turnbull, 1996). Thus making a reality of care in the community to include the on-going and unrelenting needs of the severely mentally ill (McFayden, 1996).

Psychiatric mental health nursing as identified by Peplau (1994) is still incomplete and largely undefined. This is in part as a result of new co-dependencies with other health care professionals whereby one role may rely heavily upon the good communication of and working relationship with others. Psychiatric nursing practice continues to expand, none the less. This is in response to trends within and without the nursing profession, scientific theory and on-going challenges within the changing face of mental health nursing and the models that do and will reflect changing patient need(s) past, present and future as we move boldly towards the nursing millennium.

Summary of implications for future practice

Models of nursing continue to reflect the crucial elements underpinning the focus to care; the person, the environment, definitions of health and the nurse's role. Such elements remain unchanged irrespective of time, place or priority of care.

Few new models exist, particularly in relation to mental health nursing, suggesting a universality of needs across nursing contexts. As such existing models focusing upon interaction, patient centredness, mutuality, and psychosocial need, coupled with relatively new emerging concepts such as reflection, advocacy, subjectivity and shared professional learning and control, highlight the flexibility and adaptability of some timeless, dynamic, nursing models.

The mental health nurses' role is finally being encouraged, nurtured, promoted and redefined to incorporate the changing needs of patients in the community setting as opposed to the priorities of the institution and society at large. The needs of the long-term mentally ill in particular are a high priority, not without some opposition (Barker and Jackson, 1996).

Increasing and on-going criticism of both models and the mental health system has meant that evaluation, accountability and adaptation are crucial to the way forward for mental health nurses.

The nature–nurture debate continues in the field of psychiatry and as such must be recognized in the development and utilization of nursing models (Dawson, 1994; Peplau, 1994).

The definition and scope of mental health nursing remains incomplete and as such allows the future to be shaped by nurses themselves, the models they adopt and with the empowerment of those they care for. In many respects the pages are blank and with the vision of experience, research, intuition and hindsight, the time is now for nurses to choose to write the nursing history of tomorrow.

References

Aggleton P & Chalmers H (1990) King's Model. *Nursing Times*, **86**(1), 38–39.

Andrews C (1983) Ida Orlando's model of nursing. In Fitzpatrick J & Whall A (eds) *Conceptual Models of Nursing*. Bowie, MD: Robert J. Brady.

Arnold E & Boggs K (1995) *Interpersonal Relationships*. London: W B Saunders.

Barker P & Jackson S (1996) Seriously misguided. *Nursing Times*, **92**(34), 56–57.

Beecham J, Knapp MRJ & Schneider J (1996) Policy and finance for community care. In Watkins *et al.* (eds) *Collaborative Community Mental Health Care*, pp. 40–57. London: Arnold.

Beese J & Turnbull J (1996) Mental health care – Gone astray. *Nurse Manager*, **2**(9), 16–17.

Benton D (1995) The role of managed care in overcoming fragmentation. *Nursing Times*, **91**(29), 25–27.

Bowers L (1992) A preliminary description of the United Kingdom community psychiatric nursing literature, 1960–1990. *Journal of Advanced Nursing*, **17**, 739–746.

Brearley P (1990) *Patient Participation*. London: Scutari Press.

Burrows S (1996) Community reforms: do they improve the mental health of clients? *British Journal of Nursing*, **5**(45), 918–919.

Collister B (1986) Psychiatric nursing and a developmental model. In Kershaw B & Salvage J (eds) *Models for Nursing*. London: Wiley.

Dawson PJ (1994) Contra biology: a polemic. *Journal of Advanced Nursing*, **20**, 1094–1103.

DOH (1994) *Working in Partnership: A Collaborative Approach to Care*. London: HMSO.

DOH (1995) *Building Bridges – Guide to Arrangements For Interagency Working For The Care and Protection of Severely Mentally Ill People*. London: HMSO.

Draper P (1990) The development of theory in British nursing: current position and future prospects. *Journal of Advanced Nursing*, **15**, 12–15.

Essex B *et al.* (1990) Pilot study of records of shared care for people with mental illnesses. *British Medical Journal*, **300**(6737), 1442.

Faulkner A (1993) *Teaching Interactive Skills in Health Care*. London: Chapman & Hall.

Fitzpatrick J, Whall A, Johnston R & Floyd J (1982) *Nursing Models: Applications to Psychiatric Mental Health Nursing*. Bowie, MD: Robert J Brady.

Frey M, Rooke L, Sieloff C, Messmer P & Kameoka T (1995) King's framework and theory in Japan, Sweden and the United States. *Image: Journal of Nursing Scholarship*, **27**(2), 127–130.

Gates B (1994) *Advocacy. A Nurses' Guide*. London: Scutari Press.

Gonot P (1983) Imogene M King: A theory for nursing. In Fitzpatrick J & Whall A (eds) *Conceptual Models for Nursing*. Bowie, MD: Robert J Brady.

Gourney K (1990) A return to the medical model. *Nursing Times*, **86**(40), 46–47.

Gourney K (1994) Redirecting the emphasis to serious mental illness. *Nursing Times*, **90**(25), 40–41.

Holdsworth N (1995) From psychiatric science to folk psychology: an ordinary language model of the mind for mental health nurses. *Journal of Advanced Nursing*, **21**, 476–486.

Johns C (1996) The benefits of a reflective model of nursing. *Nursing Times,* **92**(27), 39–41.

Jootun D & McGhee G (1996) Why the modern community has stopped caring. *Nursing Times,* **92**(30), 40–41.

Kenny T (1993) Nursing models fail in practice. *British Journal of Nursing,* **2**(2), 133–135.

King I (1986) King's theory of goal attainment. In Winstead-Fry P (ed.) *Case Studies in Nursing Theory.* New York: National League for Nurses.

Kwakwa J (1995) Alternatives to hospital based mental health care. *Nursing Times,* **91**(23), 38–39.

Mangen SP *et al.* (1983) Cost effectiveness of community psychiatric nurse or out patients psychiatric care of neurotic patients. *Psychological Medicine,* **13**, 407–416.

McFayden JA (1996) Assertive community treatment: a recipe for mental illness services for severely mentally ill people.

McFayden JA & Farrington A (1996) The failure of community care for the severely mentally ill. *British Journal of Nursing,* **5**(15), 920–928.

McKenna HP (1989) The selection by ward managers of an appropriate nursing model for long stay psychiatric patient care. *Journal of Advanced Nursing,* **14**, 762–775.

Onega LL (1991) A theoretical framework for psychiatric nursing practice. *Journal Of Advanced Nursing,* **16**, 68–73.

Orem D (1990) *Nursing: Concepts of Practice,* 3rd edn. New York: McGraw Hill.

Paykell ES (1982) Community psychiatric nursing for neurotic patients: A controlled study. *British Journal of Psychiatry,* **140**, 573–581.

Pearson A & Vaughan B (1986) *Nursing Models for Practice.* Oxford: Heinemann.

Peplau HE (1994) Psychiatric mental health nursing: challenge and change. *Journal of Psychiatric and Mental Health Nursing,* **1**, 3–7.

Rae M (1990) Relapse risk for psychiatric inpatients. *Nursing Standard,* **4**(23), 14.

Reed PG (1987) Constructing a conceptual frame-work for psychosocial nursing. *Journal of Psychosocial Nursing,* **25**(2), 24–28.

Reed PG & Johnston RL (1983) Peplau's nursing model: The interpersonal process. In Fitzpatrick J & Whall A (eds) *Conceptual Models of Nursing.* Bowie, MD: Robert J. Brady.

Rogers A, Pilgrim D & Lacey R (1993) *Experiencing Psychiatry.* Basingstoke: Macmillan/MIND.

Roy C (1984) *Introduction to Nursing: An Adaptation Model.* Englewood Cliffs: Prentice Hall.

Schmeiding NJ (1986) Orlando's theory. In Winstead-Fry P (ed.) *Case Studies in Nursing Theory.* New York: National League for Nursing.

Scott H (1994) Why does nursing theory fail in practice? *British Journal of Nursing,* **3**(3), 102–103.

Siegler M & Osmond H (1966) Models of madness. *British Journal of Psychiatry,* **112**, 1193–1203.

Smith L (1986) Issues raised by the use of nursing models in psychiatry. *Nurse Education Today,* **6**, 69–75.

Swinburne RG (1986) *The Evolution of The Soul.* Oxford: Clarence Press.

Whall A (1983) The Betty Neuman health care system model. In Fitzpatrick

J & Whall A (eds) *Conceptual Models of Nursing.* Bowie, MD: Robert J Brady.

Wilkinson G (1988) I don't want you to see a psychiatrist. *British Medical Journal,* **297** (Nov. 5), 1144–1145.

Woods C (1994) King's theory in practice with elders. *Nursing Science Quarterly,* **7**(2), 65–69.

Zito J (1994) Diminished responsibility. *Nursing Times,* **90**(5), 42–43.

Recommended further reading

Weller MPI & Muijen M (1993) *Dimensions of Community Mental Health Care.* London: Ballière Tindall.

Nursing Models in Oncology

Key issues to be addressed in this chapter include:

- the relationship between cancer, nursing models and holistic care;
- model-based care plans in cancer care;
- use of models in addressing the needs of a person with pain;
- models and managed care;
- models and clinical supervision.

Introduction

Nurses and nursing are at the forefront of all areas of cancer care, from promoting health and preventing cancer to its early detection, treatment, rehabilitation and palliative care. Thus, nurses care for cancer patients in a wide variety of health care settings and across all age groups. Malignancies may arise from numerous different tissues, each of which will have its own characteristic pattern of growth, progression and spread. It is within this context that nurses should be seeking to examine critically the care they deliver. To support individuals through a range of physical, emotional, social, cultural and spiritual upheavals and crises, nurses need to be what Wright (1989) described as 'questioning creative practitioners who have the essential problem solving skills enabling them to deal with masses of complex situations in a highly volatile and unpredictable setting'. Nursing models would seem to be a potential tool to enable nurses to function in such a way. They offer the practitioner a framework to assist in organizing the assessment of information, identifying a need for nursing care, the nature of the nursing intervention required and for evaluating the outcome. They also enable the nurse to internalize a perception of nursing as it is defined within the model and this will be reflected in care given be it derived from one model or several (Kershaw, 1992). This chapter aims to examine the use of nursing models in oncology. It focuses on three commonly used nursing models and critically reviews their use as a framework for care. These same models are then applied in turn to the case of a woman with the problem of pain. Finally, the potential contribution of nursing models to future developments in oncology nursing are considered.

Cancer is a major cause of death and avoidable ill-health. It currently affects one in three of the population and accounts for about 25% of deaths. A diagnosis of cancer continues to be one that is feared and dreaded. It is often likened to a death sentence, the pronouncement of which condemns the individual to a future associated with physical suffering, mental anguish and premature death. Uncertainty prevails over the length of the sentence which may be weeks, months or years, with the potential of remissions for 'good behaviour'. A more accurate and informed perspective recognizes that cancer is not one disease but many and that scientific and medical developments have significantly improved the prospects of a cure for many people with cancer. Others may have their disease controlled, giving them variable periods of relative normality but with the threat of recurrence requiring further treatment. Cancer has much in common with other chronic and potentially fatal conditions like chronic obstructive airways disease, diabetes and renal failure although the palliation of symptoms for people with advanced cancer is often achieved more sucessfully than it is for people with non-malignant diseases. How cancer differs from most other non-malignant conditions is in the extent to which it appears to threaten attitudes and beliefs and challenges the coping strategies not only of the individual concerned but also of their families, friends, colleagues and all those involved in their care.

In recent years, emphasis has been placed on the need to help those individuals who have physically responded to treatment to repair their self-esteem, adapt to a new image of themselves and generally be rehabilitated within the limits of the disease process. At the other end of the spectrum, palliative care, aimed at providing good symptom management and family-centred multidisciplinary care, has become more widely available and is being accessed earlier so the boundaries between active treatment and palliative treatment are less defined. Nurses are providing specialist input on symptom control, breast care, stoma care, lymphoedema care, etc. in hospital and in the community. Working together as part of a multidisciplinary team of doctors, nurses, rehabilitive therapists, counsellors, social workers and representatives of various faiths there is always a danger that care becomes fragmented and communication breaks down as successive experts are consulted. It is therefore essential that an individual's care is planned in an integrated and holistic way with collaboration between professional groups or we risk reinventing the reductionist approach of the medical model.

Cancer is a disease apparently influenced by a combination of social, physchological and environmental factors. For example, breast cancer is commoner in women in social classes 1 and 2 and in women who have postponed childbearing, whereas cervical cancer more commonly affects women in social classes 4 and 5 who have become sexually active and had their first pregnancy at an early age. Radon gas and ultraviolet light are examples of environmental agents associated with lung cancer and skin cancer respectively and occupational exposure to certain chemicals is known to increase risk of cancers in later life (e.g. asbestos leading to mesothelioma). Psychological research has suggested that there may be links between certain personality types and the development and progression of malignant disease. These themes of the person interacting with the environment and the person viewed as an integrated bio-psychosocial being are common to most nursing models and thus it would seem appropriate to explore in more detail how they might facilitate our care of the person with cancer.

Many nurses, because of their close and sustained contact with cancer patients and their significant others, have long realized that the social and psychological perspectives of cancer are as important to their patient as the physical. Unfortunately, all too often it is the traditional medical model of care that predominates, with its emphasis on physiological systems and anatomical structures and its distinction between mind and body. Such a reductionist approach is illustrated by the case of a woman who had undergone a radical vulvectomy. Her surgeon was delighted with the fact that a complete excision of the malignant tissue had been made and the nurses were delighted that her wound was healing without any infection. The woman meanwhile was becoming more and more depressed and the focus of this depression was the post-operative swelling of her right leg. It transpired that she had been told of the possibility of lymphoedema and saw this early swelling as a manifestation of its inevitability. She was terrified that this would progressively limit her mobility, interfere with her ability to continue with her present job as a sales assistant, her ability to wear fashionable clothes and her long standing hobby of Latin American dancing. In short, this particular visible side-effect of treatment was for this woman at least as great a blow to her self-image as the removal of her vulva and impairment of sexual function, which would be concealed from all but her husband or partner.

In recent years many cancer patients have sought out complementary therapies alongside their orthodox treatment. These therapies apparently offer individuals some means of coping with the experience of cancer and its treatment and of regaining control over their lives. Many nurses working alongside cancer patients have undergone appropriate instruction in order to incorporate therapies such as massage, relaxation, and aromatherapy into their own nursing practice in an attempt to offer more holistic care. The underlying principles of holism as described by the British Holistic Medical Association (1987), namely responding to the person as a whole in their environment, seeing the individual as a combination of mind, body and spirit; willingness to use a range of interventions including both orthodox and complementary therapies; and encouraging the patient's self-responsibility, are again themes echoed in the core elements of most nursing models. Concepts associated with particular models such as those of integration, equilibrium, roles and relationships, communication, change and progression also appeal to the nurse who is seeking to practise holistically and who acknowledges that good technical and physical care alone does not always produce healing.

McFarlane (1986) suggested that the value of models of nursing is that they:

- serve as tools which link theory and practice;
- clarify thinking about the elements of a practice situation and their relationships to each other;
- help practitioners of nursing communicate with each other more meaningfully;
- serve as a guide to practice, education and research.

In contrast, Luker (1989) suggested that the introduction of nursing models is an implicit criticism of practice as it is and that the models divert attention away from structural and contextual factors that limit the care that nurses are able to provide. As such she claims that they offer little more than an illusion that a change for the better is on the way. In the current climate where it is necessary to demonstrate the ability to provide efficient and cost-effective care which can be audited in terms of quality, implementation of a nursing model may be seen as both a carrot and a stick. Kershaw (1992) suggested that a combination of the nursing process with a nursing model enables nurses to be seen as clearly accountable for the care they give, while Manley (1992) stressed that the values and beliefs of a model need to be congruent with those of the staff involved if they are to become self-directing and motivated to participate actively in setting standards and quality assurance.

Aggleton and Chalmers (1990) also acknowledge the evaluation of a particular model's usefulness may well highlight constraints within the care environment which limit the model's ability to contribute to improved care. They emphasize the need to use this evidence to support and influence the need for change, to highlight the need for further education and research and to demonstrate the need for acquisition of specialist nursing skills. Using a nursing model should empower nurses to care for patients and not be perceived as a millstone round the neck. It is the values and concepts that are adopted to guide and direct the approach to caring which are crucially important not the documentation, which unfortunately often becomes the focus of criticism.

A more pragmatic approach to evaluating the value of a nursing model may be that proposed by Reynolds and Cormack (1991) who suggest that the following questions may be used when evaluating the relevance of a model to nursing practice:

- Does the model assist identification of the range of human responses to actual or potential health problems?
- Does the model enable a nursing diagnosis to be made?
- Does the model explain why individuals respond to health problems in the way they do?
- Does the model provide guidance on the nature of the nursing intervention required to enable optimum health to be achieved?
- Does the model provide an understanding of the desired outcome of nursing intervention?

Alternatively, Aggleton and Chalmers (1986) include the recipient of care in their evaluation of the usefulness of a model. The following key points are very relevant to caring for a patient with cancer:

- Does the nursing model provide guidelines on assessment which enable the patient's problems to be clearly identified?
- Does the planning of care and the setting of goals match the patient's expectations of care?
- Does the model suggest a range of nursing interventions that are practical in that particular care setting?
- Do the nursing interventions carried out enable the nurse to provide a standard of care acceptable to him or herself and the patient?

These questions need to be addressed if nursing models are to be used as a means of improving the quality of nursing provided.

Caring for people with cancer presents any nurse with an enormous challenge. Cancer treatment may include surgery, chemotherapy, radiotherapy, biological or hormone therapy or a combination of these. In addition to knowledge of pathological processes and treatments, the nurse is regularly confronted by ethical issues such as truth telling, informed consent, letting die (euthanasia) and autonomy. The values inherent in a particular nursing model may enable the nurse to view the ethical dilemma with more clarity. For example, the person who declines treatment exerts autonomy but the nurse is left with the dilemma that she believes that the treatment will prolong life and would therefore be beneficial to the patient and his family. The decision of a man to refuse cystectomy on the grounds that sexual function will be impaired or of a musician to decline platinum-based chemotherapy because of the risk of hearing loss will be more understandable if the nurse's assessment has explored the issue of sexuality or self-concept or analysed the self-care requisites of being normal and health deviation.

In order to confront sensitive issues such as those related to sexuality and body image, loss and grief and also problems of a spiritual nature, communication skills are essential. Trusting, supportive relationships enable such problems to be voiced and confronted. Nurses also need teaching skills to be able to inform and educate patients and families in order to enable them to become self-caring on discharge, to be treated as outpatients or to remain at home.

In addition to the knowledge and skills required to give a high standard of nursing, care of the cancer patient may require of the nurse advanced knowledge and skills related to management of pain and symptom control, wound care, intravenous therapy and nutrition, to highlight just a few areas of specialist practice. When caring for a group of people with such a diversity of needs it is inconceivable that one model can provide all the answers. Whatever model is chosen, it should empower the nurse to give better care and not control or restrict the care given. The model should fit the needs of the patient or client group and ideally reflect the values and beliefs of the primary nurse or nursing team. Adopting an eclectic approach or adapting an existing model may be a solution and is discussed later in the chapter.

In the example of the woman who had a vulvectomy, use of Roy's model in the patient's assessment might have provided more information within the physiological mode in relation to her need for rest and activity, and within the self-concept mode about body image. This could have led the nurse to anticipate a potential maladaptive problem and take steps to pre-empt it. Similarly, a patient presenting with a husky voice as a result of a laryngeal tumour who is admitted for a laryngectomy will also be subjected to anatomical changes that will be with them for the rest of their life. Use of Henderson's model when planning care for this patient might lead the nurse who is less experienced in the care of people with head and neck cancers to concentrate not only on the patient's loss of ability to express him or herself by normal speech and need to adapt to breathing through a tracheostomy but to reflect on how this will affect other fundamental needs. This would include the need to select suitable clothes, to avoid changes in the environment, and to participate in recreation, to illustrate some of the more obvious problem areas. If the nurse is unable to identify any need, this in itself might lead the nurse to examine his or her own deficiencies in terms of nursing knowledge.

An alternative approach using Orem's model (1985) could be equally useful with its emphasis on restoring the individual's ability to be self-caring following surgery that disrupts structure, function and requires the person to learn new behaviours. Application of this model would emphasize how the nurse shifts from providing wholly compensatory care to that of a supportive educative role encouraging the person to resume self-care and to meet their universal and health deviation self-care needs. This may highlight the need for the nurse to develop his or her own teaching skills. It may also indicate a need for resources and materials such as patient-information literature, videos and equipment to enable the person to become independent and self-caring more readily.

Roy's model (1984) also has much to commend its use for this individual as it places relatively equal focus on the four adaptive models covering the need for psychological and social as well as physiological integrity following mutilating surgery.

For individuals undergoing chemotherapy or radiotherapy and being intermittently hospitalized, Orem's model has the potential for readily identifying actual or potential self-care deficits and in paediatric oncology it fits well with a philosophy which acknowledges that parents with education and support can remain the primary care givers. For situations of approaching death, Roy's focus on adaptation in the four modes has a certain congruence with the ideal of a peaceful dignified death and may be applied to the family as a unit rather than the individual; however, Orem's model too may still be applicable here as many more patients are now enabled to stay at home with family as primary care agents being admitted only for respite care and perhaps the final days.

The examples that follow use conventional nursing care plans to demonstrate the application of models in caring for three fairly typical cancer patients. Critical pathways (CPs) may, however, be developed for patients with cancer and offer the obvious advantage of ensuring a co-ordinated, multidisciplinary approach, while retaining the concepts of care embedded in any one nursing model.

Example 1 — Roper's model; Sally Barlow

Sally Barlow is a 26-year-old with cancer of the cervix. Four years ago she was treated with two caesium insertions and a 6-week course of radiotherapy to her pelvic area. She has been undergoing investigations as an outpatient for a suspected recurrence involving her rectum and has today been admitted to the ward with a view to her having posterior pelvic exenteration. Sally was accompanied by Dave her partner but he disappeared quickly saying that he would come back later in the day. Roper *el al.*'s activities of living (ALs) (1996) were used as prompts during the assessment interview and information was documented in the order in which it was obtained.

Usual routines	Patient's problem	Goal	Nursing action
MAINTAINING A SAFE ENVIRONMENT Fully independent.	(1) Hazards of surgery (P).	No post-op complications	Explain need for pre-op preparation. Follow standard procedures including bowel preparation.
MOBILIZING Fully independent.			
COMMUNICATING Sally observed chatting to the lady in the next bed. Talks openly about proposed surgery and says she wants as much information as possible. Becomes tearful when discussing colostomy.	See elimination.		
BREATHING P80, BP120/80, R16. Smokes 20 per day has tried to cut down.	(2) Breathing problems post-anaesthetic (P).	Sally will stop smoking pre-operatively.	Explain why smoking increases risks of complications. Help Sally set a time to stop. Suggest alternative stress-reducing strategies. Offer support and encouragement. Reinforce breathing and effective coughing techniques.
EATING AND DRINKING Ht 1.64 m Wt 55 kg. Well-balanced diet, no special likes or dislikes.			
ELIMINATION Urinalysis N.A.D. 1–2 bowel motions a day since radiotherapy. Recently experiencing an urgent desire to defecate – usually a false alarm. Worse at night. Occasionally passes fresh blood with her motions. Low backache for several weeks.	(3) Discomfort associated with having bowels opened (A).	No discomfort.	Offer analgesia as prescribed.
Understands surgery involves removal of 'back passage', not the bladder. Says she has been told she would need to wear a bag. Doesn't know what this entails. Feels frightened.	(4) Anxiety and fear related to lack of knowledge about colostomy (A).	For Sally to be able to discuss the impact of a colostomy on her lifestyle without becoming tearful.	Refer to specialist stoma care nurse. Provide the opportunity for Sally to voice her specific fears. Provide verbal and written information for Sally. Arrange contact with ostomist of similar age if appropriate. Sally to try wearing bag filled with water. Mark suitable sites.
PERSONAL CLEANSING AND DRESSING Fully independent.			
CONTROLLING BODY TEMPERATURE T37.1°C.			

Usual routines	Patient's problem	Goal	Nursing action
WORKING AND PLAYING Croupier in local casino. Socializes mainly with her family. Is saving to buy a house with Dave.			
EXPRESSING SEXUALITY Sally and Dave live together with Sally's parents. Sally and Dave have accepted that they will not have children because of Sally's previous radiotherapy. Sally used vaginal dilators and they have been able to have vaginal intercourse. Recently Sally hasn't felt like sex because of all the examinations. She is very anxious about how the surgery will affect her sexual relationship with Dave as she knows part of the vagina will have to be removed.	(5) Uncertainty about ability to have vaginal intercourse post- surgery (A).	For Sally to be able to state the potential outcome of surgery and identify some postive coping strategies.	Facilitate discussion with surgeons about this topic involving Dave according to Sally's wishes. Ensure privacy for this. Explain to Sally and Dave the resources that exist to give them support and advice with sexual difficulties post-surgery.
DYING Devastated that the cancer has recurred. Says 'but I feel so well'. Feels there is no option but to have the operation. 'I'm much too young to die'. Is frightened that she will have the operation and still die.	(6) Fear of surgery and death (A).	Sally will verbally express confidence in her decision to proceed with surgery.	Allow Sally time to express all her fears. Ensure medical staff fully explain options and answer all her questions. Reinforce and help Sally interpret information given. Provide information about post-op care.
SLEEPING Normally sleeps 8–9 h – recently disturbed (see elimination). Finding it hard to get off to sleep since she found out she had a recurrence.	(7) Lack of sleep (A).	Sally will report 8 h sleep.	Offer night sedation. Teach relaxation techniques.

Sally's problems are related to the forthcoming surgery and are prioritized to ensure she is physically and mentally prepared for this. Problems (4), (5) and (6) are the most important. Problems (3) and (7) are related to the cancer and will be alleviated by the operation. Sally decided to proceed with surgery and problems (1) and (2) then became priorities.

Post-operatively, Sally was nursed in a high dependency unit. After 24 h she was transferred back to the ward and a reassessment was undertaken. As a result of this a revised care plan was formulated for Sally's post-operative care.

Usual routines	Patient's problem	Goal	Nursing actions
MOBILIZING Sally is reluctant to move in bed or sit out as she is experiencing pain (see Pain assessment chart – rated 8).	(1) Pain due to surgery (A).	Sally to rate pain less than 3.	Administer analgesia via epidural infusion. Titrate prescribed dose against pain. Inform anaesthetist if not controlling pain. Substitute oral analgesia as pain diminishes. Encourage coping strategies – distraction, massage, etc.
	(2) Complications of immobility – DVT, chest infections, pressure sores, etc. (P).	No avoidable complication.	Assist Sally to change her position 2-hrly while in bed. Encourage 2-hrly deep breathing and coughing when awake. Refer to physiotherapist. Promote mobilization by use of effective analgesia.
EATING AND DRINKING Sally has a naso-gastric tube; and IVI *in situ*. She is NBM.	(3) Dehydration (P).	Sally to have a fluid intake of 2–3 l/24 h.	Monitor and care for IVI. Administer IV fluids as prescribed. Aspirate NG tube. Maintain fluid balance record. Provide mouth care. Introduce oral fluids and diet as intructed by surgeon.
MAINTAINING A SAFE ENVIRONMENT Sally has an abdominal wound, a perineal wound and a corrugated drain.	(4) Impaired healing due to infection (P) and previous radiotherapy (A).	Wound will be healed in 16 days.	Record vital signs 4-hrly. Administer antibiotics as prescribed. Abdominal wound – check dressing – leave intact for as long as possible. Perineal wound – repad and redress as necessary – shorten drain daily after 3rd day post-op. Leave all sutures for at least 14 days.
ELIMINATION Catheter *in situ* and draining well.	(5) Risk of UTI (P).	No UTI.	Observe, measure and record urine output. Ensure Sally remains in fluid balance and has an average urine output of > 35 ml/h. Monitor temperature 4-hrly. Maintain closed drainage system. Meatal cleansing prn.
Newly formed left ileac terminal colostomy with drainable bag attached. Small amount of haemoserous fluid.	(6) Alteration in elimination habits (A).	For Sally to manage her colostomy independently in 14 days.	Check stoma for colour and evidence of retraction 4-hrly. Measure and chart drainage. Observe for passage of flatus and stool. Administer medication to solidify stool as prescribed. In conjunction with the stoma care nurse demonstrate change of appliance with full explanation.

Usual routines	Patient's problem	Goal	Nursing actions
			Encourage increasing level of participation. Encourage Sally to decide on an appliance system of her choice.
PERSONAL CLEANSING AND DRESSING Restricted by IVI catheter, etc.	(7) Inability to perform own hygiene needs (A).	Sally to state she is satisfied with her appearance.	Give bed bath or assist wash until Sally is independent. Encourage Sally to wear her own clothes.

By the ninth day post-surgery Sally had made very good progress and resumed independence in all of the above actitives of living with the exception of elimination. Two new problems were identified.

Usual routines	Patient's problem	Goal	Nursing actions
ELIMINATION Tearful and keeps asking to have the stoma bag changed as she thinks it smells. Has not as yet touched the stoma or undertaken a bag change herself.	(8) Reluctance to assume responsiblity for her stoma (A).	Sally to touch and clean stoma within 24 h. Sally to complete a bag change in 2 days.	Support and reassure Sally. Encourage her to start participating right away in self-care by removing bag, cleaning her stoma and preparing the new bag. To change bag with assistance tomorrow and with minimal supervision the day after. Discuss dietary changes that may help reduce flatus and discuss products that can reduce odour. Discuss arrangements for coping with the stoma at home and follow-up care.
EXPRESSING SEXUALITY Sally is worried about how Dave will react to the sight of her stoma. She feels her body had been disfigured and that she wants to cover it up even at night so that Dave will not be put off.	(9) Anxiety about altered body image (A).	Sally feels confident enough to sleep in the nude.	Encourage Sally to show Dave the stoma before discharge. Suggest interim coping strategies, e.g. wearing bag covers or a waist slip, etc.
	(10) Alteration in sexual behaviour (P).	Sally to report a satisfying sexual relationship (long term).	Get Sally's surgeon to explain what potential for vaginal intercourse exists. Identify potential problems with Dave and Sally and suggest alternative ways of love-making until healing is complete. Offer follow-up support and advice. Discuss reconstructive surgery if appropriate.

Example 2:	**Orem's model**; Jim Davies

Jim Davies is a 39-year-old man who has been admitted with non-Hodgkins lymphoma presenting with lung involvement. This diagnosis has just been confirmed following several weeks of uncertainty and numerous investigations. It is planned to give Jim his first course of chemotherapy on this admission and it is expected that he will receive further courses every 4 weeks for the next 6 months. The exact drugs he is to receive are not specified as the agents used may vary. It is important that the nurse is familiar with the potential side-effects of the specific drugs used. Some side-effects related to drugs commonly used are indicated but the reader should refer to an oncology or pharmacology text for more detail. Some of the side-effects of the therapy may only affect Jim after he has been discharged. For this reason it seems appropriate to use Orem's framework as the basis for planning his nursing care.

Normal self-care abilities	*Current self-care abilities*
AIR No breathing problems until 3 months ago when Jim started to get progressively short of breath and developed a dry unproductive cough. Breathing got worse and 2 weeks ago Jim had 'fluid drained from my lungs'.	Respirations 21. Breathing not laboured and no pain reported. Still has dry irritating cough at times.
WATER Drinks a variety of fluids – usually has 7–10 cups of tea/coffee/milk a day. Used to like to drink 5–6 pints of beer in his local on Saturday night.	Found even small amounts of alcohol started to make him feel ill, so hasn't been to the pub for several weeks.
NUTRITION Ht 1.78 m Wt 72 kg. Eats a well-balanced diet; wife does all the cooking but is 'health conscious'. Tends to eat two meals a day – no breakfast.	Has been 'off food' and has lost 4–5 kg in the last 3 months.
ELIMINATION Bowels very regular every day after first cup of coffee. No problems passing urine.	Bowels have been irregular of late but not constipated. Jim puts it down to eating less.
ACTIVITY AND REST Jim describes himself as an active man. Works as a foreman at the local factory and plays football for the works team. Says he was always on the go. Usually sleeps about 7 h at night, never in the day.	Feeling tired and listless and had to slow right up when his breathing got bad. Better now but still has little energy. Sleep has been disturbed by night sweats.
SOLITUDE/SOCIALIZATION Married to Susan for 13 years; they have 2 children, Paul 12 and Sian 9. Enjoys an active social life and 'never had a moment to myself'.	Finds people are avoiding him and don't seem to know what to say. Feels he has to keep cheerful for Susan and the kids.
HAZARDS Used to smoke but gave up 5 years ago. Drank regularly in his youth but cut down when he met Susan.	Has heard that chemotherapy makes hair fall out and makes people very sick and would like to know if this is true. Thinks the treatment might be worse than the disease.

Normal self-care abilities	Current self-care abilities
BEING NORMAL Felt life was going well and says he was just an ordinary chap, lucky to have a good job, happy marriage and lovely kids.	Feels life had become a nightmare – nothing is the same any more.
DEVELOPMENT Doesn't like asking others for help, has always been very independent. Feels his wife and children have always been able to depend on him.	Is afraid of 'letting the family down'. Scared of being an invalid and of death.
HEALTH DEVIANCY Always considered himself healthy and never took a day off sick until now. No personal experience of anyone with cancer, has only heard of people who have died.	Feels his body is out of control. Knows his diagnosis but has never heard of this sort of cancer. Has been told he will need at least 6 months chemotherapy to treat this. Jim says he wants to believe it will cure him but he is worried that the treatment is experimental and that he is just a guinea-pig.

From this assessment, Jim's self-care deficits (patient problems) are identified and prioritized to produce the following care plan. It is anticipated that care given during his initial admission and while having intravenous therapy will be partially compensatory, but as treatment progresses care will become more supportive–educative unless his disease should fail to respond to treatment. Although Jim's self-care deficits will need review on each admission for chemotherapy and new ones may be identified, it is likely that this care plan will also be relevant for each subsequent course of chemotherapy.

Self-care deficit	Goal	Nursing actions
(1) Inadequate knowledge of cancer in general and lymphoma in particular (A).	Jim will be able to discuss his condition knowledgeably and ask relevant questions.	Explain the nature of cancer and give verbal and written information about lymphomas and the treatment options. Encourage questions and answer as honestly as possible. Involve Susan in discussions whenever possible.
(2) Inaccurate knowledge of chemotherapy (A).	Understanding of chemotherapy demonstrated by:	Explain how chemotherapy works and the major side-effects of Jim's treatment.
	(1) Jim's ability to identify potential side-effects.	Explain how these are prevented or controlled, answering all questions as honestly as possible. Reinforce with written information that Jim can show to his family.
	(2) Jim's ability to describe his treatment plan.	Ensure Jim is kept informed of treatment plans, e.g. when chemotherapy is to be given. Reinforce information given by medical staff using terms Jim can understand.

Self-care deficit	Goal	Nursing actions
		Ensure Jim knows who to contact if he has questions or problems at home.
(3) Infertility (P).	Retention of potential for future paternity.	Discuss risk of infertility with Jim and Susan and offer opportunity for sperm banking.
(4) Anorexia (A).	No further weight loss.	Explain chemotherapy may exacerbate this problem. Arrange for dietitian to see Jim and Susan. Offer Jim food supplements in addition or in place of hospital food. Administer anti-emetics as required. Monitor weight on each admission.
(5) Constipation (P).	Daily motion. Soft formed stool.	Discuss dietary and fluid intake. Encourage high-fibre diet as tolerated.
(6) Weakness and lethargy (A).	Jim reports having more energy.	Reassure Jim that the treatment should not make this worse and that as the cancer responds to the drugs he should start feeling more energetic.
(7) Lack of sleep (A).	Jim reports undisturbed sleep.	Reassure Jim night sweats are a symptom of the cancer which should disappear as treatment takes effect. Ensure Jim has changes of nightwear and bedclothes. Assist Jim with washing when they occur.
(8) Difficulty accepting the reality of his condition and adjusting to 'sick role' (A).	Jim to verbalize strategies for making changes in his life during chemotherapy treatment.	Encourage discussion about potential changes Jim will need to make. Offer support for positive change and suggestions for self-care. Encourage Jim's involvement in decisions, e.g. about time of treatment, etc. Encourage Jim to accept support from others during his treatment.
(9) Anxiety about job and loss of earnings (A).	Short term – Jim and Susan to discuss changes in family budget. Long term – Jim to return to work.	Reassure Jim that many patients return to work during treatment. Suggest he contact company personnel officer to discuss arrangements. Refer to social worker if Jim agreeable.
(10) Feels isolated from friends and family (A).	Jim to report improved communication between him and family and freinds.	Encourage and provide opportunities for Jim to express his feelings. Facilitate communication between Jim and Susan by giving them information together and offering them privacy for discussion. Suggest strategies that Jim could use to make contact with friends and overcome the 'barrier' of his diagnosis.

Self-care deficit	Goal	Nursing actions
(11) Requires intravenous injection of cytotoxic drugs.	Safe administration.	Follow hospital policy and procedures for administration of IV cytotoxic drugs.
(12) Nausea and vomiting (P).	No vomiting.	Administer anti-emetics, steroids and sedatives prior to chemotherapy and as prescribed. Evaluate effect and notify medical staff if ineffective. Provide clean vomit bowls, tissues and mouth wash as precaution and as required. Give diet as tolerated. Ensure oral medication available on discharge. Teach distraction/relaxation techniques.
(13) Poor fluid intake (P).	Fluid intake of 3 l in 24 h.	Explain need for high intake in order to promote rapid excretion of drugs and metabolites. Monitor and care for IVI until hydration regime complete and Jim is able to tolerate oral fluids. Give anti-emetics.
(14) Bone marrow depression (P).	Jim will experience minimal neutropenia, anaemia, thrombocytopenia and their sequelae.	Ensure Jim and family are aware of manifestations of BMD, i.e. fevers, malaise and bleeding and bruising. Encourage good oral hygiene – need to avoid people with known infections; need to use soft toothbrush and avoid wet shave, etc. Encourage rest and conservation of energy. Explain procedures for checking blood counts and delaying treatment if count too low. Ensure Jim knows who to contact if concerned.
(15) Specific side-effects of drugs used (P).	No unexpected side-effects.	Inform Jim of these and appropriate strategy for prevention.

Example 3   **Roy's model;** Mary Carter

Mary Carter is a 44-year-old woman who has been admitted to the ward for breast surgery. She works as a midwife at a hospital some distance away and arrived unaccompanied. Mary had been attending the hospital as an outpatient for 6 years because of a history of nodular breasts and a family history of breast cancer. Mammography 12 months ago was negative but when repeated 12 days ago had shown suspicious features. Needle aspiration cytology performed at the same time also indicated the presence of malignant cells. Mary had been clerked by the surgical houseman at a pre-admissions clinic and routine blood tests and a chest X-ray had been taken. Mary had also met the nurse specialist for breast care and discussed the options for surgery. A bone scan and a liver scan were also performed to establish the presence of any disseminated disease. Mary was fully aware of her diagnosis and the intended surgical procedure, which for her was a left mastectomy. The following assessment for Mary was completed using Roy's framework.

First-level assessment	Second-level assessment

PHYSIOLOGICAL MODE
Oxygenation and circulation

RR18, BP130/85, P82.	Varicose veins (F).
No shortness of breath.	Familial problem (C).
Non-smoker.	Overweight (C).
Tortuous dilated veins both legs. Causing aching legs at the end of the day.	On her feet for long periods at work (C).

Nutrition

Ht 1.64 m Wt 75 kg increasing over last year.	Inappropriate diet (F).
	Enjoys food (C).
Looks overweight and says she finds it hard to diet.	Limited exercise (C).
Likes dairy produce.	Unaware of association between high-fat diet and breast cancer.
Cooks for her father who eats very little and says she often 'finishes things off' rather than waste them.	Belief that it is wrong to waste food (R).

Elimination
Bowels opened daily no current difficulties. Urinary – no difficulties. Urinalysis NAD.

Activity and rest
Goes to bed about 10.30 p.m. and describes herself as a lark. No current sleeping difficulty. Enjoys swimming when she has time.

Skin integrity

Skin intact – first noticed left nipple was inverted 6 weeks ago.	Malignant lump in left breast (F).
	Nodular breast for many years (C).
	Practised BSE (C).
	Negative mammography 12 months ago (C).
	No pregnancies (C).
	Mother died of breast cancer (R).

Regulation

Appears well hydrated.	Premenstrual syndrome (F).
T 37.1 °C.	Usual pattern of menses (C).
Periods regular 5/28 days. LMP last week.	Possible hormonal imbalance (C).
Gets severe premenstrual breast tenderness and	Homeopathic medication (C).
increased nodularity. Often feels tense and irritable 'before the curse'.	Cultural beliefs about female role (R).

SELF-CONCEPT MODE
Physical

Doesn't mind losing a breast if it the best way to ensure the cancer has all been removed. Does not want to have radiotherapy as she remembers what it did to her mother.	Impending mastectomy (F).
	Fears radiotherapy (C).
	Memories of her mother's reactions to radiotherapy (R).
Says she can cope with the physical disfigurement herself but says 'no man will want me now with only one breast'.	Prospect of changed body image (F).
	Has seen mastectomy scars (C).
	No current partner (C).
	Fear of being sexually unattractive (C).
	Belief about importance of breasts to men (R).

First-level assessment	Second-level assessment
Personal	
Fully aware of diagnosis and its implications. Feels angry with herself and with doctors. She believed that screening would be reliable and that she has been let down. Thinks she should have been more assertive and asked for an earlier appointment when she first noticed a change.	Breast cancer (F). Different feeling lump for about 3 months (C). Negative mammography last year (C). GP unsympathetic (C). Known greater risk of breast cancer (C).
ROLE FUNCTION	
Unmarried. One older brother. Cares for elderly and demanding father who has been admitted to the local cottage hospital for the duration of Mary's admission. Mary is tearful when she talks of her father and admits to feeling guilty for resenting the demands he puts on her. RGN and SCM. Is worried at being off sick and the extra work others will have to do.	Hospitalization (F). No support services involved in father's care (C). Conflict between brother's wife and her father (C). Assumption of her mother's role (R). Demanding job (F). Expectations of self (C).
INTERDEPENDENCE	
Has always thought of herself as very independent. Finds it hard to ask for help. Feels she should be able to cope with the surgery because she is a nurse and 'knows what it is all about'. Doesn't want to be a nuisance or treated differently because of being a nurse. Says there are many people much worse off than her.	Hospitalization (F). Familiarity with hospital staff and routines (C). First time she has been a patient (C). Breast cancer (F). Normally self-reliant (C). Perception that nurses are 'difficult patients' (R).

From this assessment the following maladaptive problems were identified:

(1) Potential risk of DVT or pulmonary embolism.
(2) Excessive weight gain.
(3) Inverted L nipple.
(4) Anxiety about (i) spread of cancer, (ii) radiotherapy.
(5) Feelings of loss related to potential altered body image.
(6) Anger that preventive actions have not been effective.
(7) Guilt about inability to continue caring for her father.
(8) Conflict between professional role and sick role.
(9) Difficulty accepting dependence on others.

Problem (3) will be addressed by surgery and problem (1) will be important in the post-operative period. Problem (2) is a long-term problem and does not have priority at this stage. All the remaining problems will be relevant throughout Mary's admission and the following care plan was devised pre-operatively.

Problem	Goal	Nursing actions
Hazards of surgery (P).	No avoidable complications.	Follow standard pre-op preparation following hospital policy.
Anxiety (A).	Mary will say (a) she is more confident the cancer has not spread; (b) she is less frightened of radiotherapy.	Encourage Mary to express her fears. Discuss route of spread and remind Mary negative scans. Provide written information on sources of support, e.g. Mastectomy Association. Reassure Mary of follow-up care. Provide written and verbal information about radiotherapy. Introduce her to a patient who has recently had radiotherapy.
Anger (A).	Mary to say she feels less angry.	Encourage Mary to express her feelings by writing them down and asking the doctors to explain why tests were negative. Teach stress-reduction techniques and encourage Mary to identify ways she could be more assertive in the future.
Difficulty accepting dependence on others (A).	Mary to accept her need for temporary dependence.	Identify Mary's previous coping mechanisms. Encourage Mary to identify her support network and to identify who might be of most help to her at this time. Identify gaps in Mary's informal support system and suggest what 'formal' help might be available.
Difficulty accepting transition from nurse to patient (A).	Mary to temporarily relinquish her 'nurse role'.	Encourage Mary to verbalize her feelings about being a patient. Establish her knowledge base prior to giving information to ensure it is pitched at an appropriate level. Encourage Mary to ask questions and facilitate her participation in decision making. Ensure nursing staff give Mary the same amount of attention as other patients while respecting her professional status.

Following surgery and Mary's return to the ward her condition was reassessed and her care plan was revised.

First-level assessment	Second-level assessment
PHYSIOLOGICAL MODE *Oxygenation and circulation* RR15, BP110/75, P74.	Narcotic analgesia (F).

First-level assessment	Second-level assessment
Nutrition and fluids NBM for over 8 h. IVI	Anaesthetic (F). Pre-op fasting (C).
Elimination Last passed urine pre-operatively.	Anaesthetic (F). Pre-op fasting (C).
Activity and rest Drowsy but can move left arm when asked.	Surgery (F). Left breast cancer (C).
Skin integrity Left Patey mastectomy scar covered in Op-Site dressing. Two Redivac drains, one to mastectomy flap and one to axilla.	As above.
Regulation IVI	Surgery (F). NBM (C).
T 36.3°C.	Anaesthetic (F). Cold operating theatre (C).
IM Omnopon and Fentazin given in recovery. Mary says she has very slight discomfort; 2 on a scale of 1–10.	Pain (F). Surgery (C).
SELF-CONCEPT MODE Asking if all the cancer has been removed.	As above.
ROLE FUNCTION Asking if her brother has telephoned.	As above. Next of kin (C).
INTERDEPENDENCE Inability to fulfil all physical needs.	Surgery (F). IVI, Redivac drains, etc (C).

Care plan problem	Goal	Nursing action
Hypovolaemic shock (P).	Systolic BP will remain above 100.	Monitor vital signs ½–4-hrly. Observe wound and drains for excessive blood loss.
Inability to use L arm due to pain (A).	Short term – Mary will say she has no pain.	Administer analgesia within prescribed limits taking account of vital signs. Evaluate using pain scale and report to medical staff if analgesia not effective. If pain is well controlled, commence oral medication once Mary is eating and drinking.
	Long-term – Mary will be able to raise her arm to shoulder level within 5 days and will have regained full range of movement in 4 weeks.	Refer to physiotherapist for instruction on exercises. Reinforce teaching and encourage regular exercises.

Care plan problem	Goal	Nursing action
		Advise Mary prior to discharge about beneficial and harmful activities. Encourage Mary to resume swimming.
InsuffICent fluid intake (P).	Mary will have a fluid intake of 2.5 l in the first 24 h.	Maintain and monitor IVI until Mary tolerates oral fluids. Check Mary does not require a blood transfusion before removing cannula.
Risk of DVT or pulmonary embolus (P).	No DVT or PE.	TED stockings until mobile. Encourage leg exercises when awake until mobile. Encourage Mary to be fully mobile within 24 h.
Nausea and vomiting (P).	No nausea or vomiting.	Provide vomit bowl, tissues and mouthwash, etc. Administer anti-emetics as required and evaluate effect. Commence oral fluids when awake and increase as tolerated.
Oedematous left arm (P).	Short-term – no post-op oedema.	Elevate arm on 1–2 pillows. Ensure left arm is not used for BP measurement, IVI or blood sampling.
Retention of urine (P).	Mary to pass urine within 12 h.	Maintain IVI and encourage fluids when awake. Offer commode rather than bed pan to promote normal micturition. Note time Mary passes urine and volume.
Impaired healing due to infection or fluid collection (P).	Wound will heal without infection or fluid collection.	Monitor temperature 4-hrly. Observe wound for oozing of blood or serous fluid. Leave Op-Site intact for as long as possible. Check wound drains hourly for 24 h then 4–hrly for patentcy, vacuum and amount and type of drainage. Remove when drainage is less than 25 ml in 24 h. Observe mastectomy flaps for any fluid collection. Remove sutures as instructed by surgeon.
Impaired thermoregulation (P).	Mary's temperature to be back to 37.1°C within 4 h.	Provide extra blankets or use space blanket to insulate Mary from further heat loss.

Care plan problem	Goal	Nursing action
Arm lymphoedema due to surgery, trauma or infection (P).	Mary will not develop arm lymphoedema.	Explain potential risks realistically without provoking unnecessary anxiety. Give advice on hand and arm care and reinforce with written information. Assess factors in Mary's life that might cause trauma to her arm, e.g. gardening or needlework, etc. Suggest strategies for avoiding truama, e.g. gloves or using thimble, etc.
Anxiety about spread of disease (A).	Mary will start to identify coping strategies to enable her to manage this.	When Mary is fully conscious, get surgeon to explain the surgery performed. Explain it will take some days to get pathology result. Encourage Mary to verbalize her anxieties about further treatment, etc. Explain how Mary's follow-up will be arranged. Encourage Mary to make plans for her future.
Change in body image (A).	Mary will look at and touch her scar; will select an appropriate bra and demonstrate her ability to fit a temporary prosthesis prior to discharge.	Be with Mary when she looks at herself in the mirror for the first time, and encourage her to express how she feels. Get Mary to wear her bra with a temporary prosthesis once the drains have been removed. Encourage Mary to wear her own clothes in the ward. Show Mary different types of prostheses available and provide her with relevant literature on prostheses and clothing. Arrange follow-up with specialist nurse for fitting with bra and swimming costume. Discuss opportunities for future breast reconstruction. Tell Mary about support groups and give her their literature.
Feeling of guilt about her father (A).	For Mary to accept her need for support as her father's carer.	Co-ordinate meeting between Mary, her brother and the social worker to discuss her father's needs.
Overweight (A).	Mary to lose 2 kg by discharge and 1 kg per week for 6 weeks.	Discuss relationships between high-fat diet and breast cancer. Refer to dietitian.

Discussion

The Roper, Logan and Tierney (1996) model is familiar to many British nurses and has been implemented in a wide variety of clinical areas. It is essentially a British interpretation of Henderson's (1966) ideas concerning the need of all individuals to perform certain fundamental activities of daily living (ADLs). Like Henderson's 14 ADLs, Roper *et al.*'s 12 activities of living (ALs) can be separated into those with a biological basis and those which, while integral to living, are non-essential, being concerned more with the quality of life. In this respect it would appear to address issues of fundamental importance to nurses caring for patients with cancer, for example the expression of sexuality and also specifically the subject of dying.

Its application to Sally's care illustrates some of the strengths and problems of using this model in practice. On admission, Sally was essentially independent in most of the ALs, and this is a feature common to many patients facing the prospect of radical treatment for cancer. The planned surgery had enormous implications for Sally in terms of potential alteration in the AL of eliminating and in her ability to express sexuality in the conventional way. Thus, the focus of Sally's care both pre-operatively, post-operatively and in the long term was the physical and psychological difficulties experienced in relation to these two ALs, while physical aspects of care related to survival and safety were the priorities of care in the immediate pre- and post-operative period.

Sally's problems that have a physical or biological basis were readily identified using the model and 'scientific knowledge' could be applied to resolve them, for example in relation to wound care or catheter care. It is less easy to apply the model when problems have a social or behavioural foundation, because Roper *et al.* (1996) address these aspects only superficially. In this example, Sally finds her stoma offensive. We can provide her with better appliances or air fresheners but we are not specifically encouraged to explore her sociocultural beliefs about elimination, environmental factors such as toilet facilities at home and at work, or how Sally can be helped to return to her previous job and disguise a colostomy bag or the gurgling noises her stoma makes beneath flimsy evening wear. With experience, the nurse would anticipate these potential problems and would explore the wider social context in which Sally lives and works. It would then have to be decided whether these problems were still related to elimination or whether they would be more appropriately considered under the ALs personal cleansing and dressing and working and playing.

This highlights one of the practical difficulties commonly experienced with this model, that the inter-relationship of many of the ALs makes it difficult to decide where to locate information. Sally was tearful when discussing her colostomy – this is part of non-verbal communication, but should this behaviour be recorded under communicating or eliminating?

Finally, in considering Sally's case there is the problem of defining the goals, especially in relation to problems that are related to fear and anxiety. Roper *et al.* (1996) state that goals should not be imposed and should wherever possible be expressed as behaviour that can be observed or measured. It may be that, after helping Sally review all the relevant information, her decision is not to proceed with surgery at all. In her role as patient advocate the nurse must support Sally in this decision with all its implications, even though the outcome is not the goal originally agreed.

Orem's model of care focuses on the role of the nurse in assisting individuals to meet their own self-care requirements (Orem, 1985). Inherent in this approach is the belief that patients participate in the decision-making process about the management of their illness and the circumstances surrounding their quality of life. This may only be achieved if patients are in possession of the facts concerning their diagnosis and prognosis. The nurse–patient relationship is perceived as being complementary. Nurses act to help patients achieve responsibility for their health-related self-care by making up for deficiencies in capabilities for self-care; by supplying the necessary conditions for patients to withhold self-care for therapeutic reasons, or by maintaining, increasing or restoring self-care capabilities in order to promote independence. This can be achieved by a variety of methods such as acting for, teaching, guiding and supporting the patient, and providing the right environment for growth and development of the patient. Emphasis on self-care and personal responsiblity suggests it could be usefully applied by nurses involved in promoting health behaviours aimed at preventing cancers although behaviour is notoriously difficult to change. For nurses caring for patients with cancer, characterized by its chronic course and often intermittent contact with the health care system, this model has much to commend it. It can also be applied to family units rather than individuals, as in the case of children or in palliative care situations. Jones (1996) has reviewed its potential value in caring for the dying but conflicts and inconsistency in the model are apparent when considering care of terminally ill and dying patients. Orem states that the aim of care in such situations is to enable patients to live as themselves, understand their illness, to approach death in their own particular way. If the patient and/or their family choose to use denial as their coping mechanism, the nurse may go along with this but would fail to assist the patient and family to understand the projected outcome of the disease or prepare for the future.

Other difficulties arise when patients are unable to comply with medically defined treatments. Take, for example, the case of a single mother with ovarian cancer who is experiencing difficulty with child care during her hospitalization for monthly chemotherapy. The mother is admitted for her treatment but is told that she needs a blood transfusion first that would delay treatment for at least 24 h.

The patient at this point wishes to discharge herself because there is no one to care for her daughter. Thus, the patient's social circumstances and the patient's own role as dependent care agent for her daughter take priority over the patient's own universal self-care requisites; care must be adapted accordingly.

In Jim's case, use of Orem's model usefully highlighted his need for knowledge and support and guidance in maintaining the ability to be self-caring throughout his chemotherapy treatment. Nurses acted for Jim during the actual administration of the treatment and provided an environment which on subsequent admissions could enable Jim to make decisions about the timing of his treatment, and the management of his symptoms, enabling him to achieve minimum disruption to his family life. Such a model could apply equally well to a patient undergoing radiotherapy.

While there is no specific assessment category that is concerned with issues related to sexuality and body image, the more objective aspects of the effects of cancer and its treatment on the individual would be considered under 'being normal' rather than under 'health deviancy', which would be concerned with the more subjective.

Roy's model considers the person to be a biopsychosocial being in constant interaction with an ever-changing environment (Roy, 1984). She identifies the recipients of nursing care as being people who have problems coping with their internal or external environment manifested by maladaptive behaviour in one of four modes, the physiological mode being concerned with structure and function; the self-concept mode with psychological needs, mental function and feelings; the interdependence mode with the need for social integrity and relationships with others; and the role function mode with psychosocial integration and expectations of society. The individual's level of or maladaption within each mode is determined by a combination of focal, contextual and residual stimuli, and the nurse's role is to promote adaptation by manipulating the stimuli appropriately. This is assumed to conserve energy, making it available for investment in the healing process and responding to new stimuli.

This model has been used successfully in the care of dying people. Responses that are considered ineffective in other situations, for example fear, denial, anger, depression, are considered to be adaptive in the process of dying (Kubler-Ross, 1969) and the model also emphasizes that the recipient of care may include the individual family or groups. Chadderton (1986) and Logan (1988) have both explained their use of this model to effectively guide care given in palliative care and hospice settings. A further advantage of this model is for the care of the patient with cancer-induced pain, as the issue of pain is specifically assessed under the regulatory processes in relation to sensory experience. Walker and Campbell (1989) suggest that Roy's model has all the elements required to make a comprehensive assessment of pain in terms of manifestation, causes, influences and consequences.

In applying Roy's model when planning Mary's care, assessment of adaptation in the physiological mode was based on the five basic needs described in Roy (1984) which includes skin integrity. This was felt to be an important need area in Mary's case as she was to undergo surgery which would disrupt the skin but also because of her anxieties related to her fear of radiotherapy and its disfiguring effect on the skin, which she remembered from her mother's treatment.

Webb (1986) and Gerrish (1989) have both commented on the difficulties experienced in separating behaviours into specific modes, and this problem was experienced when writing Mary's assessment. Was Mary's weight problem related to nutrition or to self-concept, and was her difficulty making the transfer between the role of nurse to one of patient related to role function or interdependence? It was also difficult deciding whether to classify Mary's acceptance of a mastectomy as representing adaptive behaviour in coming to terms with the potential loss of her breast, or whether it was maladaptive and indicative of low self-esteem or maladaptive because it indicated an insufficient knowledge about current methods of radiotherapy. Roy leaves adaptation undefined and this leads to problems being identified on the basis of value judgements by the nurse, unless the nurse makes strenuous attempts to validate the patient's own views of the situation.

One advantage that makes Roy's model an attractive one to use with cancer patients is the relatively equal focus it places on physiological, psychological and social needs. However, it can take considerable experience and confidence to utilize the assessment framework and, although experienced oncology nurses may find it easy to recognize and classify maladaptive behaviours within the four modes and identify the relevant stimuli; in practice, the less experienced nurse may have difficulty with this. The reader should compare the CP approach to caring for a patient undergoing mastectomy, as discussed in Chapter 4, to the conventional care plan presented here and reflect upon which would be most practical and effective to use.

Both Reynolds and Cormack (1991) and Aggleton and Chalmers (1986) suggest that in order to be relevant to clinical nursing practice a model should assist with the identification of health problems and responses to those problems. Pain is a problem frequently encountered in oncology nursing practice. Around a third of people with cancer experience pain at the time of diagnosis and it is a problem for over 70% of people with advanced disease (Twycross, 1994). Pain is a complex and multidimensional phenomenon with physiological, sensory, affective, cognitive, behavioural and sociocultural components (McGuire, 1992). Despite development of various pain assessment tools aimed at the assessment of pain and evaluation of pain relief measures there are many reports in the literature of inadequate pain assessment. Saunders (1967) introduced the concept of total pain encompassing not only physical but social, emotional and spiritual pain. Spirituality is not a topic given much attention in any of the models discussed in this chapter, but spiritual issues, of which religious belief is only one component, frequently give rise to distress and hopelessness in people with cancer. Oldnall (1995) suggests that omission of spiritual needs in existing models results in failure to deliver holistic care and may have a negative impact on a person's recovery or adaptation to an altered state of health and disease. The following case is used to demonstrate the strengths and weaknesses of the three nursing models already described in illuminating and managing the problem of total pain.

Viv is 47 years old and has spent most of her adult life in the USA. She returned to England following divorce leaving her two adult sons in the USA. Twelve years ago she had a cone biopsy and cryosurgery but she now has a large retroperitoneal mass and a laparotomy and biopsy confirmed squamous cell carcinoma arising from the cervix. She is in hospital for pain control and a course of palliative chemotherapy.

Roper *et al.*'s model does not include pain as a primary focus for assessment and it is discussed under the biological aspects of living, with only superficial mention of any social, psychological or spiritual dimension. Their solution to this difficulty is to suggest that unless the pain interferes directly with a specific AL it should be documented under communication. The justification for this is that the perception of pain requires an intact nervous system, an assumption that tends to support the opinion that the model retains a rather mechanistic approach which neglects other sources of distress and which could in theory lead to a failure to identify pain as an indirect cause of problems in other ALs.

Assessment suggests that Viv is communicating pain verbally, non-verbally and behaviourally. She describes pain in her right leg as sharp, shooting and searing and an abdominal pain as a dull ache. She is observed to wince and grimace and occasionally moans. She is reluctant to move. Her pain is assessed using a body outline to determine location, specific prompts about the nature of the pain, onset, what makes it worse, etc. and a visual analogue scale to gain some measure of intensity. Assessing pain under the activity of communicating does require the person to be able to hear, see, speak and understand the assessment tool and to this extent is appropriate only for those individuals with no impairment of these capacities. From this the nurse identifies two different pains: a deep dull constant ache in her lower abdomen and a sharp, shooting, searing pain in her right leg which penetrates down her leg to her foot and which has characteristics of neuropathic pain (pain arising from the nervous tissue itself in the absence of noxious stimulus).

Viv welcomed the opportunity to talk and expressed a variety of emotions such as fear about returning to her home alone and fear of being disabled for the rest of her life and being apart from her sons. She became tearful when discussing them and acknowledged that her pain had escalated since they had returned to the USA after visiting her. She also felt anger at the way various professionals and friends had responded to her since her diagnosis, anger with herself for contracting the disease, and some degree of guilt at sexual behaviour in her past that she felt might have contributed to her disease (noted under Expressing Sexuality). This led the nurse to assume that Viv also was experiencing social, emotional and spiritual pain. Assessment of the other ALs revealed that pain was causing relative dependence in most other ALs, notably restricting Mobilizing and Working and Playing but also Eating and Drinking – the pain is making Viv nauseous; Eliminating – Viv is constipated as a result of opioid analgesia; Personal Cleansing and Dressing – Viv's Waterlow score indicates she is at high risk of tissue damage; she has lost interest in her appearance; Dying – Viv fears the pain will get much worse and that she will lose control; Sleeping – pain keeps her awake. She is a regular church-goer and feels the cancer is punishment for past behaviour.

Goals are established with Viv to achieve physical pain control in stages: pain-free at night; then at rest and ultimately while mobilizing. Progress towards these goals will be evaluated by a reduction in pain intensity on the VAS. To achieve this the nurse will administer and monitor prescribed drugs, analgesics which will be titrated against the pain, co-analgesics and also chemotherapy. A TENs machine may be tried and comfort measures, positioning, warm baths and other non-pharmacological therapies such as relaxation and massage, will be tried.

Goals for the non-physical aspects of pain are harder to establish. They might be that Viv will not become tearful and angry although it could be claimed that these emotions are indicative that Viv is adapting to the inevitability of her situation (Kubler-Ross, 1969). More realistically, Viv should perhaps be able to feel free to express these feelings and emotions with the nurses giving her time, privacy, support and comfort. Encouraging her to explore music or art therapy as an alternative way of venting emotion is another option. Spiritual issues in particular are not addressed in the model although they have emerged in the assessment in relation to both Communicating and Dying. Viv's goal is that her faith should continue to be a support to her and this may be achieved with the assistance of her minister and opportunities to discuss her spiritual concerns. Other potential problems indirectly related to pain will met by preventive care such as pressure area care, nutritional supplements and use of aperients, etc. Social aspects of Viv's pain are not particularly well established although could be explored in more depth under Working and Playing.

Roy's model has been perceived by Walker and Campbell (1989) as having all the elements necessary to make a comprehensive assessment of pain. The relatively equal focus placed on the four adaptive modes suggests that this model may well fit with the concept of total pain and help to identify manifestations, causes, influences and consequences of pain although lack of a spiritual dimension to the model is again identified as a potential limitation. In terms of assessment, pain was originally considered in the physiological mode under regulation (sensory overload). Amendments to the model have resulted in neurological function and the senses being considered as contributory to the regulatory mechanism necessary to maintain physiological integrity. Here pain is considered under the heading of need for protection because pain can be perceived as a protective mechanism, although this does not apply to all chronic pain or to neuropathic pain. A spiritual component to assessment can be included under consideration of the personal self in the self-concept mode. Assessment would be likely to identify pain as a focal, contextual or residual stimulus giving rise to an adaptive problem in all four modes. It is worth remembering that a major difference between acute and some chronic pains is that the body adapts physiologically and behaviourally so there may in fact be little or no evidence of an adaptive problem leading to the theoretical possiblity that in some circumstances pain could be overlooked.

Viv is identified as having an adaptive problem in relation to nutrition (nausea, loss of appetite and weight loss) and elimination (constipation) where pain is a contextual stimulus, and in the need for activity and rest (immobility, difficulty sleeping) where it is a focal stimulus. Pain itself is identified as a problem under the need for protection with cancer as the focal stimulus. It is assessed fully here in terms of location, quality and intensity. Exploration of the pyschosocial modes reveals in the self-concept mode that Viv is depressed and fears being disabled for the rest of her days. She expresses sadness and frustration with her inability to do things for herself. She is angry that previous treatment had failed to prevent the cancer and feels her body has let her down. Viv believes her past sexual behaviour might make her responsible for getting cancer. She is very anxious about how she will cope physically or mentally with further deterioration. On a positive note in relation to personal self she claims that her faith is a great strength to her even though she perceives the cancer as God's punishment. Recurrent cervical cancer and pain are focal stimuli, immobility and dependence on others are contextual factors and beliefs about the cause of cancer and inevitability of pain and suffering are residual stimuli. Under role function, Viv is still coming to terms with her divorce and changed circumstances. She has not really had time since returning to this country to re-establish her career or to develop new interests and friends. She has a close relationship with both her sons and feels guilt at making her sons' lives difficult by developing cancer at this time, causing them expense and worry. Focal stimuli are divorce, move to new country, separation from her sons and friends, and sick role. Contextual stimuli are few friends, no job. In terms of interdependence, Viv is lonely at being separated from her sons and this makes the pain seem worse. She is angry with and feels rejected by some of her friends but there is one friend in particular who is giving her a lot of support. Again there is overlap between the modes with common stimuli which are difficult to tease out. Problems that emerge include fear and anxiety for the future; depression and a sense of loss of control; loneliness and isolation.

It becomes clear that as well as resolving the physical pain in ways previously described, more information has been gained about other dimensions of her pain which require long-term solutions. To enable her to go home will require establishing multidisciplinary support involving a network of carers. The goal is that Viv will feel confident to go home with comprehensive support services and that she reports feeling less isolated. Again the emotions she expresses are not necessarily maladaptive in a person approaching death and the goal is for Viv to feel able to express these feelings openly and for her to report that she feels she is still involved in making decisions about her care, for example whether or not she would wish to be sedated by drugs or admitted to a hospice for terminal care. Roy's model is criticized for restricting patient participation and being paternalistic because it is the nurse who decides that there is an adaptive problem and who manipulates the stimuli. In practice, promoting control in one mode resulted in maladaption in another. Viv refused to take amitriptyline for the neuropathic pain in her leg preferring to accept that this pain might not be fully controlled. She was demonstrating autonomy but this was seen as a new maladaptive behaviour needing further exploration.

Finally Viv's case is discussed in relation to Orem's model. Reasons for choosing this model of care would be the emphasis on self-care and the concept of partnership between nurse and client. Viv has no immediate family available to be the self-care agency; however, achieving good pain control may enable Viv to regain her independence and return home. The alternative is for her to be a recipient of partial or total compensatory care. There is little explicit guidance on how pain may be dealt with within this model. Walker and Campbell (1989) point out that pain does not appear in the index of Orem's book and suggest that failure to emphasize its importance in the assessment scheme is detrimental to the concept of holistic care.

Orem (1985, p. 203) actually refers to Saunders' (1967) concept of total pain and outlines the health requirements in relation to terminal illness. Pain is mentioned here as a focus for care but little help is given on how it is assessed. Pain is likely to emerge as a contributory cause of self-care deficits with the onus on the nurse to identify its contribution to either physical or psychological problems in any of the universal, developmental and health deviation self-care requisites. This raises the problem of where a detailed assessment would be documented. In Viv's case this is likely to be most relevant to the self-care requisite for activity and rest and prevention of hazards on the ground that pain has interfered with her well-being.

The social and psychological aspects of Viv's pain emerge in relation to assessment of maintenance of balance between solitude and social interaction, promotion of normalcy and in terms of developmental and health deviation self-care needs. As with Roy, there is no clear spiritual dimension to the model although Jones (1996) suggests that the self-care model is congruent with the concept of existential humanism. Viv's actual and potential physical problems are identified as being: Nausea (A); Loss of appetite (A); Constipation (P); Unable to get to the toilet (A); Difficulty sleeping (A); Unable to mobilize on affected leg (A); Risk of complications of immobility (P), etc. Her psychosocial problems include; Loneliness and separtion from her family (A); Fear of being disabled and dependent for the rest of her life (A); Fear of increasing pain (P); Lack of a caring supportive network of family and friends (A); Difficulty coming to terms with her diseases (A), etc. Goals are derived from Orem's health care requirements and include nursing and medical management for:

- Regulation of symptoms, e.g. Viv reports no nausea; bowels opened every other day; Viv to indicate improved pain control. < 3 on VAS.
- Meeting of the universal self-care requisites, e.g. no further weight loss; two small meals taken a day; Viv able to mobilize alone to toilet/bathroom and back.
- Assistance to control feelings of despair or rejection. This raises the question of whether these feelings need to be controlled, e.g. Viv to express her feelings anger/tears/guilt, etc.
- Assistance to understand the illness and outcome and prepare for the future, e.g. Viv to identify the agencies and individuals available to provide her with support.
- Continuing support to patient and family to enable them to sustain themselves and to have a measure of security, e.g. Viv discusses strategies for managing her life and verbalizes her preferences for future care.

Viv was referred for support to a hospice home care team who visited her weekly and arranged for her to attend hospice day care. Viv knew she could contact the team day or night. Following palliative radiotherapy to the tumour, Viv was admitted to the hospice as a inpatient but asked to return home as she felt institutionalized. This was arranged with the help of night nurses together with carers from social services who visited three times a day. Her pain level did not improve, except during a visit from her sons but it intensified when they returned home. A case conference was held at Viv's home and further support from respite carers, volunteers and night nurses arranged in conjunction with care provided by her GP and the district nurses. The intensity of the neuropathic pain was reduced slightly by medication changes and Viv reported feeling more in control, especially with the fitting of an intercom door entry system. Shortly afterwards, Viv's condition deteriorated very rapidly. She was admitted to a hospice, commenced on diamorphine and midazolam via a syringe driver and died peacefully, unfortunately before her sons were able to get to her bedside.

Viv's case demonstrates how in practice selection of the model can restrict the variety and quality of information obtained and potentially limits the opportunity to plan truly holistic care. There are other aspects of Viv's case which have not been addressed in this exercise relating to her chemotherapy and radiotherapy treatment, etc. but it is a fairly typical example of how a patient may be in receipt of acute care, home care and palliative care from a multidisciplinary team. The reader may reach a conclusion about which model performed better overall, or whether more than one model could be used for Viv's continuing care.

Cormack and Reynolds (1992) support the view that it is ill advised and possibly dangerous to attempt to apply one model to a variety of clinical situations. The alternative is that from knowledge and evaluation of a number of models a so-called eclectic approach may be adopted whereby the nurse selects a nursing diagnosis based on the model deemed most appropriate for that specific situation and applies the relevant interventions. This obviously raises the probability that the nurse may be working with several models at one time or is in effect seeking to synthesize a model from the selected parts of others. What would have been the solution in Viv's case?

Having discussed the relative value of different models in the assessment and identification of problems, it is a natural progression to examine issues related to documentation and the care plan. The care plan is a tool for documenting the process of caring for an individual. Each individual has a potentially unique set of problems identified by the model-based assessment. The nursing interventions selected to resolve those problems and achieve the agreed goals will be chosen from a range of interventions based on a combination of research-based knowledge, experience and intuition. Individualized care ideally requires individual care plans but certain groups of patients do commonly experience the same problems related to their disease or treatment which are managed according to an agreed strategy or protocol, an example being the person at risk of infection due to chemotherapy-induced neutropenia. For many problems, the repertoire of possible interventions is limited. As the throughput of patients is increased and length of stay decreases nurses spend relatively more time on documenting the care then they spend on delivering it. The task of writing almost repetitive care plans may actually obscure the individual nature of the care given. This has fuelled the move towards the use of standard and/or core care plans sometimes based on an explicit nursing model. These can be pre-written or computer generated and then individualized for a specific individual. Richardson (1992) has produced a number of such core care plans as a basis for guiding nursing care which can easily be adapted so the goals and interventions are congruent with the nursing model of choice.

The need to establish standards of care has become part of the drive to make health service provision more consumer orientated. Standards reflect the expected outcomes of care and the resources and professional multidisciplinary practice necessary to achieve care of the desired quality (Luthbert and Robinson, 1993). Against this background, it is necessary to consider the value of case management and CPs in cancer care. Currently, these approaches do not seem to have gained too much popularity in cancer care, perhaps because the course of the disease itself is often unpredictable and because it would appear to militate against the concept of individualized holistic care. As areas of specialist practice, oncology and palliative care have always prided themselves on their emphasis on multidisciplinary care. Benoliel (1995) argues the case for nurses working in the field of palliative care to take up the challenge of participating fully in cross-discipline efforts to improve the overall quality of care by thinking beyond one-to-one primary nursing, to establishing nursing as a service essential to the well-being of their clients and pivotal to the care-giving team. Already in this cost-conscious environment, palliative care teams are required to demonstrate value for money to the purchasers of their services and managed care offers one route to achieving this.

Petryshen and Petryshen (1992) describe the case management model and the development of CPs which have also been discussed in detail in Chapter 4. The following is an example of a CP developed for a woman with cervical or endometrial cancer undergoing intracavitary radiotherapy using a remote-controlled afterloading system such as the Selectron. Roper *et al.*'s model has been used as a framework because its inherent functional emphasis seems an appropriate focus for care during this medically defined treatment and because it addresses sexuality which is an activity of living specifically affected by the treatment. Nursing interventions clearly fall into the categories of preventing, comforting and prescriptive care, while assessment of dependence/independence in the ALs can identify potential difficulties caused by psychological and sociocultural factors as well as physical, introducing a more holistic approach (e.g. the needs of a woman with a communication problem such as deafness or an inability to understand or speak English would be taken into account).

	Day 1 Pre-op/admission	Day 2 Treatment	Day 3 Discharge
Assessment and personnel	Systems examination Activities of living Anaesthetist House officer Case manager Physiotherapist	Standard pre-op checklist Vital signs 2-hrly Pain Vaginal loss 2-hrly Primary nurse Radiotherapist Physicist	As Day 2 After removal of applicators VS and vaginal loss 4-hrly
	Outcome Assessments complete and documented	*Outcome* VS within normal limits Pain free Minimal vaginal loss Assessments complete	*Outcome* No temperature Minimal bleeding
Tests	Bloods Chest X-ray	Pelvic X-ray	
	Outcome Tests completed and results available	*Outcome* Applicators correctly positioned	
Medication	Normal Anti-diarrhoeal as required *Outcome* No diarrhoea	Pre-med Analgesia Anti-emetic Anti-diarrhoeal ⎫ as Anti-pyretic ⎬ required Sedative ⎭	Analgesia Entonox *Outcome* Pain-free removal
		Outcome Medication given No vomiting, pain free, no bowel action, no pyrexia, not distressed or restless	
Treatment and care	Suppositories if bowels not opened Offer emotional suport	Mattress overlay/foam wedge for buttocks O_2 post-op as required Applicators connected Assist 2-hrly to change position and perform deep breathing and leg exercises Check catheter draining freely	Disconnect applicators when treatment ends Remove sutures, packing and applicators Assist with bath/shower Remove catheter
	Outcome Care given Empty rectum	Information and reassurance on progress Monitor and communicate via CCTV and intercom	*Outcome* Treatment completed and care given

	Day 1 Pre-op/admission	Day 2 Treatment	Day 3 Discharge
		Outcome Treatment commenced. Care given Patient knows approx. length of treatment Passing urine Pressure areas not red Minimum number of interruptions to treatment	
Diet	Normal	Normal	Normal
Activity	Normal	Confined to bed for duration of treatment No visiting	May mobilize after removal of applicators
		Outcome Pt occupied with TV/radio, etc. or sleeping	*Outcome* Normal mobility restored
Teaching	Orientate to unit Review with patient and significant other the critical path Explain pre- and post-op care; radiation precautions Leg exercises Use of entonox		Advise on potential reaction to treatment Discuss sexual activity and teach use of vaginal dilators if appropriate
	Outcome Patient will be able to describe treatment plan Pt will demonstrate leg exercises Pt can use entonox equipment PT understands need for isolation and precautions		*Outcome* Pt will be able to identify side-effects and management Information sheet given
Discharge	Discuss provisional discharge arrangements Discuss long-term effects on fertility and sexuality if pre-menopausal		TTOs OPD appt.
	Outcome Discussion occurs Pt understands and accepts loss of fertility		*Outcome* Arrangements for follow- up completed

NB Treatment will vary according to local policies and practice. The pathway could be incorporated into a longer
version covering 6 week's pelvic radiotherapy as an outpatient and one or more intracavitary treatments.

Finally, the use of models may facilitate the nurse's own professional development. Reflective practice and clinical supervision have become important concepts in the 1990s. Under the umbrella of life-long learning, the concept of relective practice and the process of reflecting on practice situations encourages us to 'draw upon theo-rectical knowledge in a creative way to address and solve problems in everyday professional practice, generating practice from theories and theories from practice' (ENB, 1994). Even where a model has not been used to guide practice in a particular situation, they can retro-spectively be used as a framework for analysing the case or incident to add insight and understanding and facilitate learning and self-awareness. Tolson and McIntosh (1996) comment on this process in relation to Roy's model and the hearing impaired. In oncology, it is not unusual to find individuals who reject the multidisciplinary team's efforts to control their symptoms and/or disease or, conversely, people whose need is to pursue until the end every possible avenue of treatment, both orthodox and non-orthodox. While respecting the individual's need for autonomy, such situations typically engender considerable disquiet and unease in carers. Clinical supervision and the use of reflective practice is one means of exploring clinical experiences whether on a one-to-one basis or by group peer review. Jones (1996) suggests that nursing models and clinical supervision have much in common and that nursing models could provide the basis for models of supervsion.

Reflective practice is itself likely to generate questions about practice issues and stimulate a search for more effective ways of achieving results. Use of the conceptual framework of a model may offer direction on the search and suggest areas for research. So, for example, the development of coping strategies for management of breathlessness could be underpinned by belief in the value of self-care, whereas the management of fungating wounds or lymphoedema is more likely to involve the nurse in finding ways of manipulating stimuli to promote adaptation. The use of models as conceptual frameworks for developing research studies still has potential (Fraser, 1990; Tulman and Fawcett, 1990; Tolson and McIntosh, 1996) and oncology is a fertile field for nursing developments.

To summarize, it is hoped that this chapter has demonstrated that nursing models can provide a framework for the delivery of nursing care throughout the continuum of cancer care. Nurses looking after people with cancer in non-specialized settings may find a model-based approach invaluable in reassuring themselves that they are giving their patient holistic care. Experienced and specialist oncology nurses are more likely to be creative in their use of multiple models, moving between models and using their conceptual frameworks as a stimulus for reflection, developing new approaches to patient care and extending their own professional expertise.

References

Aggleton P & Chalmers H (1986) *Nursing Models and the Nursing Process.* London: Macmillan.

Aggleton P & Chalmers H (1990) Model future. *Nursing Times,* **86** (3), 41–43.

Benoliel J (1995) Palliative nursing and managed care. *International Journal of Palliative Nursing,* **1** (2), 64–66.

British Holistic Medical Association (1987). In *Lampada Spring (II),* p. 46 London: Royal College of Nursing.

Chadderton H (1986) A stress adaptation model in terminal care. In Kershaw B & Salvage J (eds) *Models for Nursing,* pp. 69–71. Chichester: Wiley.

Cormack DFS & Reynolds W (1992) Criteria for evaluating the clinical and practical utility of models used by nurses. *Journal of Advanced Nursing,* **17,** 1472–1478.

ENB (1994) *Using your Portfolio: A Resource for Practitioners.* London: English National Board for Nursing Midwifery and Health Visiting.

Fitzpatrick J & Whall A (1983) *Conceptual Models of Nursing: Analysis and Application.* Bowie, MD: Robert J Brady.

Fraser M (1990) *Using Conceptual Nursing in Practice: A Research Based Approach.* London: Harper & Row,

Gerrish C (1989) From theory to practice. *Nursing Times,* **85,** (35), 42–45.

Henderson V (1966) *The Nature of Nursing.* New York: Macmillan.

Jones A (1996) Orem's self-care model and clinical supervision. *International Journal of Palliative Nursing,* **2** (2), 77–83.

Kershaw B (1992) Nursing models. In Jolley M & Brykczynska C (eds) *Nursing Care: The Challenge to Change,* pp. 103–137. London: Edward Arnold.

Kubler-Ross E (1969) *On Death and Dying.* London: Macmillan.

Logan M (1988) Care of the terminally ill includes the family. *The Canadian Nurse,* **84** (5), 30–34.

Luker K (1989) This house believes that nursing models provide a useful tool in the management of patient care. In Pritchard AP (ed.) *Cancer Nursing. A Revolution in Care,* pp. 157–159. London: Macmillan.

Luthbert JM & Robinson L (eds) (1993) *The Royal Marsden Hospital Standards of Care.* Oxford: Blackwell.

Manley K (1992) Quality assurance – the path to nursing excellence. In Jolley M & Brykczynska G (eds) *Nursing Care: The Challenge to Change,* pp. 175–209. London: Edward Arnold.

McFarlane J (1986) The value of models for care. In Kershaw B & Salvage J (eds) *Models for Nursing,* pp. 1–6. Chichester: Wiley.

McGuire D (1992) Comprehensive and mutidimensional assessment and measurement of pain. *Journal of Pain and Symptom Management,* **7** (5), 312–319.

Oldnall AS (1995) On the absence of spirituality in nursing theories and models. *Journal of Advanced Nursing,* **21,** 417–418.

Orem DE (1985) *Nursing. Concepts of Practice.* New York: McGraw-Hill.

Petryshen PR & Petryshen PM (1992) The Case Management model: an innovative approach to the delivery of patient care. *Journal of Advanced Nursing,* **17,** 1188–1194.

Reynolds W & Cormack DFS (1991) An evaluation of the Johnson Behavioural System Model of Nursing. *Journal of Advanced Nursing,* **16,** 1122–1130.

Richardson A (1992) *The Royal Marsden Hospital Manual of Core Care Plans for Cancer Nursing.* London: Scutari.

Roper N, Logan WW & Tierney AJ (1985) *The Elements of Nursing*, 2nd edn. Edinburgh: Churchill Livingstone.

Roper N, Logan W & Tierney A (1996) *The Elements of Nursing*, 4th edn. Edinburgh: Churchill Livingstone.

Roy C (1984) *Introduction to Nursing: An Adaptation Model*, 2nd edn. Englewood Cliffs, NJ: Prentice-Hall.

Saunders C (1967) *The Management of Terminal Illness.* London: Hospital Medical Publications.

Tolson D & McIntosh J (1996) The Roy Adaptation Model: a consideration of its properties as a conceptual framework for an intervention study. *Journal of Advanced Nursing*, **24**, 981–987.

Tulman L & Fawcett J (1990) A framework for studying functional status after diagnosis of breast cancer. *Cancer Nursing*, **13**, (2), 95–99.

Twycross R (1994) *Pain Relief in Advanced Cancer.* Edinburgh: Churchill Livingstone.

Walker J & Campbell S (1988) Pain assessment, and the nursing process. *Senior Nurse*, **8**, (5), 28–31.

Walker JM & Cambpbell SM (1989) Pain assessment, nursing models and the nursing process. In Akinsanya JA (ed.) *Recent Advances in Nursing 24: Theories and Models of Nursing*, pp. 47–61. Edinburgh: Churchill Livingstone.

Webb C (1986) *Women's Health: Midwifery and Gynaecological Nursing.* London: Hodder & Stoughton.

Wright S (1989) This house believes that nursing models provide a useful tool in the management of patient care. In Pritchard AP (ed.) *Cancer Nursing. A Revolution in Care*, pp. 154–157. London: Macmillan.

Further reading

Lutjens LRJ (1991) *Callista Roy: An Adaptation Model.* Newbury Park, CA: Sage.

Newton C (1991) *The Roper–Logan–Tierney Model in Action.* London: Macmillan.

10 What Next?

It is tempting, when writing a book to be published in 1997, to give it a rather grandiose title such as 'Towards the Next Millennium' or 'The Future of Nursing Models after the Year 2000'. However, it is not difficult to resist such temptation and opt for a more prosaic title such as 'What next?' as it is essential that those who write about nursing should not get carried away with fanciful flights of prose.

The question 'What next?' may be asked in rather resigned and weary tones by many nurses fed up with the ever-accelerating rate of change that has characterized the last decade or so. This may lead to the perception that models were just another passing fad that have had their day. Alternatively, the question may be asked in anticipatory tones – implying that the person is looking forward to the future in a positive way, in which case nursing models may be viewed as useful tools to help guide practice.

Nursing models were probably seen by some as recipes for nursing, to be followed devotedly, like a Delia Smith book. There was perhaps a naïve assumption that if the detailed steps laid out by the author were followed, the nursing model would be implemented and care would move forward. This view of nursing models has indeed become discredited and seen in that light, perhaps they were a passing fad, justifying the resigned scepticism of the nurse who might well ask 'What next?' in such a negative tone. But it does not have to be like that for if nursing models are seen as conceptual frameworks, connected sets of ideas about nursing that make a coherent package and hence provide a philosophy of nursing care, then they make a positive contribution to the future. This approach challenges the nurse to think creatively and to interpret models as guidelines.

A flexible style of working, utilizing different models to underpin the care needed by different patients is needed and this requires an education that differs from the traditional nurse training that the large majority of nurses have undergone. Ford and Walsh (1994) have written extensively of the difference between training and education, the former producing a skilled person who can follow orders without questioning why, the latter leading to an informed practitioner able to question practice and therefore be truly accountable. A major sea change in nursing education has occurred in the 1990s with the increase in numbers of students undertaking pre-registration degree courses and of course the replacement of traditional training with the Dip HE Nursing Studies course (Project 2000). Nurses with the benefit of this new approach to education should therefore be better equipped to see nursing models as the conceptual frameworks that can underpin nursing care. The days of the blanket 'implementation' of a single model, usually Roper, might therefore be coming to an end as nurses increasingly take a broader view of the needs of patients.

The holistic concept that now underpins nursing education is consistent with the holistic view of the person that is central to nursing models. Perhaps nursing models helped influence this change in approach away from the reductionist medical model that tended to focus more on the part of the body that was malfunctioning than on the whole person? Most of the mainstream models referred to in this book have been around since the 1970s and before; they therefore pre-date the development of this holistic approach to education and nursing in the UK. This underlines their importance in contributing to modern nursing thought and educational curricula.

At this point, reference should be made to the criticisms of Pender (1984), who has suggested that many nursing models fail to pay due attention to health promotion. Pender (1987) further considered that health promotion was a dynamic process directed towards growth and improvement in well-being; she also saw it as intrinsically different from disease prevention. Detailed analysis by Hartweg (1990), comparing the work of Pender and others (notably Brubaker, 1983) with Orem's work, has demonstrated that these concepts are consistent and that health promotion is readily seen as self care activity. Dunn (1990) has confirmed the value of the Orem model in health education by showing how it is used for health promotion in alcohol-dependent patients.

Such rigorous analysis is needed for all models of nursing if they are to be considered appropriate components of Project 2000 education. Roy's ideas, for example, of patients actively striving to adapt to stressors in their environment, implies a dynamic process (Rambo, 1984) but also suggests a reactive rather than a proactive view of the person. However, successful adaptation can be seen as an essential pre-requisite for growth and an improvement in well-being. Roy herself suggests that one of the main aims of nursing is to promote adaptation in order that the patient may free energy and resources to deal with other stimuli in their life. Growth and achievement of well-being may be thought of as maximizing human potential, a process that requires the individual to consume considerable amounts of energy and resources.

Two examples might help. Consider first helping the patient to adapt to giving up smoking; this improves cardiopulmonary function, giving the patient more energy and resources to develop greater levels of fitness and generally feel better. By the same token, helping the patient to adapt successfully to the changes in self-concept involved in stoma formation liberates the patient to resume normal life and develop new roles with confidence. From this standpoint, Roy's model, despite its reactive nature, can be seen as a promising tool for health promotion.

The emphasis of the Dip HE Nursing curriculum on community care also has implications since the way nursing is taught must at least in part be applicable to the non-hospital situation. This requires an approach to nursing that recognizes the importance of the patient as at least an equal partner in care and underlines the importance of family and social networks, self-care, independence and successful adaptation to life again after leaving hospital. These of course are the sorts of philosophies that guided King, Orem, Roper and Roy in their models of nursing. This body of ideas is therefore very appropriate to the new curriculum.

The overwhelming view of the literature is that in introducing models a multi-model approach is required (Hardy, 1986; Hoon, 1986; Field, 1987; Kristjansen *et al.*, 1987; Botha, 1989). The nursing curriculum must therefore reflect the full spectrum of models that are in the process of development in order that nurses have the conceptual repertoire they need to deal with the almost unlimited variety of patients and problems that they will encounter in their professional career. To plan a curriculum according to one model only is to invite dogma in through the front door and kick professional freedom out the back. The same comment applies to the delivery of nursing in any care setting.

This of course raises the question of who teaches the teachers? Morales-Mann and Logan (1990), in discussing the introduction of a model-based curriculum, have emphasized the need for those teaching models to be fully conversant with them, and highlighted the problems encountered by students who then find themselves in clinical areas which are neither using models nor showing any interest in them. In the UK, this underlines the need for nurse tutors to get to grips with models and how to use them as vehicles for teaching different aspects of nursing. Tutors must avoid a dogmatic recipe-book approach, however, and instead use models as the conceptual frameworks they are intended to be.

In order that a model-based curriculum may be developed, teaching staff need to develop new tools and methods. There needs to be recognition, as Aggleton and Chalmers (1987) point out, that a developmental model requires a different approach to curriculum design from a systems or interactionist model. For example, the developmental approach is concerned with locating blocks to development and other factors that hinder growth and maturation, as well as considering the normal process of ageing from cradle to grave. Social-science teaching needs integrating with the nursing to reflect this approach, while on the other hand anatomy and physiology need teaching with the focus on development (growth and degenerative changes with age) rather than a pure systems approach. Students need to look at their own development in order to better understand that of their patients, which has implications for teaching methods; reflective group work is required rather than formal lectures.

Aggleton and Chalmers have similarly shown the need for systems models to be taught with emphasis on concepts of homeostasis and how systems relate to each other and to nursing care, while the interactionist approach calls for work to identify how individuals feel about their own health, how they construct meaning out of experience, and how they see themselves. This latter approach leans much more heavily on small-group work than the former.

In conclusion, we can see that educationalists need to introduce a variety of models as part of the reform of pre-registration nursing, but should be aware that a lot of careful attention to curriculum design is needed. Integration with practice will be difficult, but is a necessary goal to be striving for since models, and the approach they represent, are a fundamental component of Project 2000. There is no point in practising that which is not taught (traditional medical model) or in teaching that which is not practised (holistic nursing models).

Models and the development of nursing as a profession

Being able to perform a technical procedure is only half the job. It is not valuable until we do it in a way that is good for the patient through care, thoughtfulness and respect. Norwegian Nurses Association (1993)

This key statement encapsulates so much good common sense about nursing. Simply being able to perform tasks is only half of the job, even if we expand our roles dramatically as the UKCC *Scope of Professional Practice* document potentially makes possible (UKCC, 1992). No matter how complex and advanced the task may be, the task alone does not make it nursing. However, it is the location of that task within a nursing framework of care, thoughtfulness and respect that turns it into nursing and nursing models provide that framework. They map out the key dimensions of the person, health, the environment and nursing itself that then allows the nurse to describe and discuss the care he or she gives; in short, the model allows the nurse to say exactly what *care* consists of and to do so in a way that demonstrates *respect* for the individual. Being accountable for that care involves the notion of *thoughtfulness* which means having the knowledge to justify and defend care decisions while reflecting critically upon practice. The Norwegian Nurses Association statement therefore helps answer the question of what nursing is about in a very common-sense way that is congruent with the notion of conceptual frameworks or nursing models.

Gruending (1985) has suggested that the development of nursing models can be seen as a way of professionalizing nursing, although she readily acknowledges that there is little consensus on what exactly constitutes a profession in the first place. On the basis of an analysis of the literature, Gruending offers as a working definition the view that a profession may be seen as a complex, organized occupation whose practitioners have engaged in a lengthy training programme aimed at the acquisition of a specialized body of knowledge. A code of ethics is a key determinant of practice together with regulations enforced by members of the profession which reflect the wishes of the profession. Competence is tested and licensed in the same way.

If this work is set against the views of writers such as Aggleton and Chalmers (1987), who see nursing models as attempts to establish the foundations of a systematic body of knowledge that is uniquely nursing and which has common meaning among nurses, then nursing models are an integral part of the definition of professionalism. The 'specialized body of knowledge' referred to in the preceding paragraph is the stuff of nursing. Nursing models seek to extend knowledge of nursing across nurses, rather than have the situation where each individual practitioner has their own idiosyncratic view of nursing which is not readily accessible to others. For example, saying that Orem's model is probably suitable for planning care for Mrs Smith conveys in a phrase the whole concept of how care should be approached for this patient. However, to describe the Orem model from first principles would take a long time – as long as it might take to describe any other nurse's individual model of care. Nursing models, therefore, are a key ingredient of professionalism in that they give nurses a common set of ideas and concepts that define nursing.

In the course of this book we have seen there are major changes beginning to happen in health care delivery whether it be the switch to primary health care, the development of nurse practitioners, the introduction of critical pathways (CPs) to replace nursing care plans and the development of multi-skilling in the name of the patient-focused hospital. All these changes present threats to nursing but also offer great opportunities to move practice forward in a way that is beneficial to patients. For this to happen, we have to adapt to change but be able to maintain that approach to care that is uniquely nursing or else risk becoming substitutes for others, particularly doctors.

Richmond and Keane (1996) present evidence from their study in the USA suggesting that some acute care nurse practitioners

(ACNPs) do see themselves very much as substituting for junior doctors while others did recognize that because of their background and education they could offer a different and greatly enhanced service. These ACNPs must have some medical as well as nursing clinical expertise in order to practise in such an expanded role but the combination of the two sets of skills within a nursing framework allowed them to make a much greater contribution to nursing care demands. The message from studies such as this is that nurse practitioners can deliver a quality-enhanced service but they must remain rooted within a nursing conceptual framework to do so. Nursing models therefore have a significant contribution to make whether it is to guiding the development of multidisciplinary critical pathways or the practice of nurse practitioners in acute or primary health care settings. Nursing models provide the philosophy and framework which defines practice as essentially nursing, not medicine. With the sort of multi-skilling changes outlined in the preceding paragraph the focus on nursing is essential but it must involve the use of nursing models as conceptual frameworks not recipe books.

The views of Gruending (1985) are particularly relevant here, for she has argued that nursing theory works at two levels: the micro and the macro level. Consider an elderly male diabetic patient who, for example, has just returned from theatre after a below-knee amputation. The nurse who carries out a pressure-sore risk assessment using the Norton or Waterlow scale, decides that the patient is at risk, and institutes a 2-h turning regime with particular attention being paid to pressure relief of areas such as the heel is acting in a logical problem-solving and independent way. This nurse is acting at the level of nursing micro-theory using nursing knowledge to act independently.

Models act as broad organizing concepts, as philosophies or frameworks of care, and in that sense operate at the large-scale or macro-theory level. In the example above, whether the nurse was using Roy, Orem or any other model to plan care, the problem, goal and interventions would have been largely the same initially. Over a slightly longer time scale Orem's philosophy might have led to more emphasis on encouraging the patient to move himself, whereas Roy's approach might have led to using a ripple mattress to help the patient adapt to his immobility. It could be argued, though, that using a ripple mattress also constituted the nurse carrying out the self-care the patient would normally do for himself, if able. When considered on the macro-scale, models incorporate a substantial amount of nursing micro-theory which remains constant from model to model; what differs is the nurse's approach to implementing that theory. In addition, models also take the nurse into broad tracts of territory that do differ with the model, particularly at the assessment stage. For example, Roy leads the nurse to explore self-concept, role function and interdependence but has much less emphasis on the developmental side of the patient that is highlighted by Orem.

In summary, we can say that at the macro-level of theory different models place differing emphases on areas of the patient for the nurse to explore. Each model also has its own unique philosophy of care. At the micro-level, nursing theory remains an independent body of knowledge, applicable under any model of nursing, but which may be implemented in different ways, subject to the approach of that model. We return to this issue later as it is of fundamental importance in trying to decide whether models of nursing bring about any improvement in standards of care.

Models, therefore, are essential in defining nursing. Only by saying that 'This is nursing' and that only a trained qualified nurse can do whatever nursing consists of will we be able to hang on to the domain of nursing. Once that is lost an army of low-paid health care assistants (HCAs) acting as 'basic carers' and 'physician's assistants' can be employed to take over. This would be detrimental both to patients and, obviously, to nurses. The huge amount of care provided by informal carers, for example family, should not be overlooked in this discussion, and neither should the emphasis placed by some models on the importance of nurses teaching family and others to care for patients. That too becomes part of nursing.

Cost-cutting management with little knowledge of nursing can cause untold harm. Nursing must stand up to the accountants in defence of itself and patients. Clichés like 'We've always done it that way' are no longer any defence. Nursing micro-theory and macro-theory must be deployed together, for example, to justify the need for registered nurses to spend time on a busy surgical ward teaching patients pre-operatively. Pre-operative teaching promotes post-operative recovery by reducing anxiety and pain levels (micro-theory); this is a desirable goal when an adaptation model of nursing is used (macro-theory). If the nurse can support the micro-theory argument with some hard numbers in terms of an estimated reduction in post-operative inpatient days of care required per year and the cost savings involved, he or she is in a very strong position to argue with any manager who wants to know why the ward needs more than one staff nurse on duty for any shift. The alternative argument, 'We've always had two RNs on an early' will not get very far in protecting staffing levels.

The issue of professionalism is therefore not about prestige and higher salaries, but rather the survival of nursing itself in an increasingly hostile health care environment. Nurses must be able to show that skilled nursing actually benefits patients; in short, that nursing makes a difference.

It can be pointed out that nobody has shown that implementing a model of nursing has improved nursing care. This is true, although nobody has shown that a model makes care any worse either!

Demonstrating improvements as a result of model implementation is a very difficult task as it involves measuring the quality of nursing care, which still has a large component of subjectivity and is subject to many confounding variables, despite all the work of the past few years on quality control. The problem of a confounding variable is understood as something that might influence the results of a study other than the matter under investigation, in this case a model of nursing. Examples might be differences in patient characteristics or the attitudes and abilities of nursing staff, all of which can affect the outcome of care.

The work of Faucett *et al.* (1990) shows just some of the problems inherent in this work. They discovered that what nurses wrote in their care plans varied little between an experimental ward that was using Orem and a control ward that continued with the institution's traditional methods of nursing. This might mean that the nursing model made no difference to care. There are, however, other interpretations, such as that this merely showed that the institutional habits, conventions and legal requirements were more powerful factors in the writing of care plans than a newly introduced nursing model. Another point of view might be to question the nature of the relationship between what is written and what is done. How closely does a written care plan reflect the care actually given? Might the study have been better observing the nursing care as practised, describing it from a qualitative point of view and then measuring it quantitatively against outcome standards?

Consideration needs to be given to the point of view that perhaps because of the general, philosophical macro-level at which nursing models operate, they might not produce change which is readily measurable in patient terms. This is certainly the view of Gruending (1985). There are certainly a great many confounding variables which make such testing a daunting task!

However, at the micro-level of nursing theory, empirical testing is possible. The example of the Waterlow pressure-sore risk assessment referred to earlier is a good example; it is an empirically derived tool, and its use can be tested to see whether it improves care by reducing incidence of pressure sores. The reader can think of many examples, such as the care of wounds or patient education and teaching, which comprise discrete pieces of nursing theory, the value of which can usually be demonstrated. Thus, aspects of nursing theory at micro-level can be empirically tested, but perhaps the larger macro-scale of nursing models is not amenable to such methods.

This view leads to the conclusion that nursing models are not models in the conventional scientific sense of the word, as then they should be amenable to empirical testing. It seems a paradox that small-scale components of nursing theory can be tested but not the larger-scale ones. But this is not necessarily so; consider the analogy of socialism and capitalism as competing models of political and economic thought. What truly objective data are there to demonstrate that one is better than the other? If the case was 'provable', perhaps the issue would have been resolved by now, given the passionate arguments of the proponents of these two competing models. If socialism and capitalism represent models of economics on a grand scale (macro-theory), it is also true that on a smaller scale there are elements of economic micro-theory that actually are demonstrable and subject to empirical testing and which apply equally well whatever the political ideology of the government. For example, inflation leads to increased wage demands, cutting the price of a product usually increases sales, and raising interest rates usually suppresses demand and cools off an economy.

Perhaps nursing models may best be thought of as subjective views of nursing which by virtue of widespread discussion become generally accepted by nurses, leading to a series of coherent frameworks which have consistent value systems applicable to the delivery of care. There is a nucleus of nursing micro-theory applicable under any model of nursing, for example 2-hourly turns to relieve pressure, but the way that theory is applied will be influenced and directed by the model of nursing in use. Each model should also lead to the development of its own micro-theory. The result is a core of common nursing theory which can be utilized in differing ways according to the model in use, and areas of theory unique to each individual model (see Figure 1).

It seems unlikely that major trials either could or should be set up to evaluate whole nursing models such as is the complex nature of nursing that it simply would not be possible to demonstrate any statistically significant differences in patient outcomes that could be confidently attributed to the use of one nursing model rather than another. The nursing model is not a tightly knit set of related concepts with the ability to generalize and make predictions that we have seen is characteristic of theory in the natural and social sciences. The conceptual framework that is a nursing model provides a focus and influences our perceptions of what nursing is about, according to Fawcett (1995). This is not the same as a theory that is amenable to testing in the conventional scientific hypothetico-deductive methodology. Even if it were, there are too many intervening variables that affect the outcomes of care and too much uncertainty in measuring the quality of care with reliability and validity to make such studies possible.

In order to try and work around this problem, Fawcett (1995) suggested models could be evaluated by comparing them with a set of criteria and seeing how they measure up to the tests involved. This could be criticized as it lacks the strength of testing in practice; however, as we have argued it is inherent in the nature of models that they cannot be tested in this way. Fawcett therefore sets a series of criteria which can be summarized as follows:

Figure 1 The rectangle represents all the problems patients may have in their lives. A series of nursing models (macro-theories) are applied to these problems, for simplicity in this diagram only three are used but more could be used. As can be seen, the three nursing models cover various areas of the problem field with a large amount of overlap. The overlap area represents a common core of problems that would be discovered by any of the three models. The goals and interventions for each problem (micro-theory) would tend to show differences depending upon the philosophy that drives the model (e.g. self-care or adaptation). There are also areas covered by one model only, indicating that some patient problems would only tend to become explicit with a certain approach to care. Three models cover a lot more of the problem field than only one, indicating that a series of nursing models is required to deal with the large range of problems a person faces as they pass through

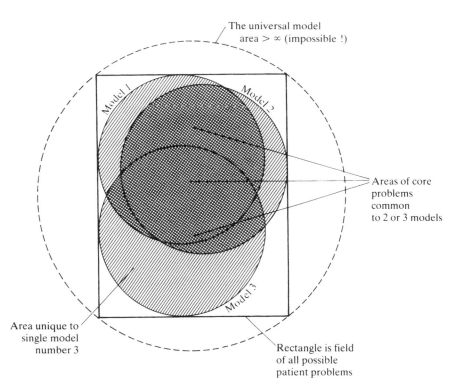

their life. It can be seen, therefore, that this approach is preferable to the single-model approach that would leave large areas uncovered.

A universal nursing model would have to encompass the entire rectangle as shown by the dotted circle. However, as the field of possible problems is infinitely large, so the circle drawn around it would have to have an area larger than infinity, which is impossible by definition, as nothing can be larger than infinity. Whether the nurse uses a common-sense definition, or engages in a little geometry, the result is the same, a universal model of nursing is impossible!

- There should be an explicit philosophical origin for the model.
- The model has sufficient depth and breadth of content. The term 'sufficient' is of course vague and can mean different things to different people. There is therefore a significant element of subjectivity here. However, this is akin to the notion of content validity in research whereby a questionnaire, for example, is assessed for the comprehensiveness of its coverage. A nursing model that ignored the psychosocial aspects of care or the issue of pain, for example, would be clearly lacking in vital areas of content and would therefore be judged inadequate by most nurses.
- There should be an internal consistency between the philosophy and assumptions underpinning the model and the content of the model. A model stressing independence as a key component of its

basic thinking which then ignored coping mechanisms and care in the community would clearly be inconsistent (or lack congruence) and fail this test.

- Although not a theory in the conventional sense of the word, models should be capable of generating ideas which are testable, or in other words hypotheses. For example, a model which espouses patients being partners in care leads to the hypothesis that patients would show evidence of wanting to be fully involved in their care.

- The model has to show credibility in a range of settings. This cannot be demonstrated directly according to Fawcett (1995) but judgements can be made about how relevant the main concepts and propositions are to the real world of nursing; in other words, does this model fit this real situation?

- The final criteria is whether a model makes any contribution to the discipline of nursing. This is not a comparative exercise, comparing one model with another, but rather taking each on its own merits.

These tests at least give some kind of structure to any discussion concerning models or conceptual frameworks although it has to be said they remain an essentially subjective set of criteria. Opinions may therefore vary considerably between nurses as to how well any particular model may perform when evaluated in this way. Perhaps the most objective criteria concerns the generation of hypotheses that may be tested as the notion of testing does give more confidence in the reliability and objectivity of this criteria.

The author is therefore indebted to the staff of ward Medisin 4 at the Regional University Hospital of Tromsø (RiTø) in Norway for sharing their recently completed research (Er Åpne Plcicplaner et Middel Til; Å Oppnå Medbestemmelse I Pleien) which is as yet unpublished in English (Forsdahl, 1996). The study investigated the implementation of their own new approach to care which blended Orem's self-care model with Orlando's interactionist perspective on their nine-bedded infectious disease unit. This established the patient as a partner in care planning, to the extent that the patient even had their own page in the care plan to write in whatever was important for them. This approach led to the hypothesis that the patient would be happy to be involved as a partner in care. Interviews with a sample of 30 patients on admission found that they wished to be fully involved as partners in planning their daily care, while on discharge 26 patients agreed that they felt that doctors and nurses had listened to what they had to say and that it had mattered. Twenty of the 30 patients agreed that they had felt fully involved in the written planning of their care while on the unit.

This is only a single small-scale study, but it does show nurses developing their own approach to care out of Orem's model with the addition of a strong partnership in care theme derived from Orlando's work (see Chapter 8). This eclectic model was used to generate a hypothesis about patient involvement in care which was testable and which upon testing, was supported by the evidence gathered.

This book has argued for models to be used as guidelines and frameworks for care. It has also argued for flexibility, creativity and bottom up change. Models imposed by management will make little difference; however, models of care developed by the staff themselves can have far more meaning as guiding frameworks for care. It is therefore appropriate to conclude this book with a case study (Chapter 11) which both demonstrates the difficulties of a 'do it yourself' model development exercise but also shows the potential benefits of such a liberating approach to nursing models.

References

Aggleton P & Chalmers H (1987) Models of nursing, nursing practice and nurse educations. *Journal of Advanced Nursing*, **12**, 573–581.

Botha E (1989) Theory development in perspective; the role of conceptual frameworks and models in theory development. *Journal of Advanced Nursing*, **14**, 49–55.

Brubaker B (1983) Health promotion: a linguistic analysis. *Advances in Nursing Science*, **5**(3), 1–14.

Dunn B (1990) Health promotion and Orem's model. *Nursing Standard*, **4**(40), 34.

Fawcett J (1995) *Conceptual Models of Nursing*, 3rd edn. Philadelphia: F Davis.

Fawcett J, Ellis V, Underwood P, Naqvi A & Wilson D (1990) The effect of Orem's self care model on nursing care in a nursing home setting. *Journal of Advanced Nursing*, **15**, 659–666.

Field PA (1987) The impact of nursing theory on clinical decision making process. *Journal of Advanced Nursing*, **12**, 563–571.

Ford P & Walsh M (1994) *New Rituals for Old? Nursing Through The Looking Glass*. Oxford: Butterworth Heinemann.

Forsdahl T (1996) *Personal Communication, Medisin 4*, University Hospital, Tromsø.

Gruending DL (1985) Nursing theory: a vehicle of professionalisation. *Journal of Advanced Nursing*, **10**, 553–558.

Hardy L (1986) Identifying the place of theoretical frameworks in an evolving discipline. *Journal of Advanced Nursing*, **11**, 103–107.

Hartweg D (1990) Health promotion self care within Orem's general theory of nursing. *Journal of Advanced Nursing*, **15**, 35–41.

Hoon E (1986) Game playing; a way to look at nursing models. *Journal of Advanced Nursing*, **11**, 421–427.

Kristjansen L, Tamblyn R & Kuypers J (1987) A model to guide development and application of multiple nursing theories. *Journal of Advanced Nursing*, **12**, 523–529.

Morales-Mann ETG & Logan M (1990) Implementing the Roy model; challenges for nurse educators. *Journal of Advanced Nursing*, **15**, 142–147.

Norwegian Nurses Association (1993) *Nursing 2010*. Oslo: NNA.

Pender NJ (1984) Health promotion and illness prevention. In Wevley H & Fitzpatrick J (eds) *Annual Review of Nursing Research*, vol. 2, pp. 83–105. New York: Springer.

Pender NJ (1987) *Health Promotion in Nursing Practice*. Norwalk, CN: Appleton & Lange.

Rambo BJ (1984) *Adaptation Nursing: Assessment and Intervention*. Philadelphia: WB Saunders.

Richmond T & Keane A (1996) Acute care nurse practitioners. In Hickey J, Ouimette R & Venegoni S (eds) *Advanced Practice Nursing*, pp. 316–326. Philadelphia: Lippincott.

UKCC (1992) *Scope of Professional Practice*. London: UKCC.

11 Changing Practice: A Case Study

Introduction

The case study that follows is based in a care of the elderly unit located in an ordinary provincial general hospital and took place without the benefit of any special nursing development unit status or extra resources. It therefore demonstrates that ordinary nurses can change practice for themselves if they are willing to reflect critically upon what they are currently doing and are willing to set their own agenda for change rather than wait for change to be imposed upon them. The unit in question had had a typically negative experience with the nursing process and felt frustrated at not being able to deliver care to the standards it aspired to.

Staff found when they began to discuss their aspirations for care that they each had their own independent approach to nursing based upon their own individual value system. The bringing together to this wide range of values and beliefs into a commonly held view that the elderly people who made up the patients in the unit wished to live as normal and independent a life as possible within society established the bedrock upon which model development could proceed. It allowed the staff to develop a common philosophy of care which is the most important aspect of nursing within a coherent conceptual framework. The staff also wanted their model to be based firmly in the real world and to grow out of experience. They rejected the idea of borrowing bits from other models and assembling them to make their own model as this felt wrong and too complicated. The analogy they gave us was that it was like trying to make a complete outfit by taking separate items from different people's wardrobes. Instead they wanted the cohesion of their own approach to care that they had developed together as a team based upon their own philosophy.

The following section outlines the initial steps in developing the model and is reproduced from the original text with the permission of the authors (Ford and Walsh, 1994) and Butterworth Heinemann publishers.

Since the early days of trying to implement the nursing process staff in the elderly care unit have worked hard, struggling to document individual client needs amongst familiar mutterings to the effect: 'But this is nothing new, we have always given individualized care'.

For some this was indeed true; skilled, perceptive and sensitive nurses did give a substantial amount of individualized care within the constraints of service provision. It was apparent, though, that continuity in care was not being achieved, however this care was documented. The situation was exacerbated by the differing and idiosyncratic interpretations that various nurses placed upon the nursing process, which resulted in a variety of styles of care plan documentation, few of which stated specific objectives in achievable steps. This led to confusion amongst staff, fragmentation of care and loss of motivation and commitment.

As a forward-looking department, methods of clinical practice and management were being continually evaluated and updated, with the result that when discussions about nursing models began in the UK, the staff wondered if models could assist with the nursing process difficulties. A very searching visit from the English National Board convinced the department that they could no longer just complacently accept the 'problems with the process' – something had to be done. After all, the department had well-motivated and keen staff who read extensively and who discussed current issues in nursing, including the emerging nursing models literature. Was this the answer?

At the time some of the wards were using a guide based around common daily living activities to facilitate care plan completion. The following familiar headings made up the guide:

- Transfers.
- Mobility.
- Washing.
- Dressing.
- Toileting.
- Clothing management during toileting.
- Eating.
- Drinking.
- Pressure areas.
- Communication.
- Mental state.

Although very physically biased, the staff had the beginnings of an approach to care in so far as there was a framework which placed some structure upon practice. There was of course no philosophy of care as yet, just a list of headings, but it was a beginning.

As staff began to explore the skills and values of nursing at this time in informal discussions, it became apparent that the whole 24 hours of the patient's day needed to be considered in terms of patterns of care. What did nurses do and when? How did they relate to the multidisciplinary team? What resources were used and to what ends? Questions such as these led to the identification of ritualistic and rigid practice. Uppermost in the minds of those staff engaged in this reflective and critical process was the realization that individualized care had been a struggle because they had never before truly examined their role as nurses, nor had they considered whether they shared a common philosophy of care. Staff realized that they had no coherent framework or agreed philosophy to guide practice; it was like trying to drive from Lands End to John O'Groats with no idea of the route.

This demonstrates how sharing views and experiences in an open and equal framework within which critical reflection upon practice is encouraged can lead to real progress, change and both personal and professional growth. Staff now began exploring models as potentially helpful and useful ways of improving care if they could rectify some of the problems that had been identified. They were not seeing them as yet another 'North American flavour-of-the-month fad' being imposed by the management.

Discussion led to the realization that there were elements in several different models which were very attractive, with Orem's self-care model seeming to have the most relevance. In the subsequent development work it can be seen that Orem's work had the biggest single influence on the team. The preference, however, was to try and develop an approach to care unique to the unit in question, as this would give all the staff a sense of ownership and achievement, in addition to being customized to meet the needs of patients on the unit. Staff were aware that growing their own model was a huge undertaking in terms of time and effort but were excited at the challenge and aware that this represented a tremendous learning opportunity for all.

The approach taken consisted of attempting to build a model out of clinical experience rather than theoretical abstractions. This model would be one firmly rooted in practice rather than relying upon academically rigorous knowledge.

The first attempts at brainstorming values and beliefs in order to arrive at a common philosophy were stimulating but failed to achieve an early agreement. However, there was a consensus around Virginia Henderson's well-known philosophy:

The unique function of the nurse is to assist the individual, sick or well, in the performance of those activities contributing to health or its recovery (or to a peaceful death) that he would perform unaided if he had the necessary strength, will or knowledge and to do this in such a way as to help him gain independence as rapidly as possible (Henderson, 1966).

With agreement reached upon this as a first stage in developing a philosophy, the next step was to arrive at a consensus view of what was understood by a model. The following definition emerged: 'a model is a collection of ideas about people's needs and how best to fulfil them'. In addition a model could act as an overall plan which would guide nurses' thinking. The function of the model would be to enable the nurse, in partnership with the patient and family, to carry out a thorough assessment of health needs and produce a meaningful plan of care. This was the view that the staff worked with throughout and what mattered was that the staff had a definition that they could agree on rather than an imposed textbook definition which may not command universal support.

In this section on the development of the model several key points can be discerned, the most important of which can be summed up by saying the staff lacked a coherent and consistent approach to guide care. Coherence is important as it means that the components of care fit together while consistency means that it does so in a logical pattern and that pattern of care is shared by all members of the nursing team. The wide range of different and sometimes idiosyncratic approaches that nurses can bring to care may lead to a situation where the whole is less than the sum of the parts. Nurse A who is on duty this morning may have a different approach to nurse B who is on this afternoon. The result is that the patient finds that they are helped with dressing in the morning but expected to undress unassisted in the evening before going to bed. Nurse A may engage the patient in conversation and be a good listener, using counselling skills to help the patient explore their feelings at coming to terms with hemiplegia but nurse C on the night shift may feel uncomfortable in this role and see this as an area for a counsellor or a mental health nurse. The patient therefore finds nurse A willing to listen but when they try to talk to nurse C, the nurse quickly finds an excuse to go off and do something else, possibly leaving the patient feeling rejected.

The team in this case study therefore were seeking to harmonize their care within a consistent framework that also included night staff. The inclusion of night staff is very important as they are responsible for the patient's care for approximately 40% of the time the patient is in hospital and yet they are often forgotten.

The developmental stage shows the influence of academic models in shaping the thinking of the staff as they draw upon both Orem and Henderson to guide the development of their own philosophy of care. This demonstrates a key function of formal nursing models in that even if they are not implemented in their original entirety, and we have already seen that the recipe-book approach to model implementation is not a helpful approach, they have a vital role as guides to reflection and thought about care. The staff here are developing their own model not as a formal academic structure but as a set of ideas and shared beliefs that can guide practice. This seems a wholly appropriate approach to take if we are to achieve the balance between a rigid imposition of a model that constrains practice (as we have seen has happened with Roper) and having a lack of coherence caused by nurses each following their own personal beliefs about nursing without reference to any set of agreed guiding principles or philosophy.

Action to develop the model

At this stage the staff had achieved a consensus upon the following:

- An understanding of what models of nursing are.
- Models could facilitate individualized patient care.
- The need to develop a model unique to the unit.
- A first step in developing a philosophy of care would be Virginia Henderson's definition of nursing.

The starting point for developing the model was a consideration of human needs within society. This had to be health- rather than ill-health-oriented, which was a problem for some members of staff, who were still strongly influenced by the medical model of illness. The whole group were involved in brainstorming sessions that consumed large quantities of flipchart paper and pens in a stimulating and creative exercise. Great care was taken to ensure a secure and safe environment for this work.

Six main patient needs emerged from this work:

- Psychological.
- Social.
- Economic.
- Physical.
- Environmental.
- Spiritual.

To maintain the momentum and expedite the work on these headings the group divided into six subgroups, each taking a topic to explore before the next meeting. Much frantic activity ensued during the following week, with many members of staff contributing their thoughts to the subgroup's deliberations.

When the subgroups reconvened, the discussion was led by a staff nurse in each case. All the presentations were constructively questioned and debated until a consensus emerged about the principal needs identified by each subgroup. At this stage it was apparent that there was substantial overlap between the topics. The team were also aware of the criticism that, whilst striving to achieve a holistic view of nursing care, the work was fragmenting the patient into different areas.

In order to resolve the problems of overlap and fragmentation, the next step was to convene a meeting at which the flipcharts were spread on the floor so that all participants could see at once what the other subgroups had achieved. This was followed by an examination of the nature of the nurse–patient relationship in order to identify specific needs which flowed from this interaction. These could then be compared with the list of general needs outlined above. The team identified the following patient needs:

- Individuality.
- Freedom of choice.
- Security and safety.
- Comfort.
- Dignity.
- Self-esteem.
- Uniqueness.
- Maintenance of health.
- Continuity of care.

The less-experienced members of the group began to realize the full importance of individualized care as they tried to reconcile these two sets of needs. Consideration of the second list led to the realization that there were three key concepts that the nurse had to recognize before making any significant interventions in these areas of need. These were:

- Observation.
- Communication.
- Orientation.

Observation

The act of observation involves the collection and recording of information. Criticism has been levelled against the nursing process because of the substantial amount of time required for this activity. The team therefore believed in the importance of recording only relevant, concise, understandable and usable information concerning the patient's needs.

Communication

It became apparent that the concept of communication was crucial as, without it, information concerning the patient's needs could neither be transmitted nor received. Communication (both verbal and non-verbal) was also noted to involve all the senses.

Orientation

Unless patients were familiar with their environment, they could not be expected to feel at ease and derive maximum therapeutic benefit from their hospital stay. This concept should be extended to ensure that the patient is oriented in time and, most importantly, to person. Orientation ensures that the patient feels secure in an environment that could otherwise be very alien and intimidating. Security thus facilitates meeting patient needs.

Having identified these three key concepts that would underpin their approach to care, the team then went on to develop four key statements of belief about the care of elderly people. These statements may be summarized as a belief in:

- Acceptance of the person as an individual and recognition of his/her needs.
- The individual's freedom of choice within the confines of a therapeutic environment.
- The promotion of health, self-esteem and well-being of the individual.
- A joint nurse–patient approach to the identification and solution of problems.

It was now possible to identify a philosophy that would underpin the evolving model of care and which encompassed these beliefs. This philosophy may be summarized as follows:

The individual is a unique being who responds to environmental stimuli in such a way as to meet his/her needs. These needs are not reduced by illness. The nurse/carer must accept the individuality of the patient and, through partnership, assist the individual in meeting his/her requirements, thereby promoting health.

As work progressed, the initial lists discussed above changed and altered, becoming absorbed into new concepts which finally grew into a new approach to care on the unit.

Before considering how these concepts subsequently evolved, it is worth noting that this philosophy was a straightforward statement of commonly held beliefs that all the team could support. To criticize it as merely a statement of the obvious is to miss the point. It was an essential step in developing care on the unit as previously, when staff had each followed their own views, the result had been confusing and at times contradictory. Such a statement therefore gets all the staff pulling in the same direction at the same time.

Working from the insight that orientation, communication and observation were three key nursing activities, the next step was to ask what might be seen as key patient activities? The empowering philosophy discussed above would provide the link between the two.

Some lateral thinking and brainstorming from experience suggested two broad headings – dynamics and mechanics. Dynamics represented to these nurses the everyday processes of our intellectual and emotional selves: moods, emotions, feelings and thoughts. They are things which flow and change, sometimes with the unpredictability and turbulence of the eddies and whirlpools seen in the flow of a river. The river can do something else, however; it can work a waterwheel. It was this notion of the everyday work of life that led the group to conceptualize mechanics as meaning movement and effort. Such work needs fuel such as food, fluids and the intake of oxygen, which in their turn produce the waste products of metabolism which have to be disposed of by elimination. Health problems of course affect our abilities to carry out these functions and at this stage the nurses working on the project acknowledged their debt to Dorothea Orem's concept of self-care abilities, which fitted their philosophy and was consistent with the view of nursing for the older person that the team were trying to develop.

Slowly but surely, the broad outlines were emerging of an approach to nursing that met the requirements of the team and which seemed consistent with the needs of their client group. It was apparent, though, that so far the team had not addressed the issues of personal choice for the client and also the safeguarding of privacy, dignity and personal space, or, to summarize, the client's own territory while in hospital. By now the group had almost made a word with the initial letters of these various concepts – CCOMODAT. It was easy to see that if an A was added on the front to represent the first thing that happens to a patient, admission, and an E to the end to represent the hoped-for destination of the patient, the home environment, the nursing team could easily summarize their view of the keys to successful nursing care for the older person by the mnemonic ACCOMODATE.

A Admission – the entry into hospital care which must be handled sensitively and which links to other concepts such as observation and orientation.

C Communication – important at admission and at all stages thereafter if there is to be a true partnership with the patient which addresses individual needs.

C Choice – something the patient must have at all times as part of the empowering, equal partnership approach to care that characterizes the chosen philosophy.

O Observation – continual observation of the whole patient is essential. This means much more than vital signs monitoring.

M Mechanics – the physical work of life, movement, dexterity and the fuels they require: nutrition, fluid and air intake, eliminatory functions.

O Orientation – to time, place and person. This is a major concern in care of the older person.

D Dynamics – the emotional, intellectual and spiritual aspects of the patient are conceptualized under this heading.

A Abilities – independence and self-care ability in terms of personal hygiene, feeding, etc.

T Territory – personal space and integrity, belongings and memories, the recognition of personal dignity.

E Environment – particularly outside hospital, the importance of where the patient has come from and where he or she is returning.

The section above shows how the staff were able to take the philosophies of others and move from them to develop their own. This could only be achieved by a lot of hard work and the participation of everybody in the brainstorming sessions which took place largely out of work hours. This raises an important point as, realistically, staff who wish to work on projects such as this must be prepared to put a significant amount of their own time into the exercise. It requires a commitment during the developmental stage to more than 37.5 h per week as employers are unlikely to be able to give large amounts of study time to staff to undertake such work. However, such activity can be enjoyable and stimulating and if at the end of the project, the working environment is a happier place because of greater job satisfaction and improved patient care, then it is time well spent.

The influence of Orem's thinking about nursing is acknowledged by the staff as they incorporate the self-care philosophy that she made explicit into their work. However, the conceptual framework evolved out of the nurses' own personal experience of working with older people and was culturally relevant to the older population of Suffolk where the unit was based, while Orem's model grew out of the wide diversity of North American culture. The model developing here therefore should be more likely to achieve cultural specificity for the client group involved. It is interesting to note that in Chapter 4 we saw examples of critical pathway (CP) development involving patient self-help groups, perhaps the nursing staff in this example might have followed the same line and involved groups such as Help the Aged in their model development?

The authors make no claims that the model conforms to the category of model associated with the natural sciences, nor is it a theory that makes predictions from which hypotheses can be tested. Nursing models do not belong in that world as we have stated earlier in the book. However, the authors of this model have come up with something that is firmly rooted in reality and derived from reflection upon experience. It is clearly a coherent philosophy of care that guides nursing practice in a holistic way and is capable of further development.

A crucial aspect of this development is that it works in practice and keeps on working; it has not fizzled out after a few months once the initial enthusiasm has waned. Evaluation has shown that it meets the needs of patients and staff. Students, interestingly, are typically critical of ACCOMODATE when it is first introduced because it lacks an obvious theoretical base, unlike other models they might encounter. Experience brings about a marked change in attitude as they find it user-friendly and appropriate for the needs of the patients. Perhaps this is an example of cognitive dissonance theory at work?

A key observation about this initiative is that the nurses had empowered each other in carrying out this work whose conclusion was an approach to care that stressed empowering the patient. This linkage is no coincidence.

The staff have since developed care-planning documentation which reflects the above main areas of concern. They are characterized by putting the most important things first, so the first thing a nurse sees when picking up an individual's care plan is information concerning orientation, principal facts concerning admission, such as next of kin, previous hospital admission and the individual's perceptions of the need for hospitalization and key nursing observations, according to the client's needs. Within the plan of care, an enabling philosophy, focusing upon self-care abilities is apparent whilst the assessment of the client moves into the areas of choice, communication, mechanics, dynamics and self-care abilities. These principles, along with respect for the individual as an equal partner, drive the nursing care on the ward from admission to discharge planning.

A great deal of change was involved in the way the unit worked as these ideas were implemented. This change from removing the obvious ritualistic and time-wasting aspects of care through to completely changing the care documentation forms. Crucially, though, there was a change in the way staff thought about and planned care, now placing the patient at the centre of activity. Nurses took responsibility for patients by utilizing the concept of primary nursing. Education of staff concerning the new ideas was greatly facilitated by the fact that the staff felt they owned the ideas, as indeed they did, having assisted in their development. Workshops were arranged on a unit basis for the benefit of trained staff and then, utilizing the cascade concept, they in their turn organized ward-based workshops for nursing assistant staff. Change has occurred in this unit with the active participation of all grades of staff utilizing an educative–normative process. The old system was unfrozen by the recognition of the need for change, which then took place by the process of involving as many people as possible.

The authors of this work would not claim that their work has progressed smoothly and is a model of excellence. However, there has been real change and a great sense of progress in the unit which has been achieved by clinically based nurses using expertise derived first-hand from practice, coupled with the will to succeed in their aim of improving services for older people.

Evaluation of staff attitudes and morale before and after the changes were implemented over a 12-month period and has been very encouraging. Staff in the unit were asked to rate their satisfaction on a scale of 0–10 for a wide range of aspects of their work. Response rates were 70% on the questionnaires for both studies and the mean scores were 4.8 before the implementation of the new approach to care: 6 months after, this had risen to 7.7. Of interest was the observation that the care characteristic that improved most referred to the degree of patient orientation; this went from 3.3 to 7.9, while in the area of choice that was available, ratings here went from a mean of 3.9 to 7.3. The dramatic improvement in staff morale revealed by these figures needs to be monitored on an ongoing basis, however, for there is bound to be a degree of novelty which is exerting a favourable influence on these ratings. Attitudes also showed a marked shift towards a greater recognition of client choice, dignity and privacy, which fed through into a more positive feeling about the value of individualized care-planning.

This account demonstrates that clinical staff can change practice providing they work in a mutually supportive and empowering way that involves honest and critical reflection upon practice. In the previous chapter we suggested that the intelligent use of computer-generated care plans may be of benefit in improving individualized care. The nurses in this study have achieved a major improvement without such computer resources. It must be acknowledged that unthinking and ritualistic following of computerized care plans will not improve individualized care.

If staff feel secure in a group, they will dare to be different and throw up unconventional ways of thinking and conceptualizing patient care, as the nurses did in this account. A new approach to care can be developed out of practice rather than textbooks and because staff feel they are stakeholders in this innovation, they are likely to be more willing to accept any associated changes. Perhaps this is a case where the process of change is at least as informative as the outcome.

The work described here has not been the subject of a major formal evaluation, but if readers wish to know more they may contact Helen Peace, Senior Nurse, Elderly Services Directorate, Ipswich General Hospital, Ipswich, Suffolk. She will be happy to supply a detailed resource pack with details of documentation. Please enclose an A4-size stamped addressed envelope and a cheque for £10, payable to the Elderly Services Directorate, to cover the expense of the pack.

This final section of the account raises three important issues: evaluating the impact of change, care planning and the importance of in-service education. Taking the last point first, no changes in care, whether it be the development of CPs or a conceptual framework of nursing, will be successful unless there is investment in staff education. Participative workshops, rather than formal lectures, are essential to ensure that all the staff fully understand what is happening and why. They also give staff the opportunity to talk through misgivings or anxieties and clear up misunderstandings.

The unit team came to the need to develop their own conceptual framework partly from dissatisfaction with the nursing process. The mechanism of implementing their ACCOMODATE model remained the conventional nursing process. Computerized care planning is increasingly advocated as a means of saving time but the weaknesses of such an approach are well illustrated with the ACCOMODATE project. Ford and Walsh (1994) have already commented on the inadequate nature of the software packages available and the fact that unless the nurse learns to touch type, the savings in time will be illusory. A further problem is that the standard problems and interventions that can be pulled out of a standard computer software package will *not* have been written with reference to ACCOMODATE, therefore care plans will be produced which are independent of the nursing model that the team are trying to use. Goals and interventions may not reflect the aspirations and philosophy of the staff as expressed in the model. Such a major dislocation between the computer generated written care plan and the staff's own ideas about nursing, as expressed in the model, cannot continue for long without the risk of either the model or the care plans falling into disuse as they are likely to be incompatible. On the other hand, a home-grown model such as ACCOMODATE could be adapted and integrated into CPs should the unit decide to take this multidisciplinary route to care delivery which also promises significant savings in nursing time spent writing out plans of care.

The final point concerns evaluation of care. As we have already suggested, there are major problems with demonstrating that a new nursing model has improved care. These stem from the fact that measuring the quality of nursing care is extremely difficult, although the Newcastle Nursing Satisfaction Scale (available from Bond S and Thomas L at the University of Newcastle Centre for Health Service Research) is claimed to be able to produce much more sensitive and valid results than the simple patient satisfaction questionnaires that have been used in the past. The other major problem relates to the wide range of confounding variables that could affect the quality of care besides simply introducing a new nursing model.

It is unlikely, therefore, that research will ever be able to demonstrate the case for or against a model of nursing by showing that with a high degree of confidence that it did or did not make a *significant* difference to the quality of care.

However, research can study different aspects of the clinical environment to investigate care after the introduction of a nursing model. In this case the team looked at staff views about care using a questionnaire which appeared to show a much more positive attitude. This is a good example of breaking a big problem down into smaller problems which can be studied. It would be interesting to know how staff attitudes have varied a year or two later, although changes could now be attributed to other factors than the model of nursing such as staff morale within the Trust and NHS in general. The analysis of the data could have been carried out more rigorously as there is no mention of statistical significance testing in the report. As the phrase 'evidence-based practice' assumes more and more importance in health care, this lack of formal rigorous evaluation will become less and less acceptable.

In conclusion, this case study illustrates what can be achieved by an ordinary group of nurses working within existing resources in an ordinary hospital. It is possible to change practice, to empower nursing colleagues and to develop a philosophy and model of care that suits local need. This process involves drawing upon the more formal nursing models to stimulate and guide thinking but it also involves imagination and creativity. It is an excellent example of bottom-up change succeeding with encouragement from management and that is perhaps the final lesson to draw from this case study, management has to encourage staff to try out new ideas but not expect every one to be a winner.

References

Ford P and Walsh M (1994) *New Rituals for Old: Nursing Through the Looking Glass*. Oxford: Butterworth-Heinemann.
Henderson V (1966) *The Nature of Nursing*. London: Collier-Henderson.

Index

Roy adaptation model *cont.*
  surgery 152–61, 161–5
  vulvectomy 230–1
Royal Derby Children's Hospital 108

Safe environment
  activities of living 232, 234
  elderly 170
  medical nursing 173
San Diego
  Sharpe Memorial Hospital 125
  Women's Centre 125
Science
  history of 9–10
  uncertainty 10
Selectron 256
Self-actualization 53
Self-care
  ability 138–9
  agency 117
    Orem's model 116–17
  deficit 117, 138–9, 193–5, 254
    non-Hodgkins lymphoma 237–9
  developmental 105, 118
  health deviancy 118–19
  myocardial infarction 145, 146
  Orem's model 27, 48, 49, 55, 104, 115–21
  patient 30, 136
  requirements 30
  therapeutic 116
    practising 117
  universal 118
Self-concept 123–4
  assessment 153, 155, 162, 163
  King model 215
  mastectomy 240–1, 243
Self-medication 59, 131
  Orem's model 143
Self-neglect 116
Service users, language of 207
Sexuality
  activities of living 233, 235
  cancer 230, 248
  elderly 171
  mobility 173
Shock
  goal 169
  intervention 169
  post-operative assessment 156
Skill mix 108–9
Skin integrity 249
Sleeping
  activities of living 233
  elderly 171
  mobility 173
Slurred speech, elderly 171

Smoker, care 174
Smoking, giving up 263–4
Smoking habits, post-operative assessment 156
Social
  classes, cancer 227
  networks, patient support 195–6
  sciences
    and education 49, 50, 51
    teaching 265
  workers, mental health 206
Socialization 139
  non-Hodgkins lymphoma 236
  Orem 178
  trauma 147, 193
Spirituality 250, 252
Spread of disease, cancer 245
Staff
  absenteeism 40
  morale 40
  recruitment 40
  retention 40
Staffing levels 22
Stages theory
  assessment 77
  care planning 77
  evaluation 77
  planning implementation 77
  planning interventions 77
  problem identification 77
Stimuli 122, 199, 253
Stoma
  acceptance, post-operative care 164
  care 38
  functioning 199
  surgery 104
Stressors 211
  adapting to 121, 263
Stroke, hemiplegia 117
Stroke patients, CPs 97
Subjectivity 7, 37
  interactionist models 30
  theory 21
Substance abuse 53
Surgery
  Roy's adaptation model 152–61, 161–5
  vomiting after 123
Symptom control, cancer 230
Symptoms, regulation of 254
System models 29–30
Systems, homeostasis 31

Task environment, problem solving 77
Teaching
  CPs 83
  elective amputation 158, 160, 161
  myocardial infarction 145, 146